Depression in New Mothers

Maternal depression is the number one cause of disability in developed countries and results in adverse health outcomes for both mother and child. It is vital, therefore, that health professionals are ready and able to help those women that suffer from perinatal and postpartum depression (PPD).

Now in its third edition, *Depression in New Mothers* provides a comprehensive approach to treating PPD in an easy-to-use format. It reviews the research and brings together the evidence base for understanding the causes and for assessing the different treatment options, including those that are safe for use with breastfeeding mothers. It incorporates a new psychoneuroimmunology framework for understanding postpartum depression and includes chapters on:

- negative birth experiences
- infant characteristics
- psychosocial factors
- antidepressant medication
- therapies such as cognitive-behavioral therapy
- herbal medicine and alternative therapies
- suicide and infanticide.

This new edition incorporates new research findings on risk factors, the use of antidepressants, and complementary and alternative medicines, as well as updated, international perspectives and research into ethnic minority differences. Rich with case illustrations and invaluable in treating mothers in need of help, this practical, evidence-based guide dispels the myths that hinder effective treatment and presents up-to-date information on the impact of maternal depression on the mother and their infants alike.

Kathleen A. Kendall-Tackett is a health psychologist and International Board Certified Lactation Consultant, and the Owner and Editor-in-Chief of Praeclarus Press, a small press specializing in women's health. Dr. Kendall-Tackett is Editor-in-Chief of two peer-reviewed journals: *Clinical Lactation* and *Psychological Trauma*. She is a Fellow of the American Psychological Association in Health and Trauma Psychology, Past President of the APA Division of Trauma Psychology, and a member of the Board for the Advancement of Psychology in the Public Interest. Dr. Kendall-Tackett is Clinical Professor of Nursing at the University of Hawaii at Manoa and Clinical Associate Professor of Pediatrics at the Texas Tech University School of Medicine, USA.

Depression in New Mothers

Causes, consequences and treatment alternatives

Third edition

Kathleen A. Kendall-Tackett

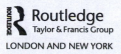

Routledge
Taylor & Francis Group

LONDON AND NEW YORK

Third edition published 2017
by Routledge
2 Park Square, Milton Park, Abingdon, Oxon OX14 4RN

and by Routledge
711 Third Avenue, New York, NY 10017

Routledge is an imprint of the Taylor & Francis Group, an informa business

First edition published 2005
Second edition published 2009

British Library Cataloguing in Publication Data
A catalogue record for this book is available from the British Library

Library of Congress Cataloguing in Publication Data
Names: Kendall-Tackett, Kathleen A., author.
Title: Depression in new mothers : causes, consequences and treatment alternatives / Kathleen A. Kendall-Tackett.
Description: Third edition. | Abingdon, Oxon ; New York, NY : Routledge, 2016. | Includes bibliographical references and index.
Identifiers: LCCN 2016010204 | ISBN 9781138120754 (hardback) | ISBN 9781138120778 (pbk.) | ISBN 9781315651521 (ebook)
Subjects: | MESH: Depression, Postpartum–etiology | Depression, Postpartum–diagnosis | Depression, Postpartum–therapy | Maternal Welfare–psychology | Risk Factors | Socioeconomic Factors
Classification: LCC RG852 | NLM WQ 500 | DDC 618.7/6–dc23
LC record available at http://lccn.loc.gov/2016010204

ISBN: 978-1-138-12075-4 (hbk)
ISBN: 978-1-138-12077-8 (pbk)
ISBN: 978-1-315-65152-1 (ebk)

Typeset in Times New Roman
by Out of House Publishing

Contents

Foreword

The first time I heard Kathleen Kendall-Tackett speak on postpartum mood disorders (PPMDs) in the early 2000s, I was impressed and flabbergasted. I was unprepared for how riveting it was, and how much I didn't know. She was and is a gifted, empathic and very clear speaker who can hold a group's attention, even though the topic is challenging for many. She touched me deeply. I had thought I was knowledgeable and fairly up to date on this topic. I knew about hormonal changes that occur abruptly after birth; I knew that profound role and identity changes occur as one becomes a parent—especially a breastfeeding parent; I even knew about a study that identified a higher risk of postpartum depression after the birth of a third child (Larsen, Evans, & Martin, 1967)! I also knew that my own profound postpartum mood disorder in the mid-1960s after the birth of my third child had been life-threatening. At the time, I was obsessed with figuring out ways I could disappear from the Earth without anyone noticing. Even after my depression had lifted, which happened spontaneously after some months (thankfully), I felt that I would never be the same. I watched my child for signs that my depression had adversely affected her mental health. I was terrified when I became pregnant with my fourth child that I would go through another horrifying depression. Years later, when my third child became a new mother, I again watched her for signs of depression. (As it turned out, none of my fears materialized, thankfully.)

Out of shame and the stigma associated with mental illness at the time, I kept my depression a secret for years from family and friends. Even when I briefly mentioned PPMD in my childbirth classes as an occasional complication of the postpartum period (because it was required as part of the curriculum), I couldn't bring myself to disclose my own depression. It was a painful and perplexing memory, and I had no idea how to bring it up without shame and loss of composure. Finally, after many years of teaching, one of my students suffered from a severe PPMD (perhaps a psychosis). Her husband wanted me to tell her to get a part-time job to cheer her up (when she heard the television set talking to her and telling her to kill herself)! This jolted me to rethink my silence on this issue. Though it felt risky to me to "disclose" what I perceived as a shameful defect, I realized I had to do so. I began discussing the prevalence of PPMD in class, and to get people to listen to me, I disclosed my own story with the message that we **can** recover from PPMDs.

How I could have used Kathleen's book at that time! When I did become aware of the first (1990) edition, I found it most helpful as I tried to prepare my expectant students realistically and positively. To this day, in class, I tell my story and give my students an adaptation of the Edinburgh Postpartum Scale. The purpose is to assist people (mot͵ fathers, and co-parents) to recognize and seek help for this disturbing condition. A knowing how difficult it is to reach out when one is depressed, I invite my students to ͼ me if they are feeling depressed, confused, or otherwise unhappy. I will listen witho͵ judgment or false assurances, and help them figure out where to go from there. I try t͵ help them get into care, which is sometimes challenging due to a shortage of appropriate services. My own experience with a postpartum mood disorder provides me with a lens through which to approach this subject. I like to think I have grown from this experience and can be helpful to today's depressed mothers; much of my confidence has come from the knowledge I gained from earlier editions of this book.

I tell you my story as a reminder that the impact of a PPMD is deep and lasts long after recovery, partly because it is so debilitating and frightening for the sufferer, and also because of widespread ignorance, social pressures, and general lack of adequate mental health services.

The rapid growth of evidence-based knowledge and understanding shows that PPMDs are not simple; they have numerous etiologies and presentations, and, fortunately, there are many ways to promote recovery. My first exposure to Kathleen made me hungry to learn more, and I read voraciously as much as I could of what she had written on the topic. It turns out that her prose is as riveting as her speaking! Her thoughtful, up-to-date descriptions of relevant studies provide accurate and convincing evidence for the conclusions she reports. I believe that you, the reader, will be as impressed as I am with Kathleen's striking breadth of knowledge and the clarity and accuracy of her engaging writing style as she discusses complex phenomena. Whether discussing such topics as historical perspectives on PPMD; adverse childhood experiences and how they impact perinatal mental health; symptoms of various PPMDs; methods of diagnosis and assessment; the impact on the sufferer's own health and her baby's; the social and emotional development of the growing family; relationships with her child and loved ones; treatments, both nonpharmacological and pharmacological; the physiology of postpartum mood disorders; practical advice on how to communicate effectively with others about this topic; and much more, you will appreciate the breadth of coverage and the scientific rigor she demonstrates in her explanations.

This new edition is divided into three sections, which provide up-to-date encyclopedic coverage of postpartum depression and all other postpartum mood disorders: (1) Symptoms, incidence, and consequences; (2) Risk factors for PPMD; and (3) Treatment options. Her Epilogue, "Some final thoughts," gives very practical and doable suggestions to the counselor or the listener with whom the depressed person shares her story. It's all here!

The list of references at the end of the book is 42 pages long! The findings of relevant studies are summarized throughout the book. This is a veritable gold mine for researchers who want to investigate specific aspects of this field and for those clinicians who seek more information for their work in the field.

In this new edition, Kathleen has added much on infant feeding methods and their impact on maternal depression. Loaded with practical information and advice for lactation consultants, nurses, physicians, postpartum doulas, and other helpers, she makes a strong case for the value of breastfeeding in increasing maternal sleep and restoring mental health and empowerment to those with previous sexual or other trauma. Furthermore, I think the reader will be impressed with the amount of research support that exists for breastfeeding as an aid to maternal and infant sleep, as a buffer against depression, and as a healing practice for those women who have experienced sexual trauma and worry about bonding with their baby.

One of the fastest growing areas of interest in maternity care today is the high prevalence of birth trauma (approximately one in four births are described as traumatic by American mothers), and the detrimental effects of traumatic childbirths on the mother, baby, and family. Trauma can be physical (i.e., including death or injury to mother or baby) and it can also be psychological (i.e., disrespectful treatment; rude or insensitive words; coerced or forced unwanted interventions; criticism of the mother; ignoring the parents' wishes, etc.). Though the field is changing and the definition of posttraumatic stress disorder has changed, Kathleen's expertise is evident in her analyses of the many facets of birth trauma: predisposing factors, diagnosis, prevalence, and symptoms. Furthermore, she provides much insight and discusses practical evidence-based ways to promote recovery.

I have had the pleasure of working with Kathleen on the Board of Directors for PATTCh (Prevention and Treatment of Traumatic Childbirth); I deeply appreciate her passion, knowhow, and generosity in assisting PATTCh to become an effective agent for change. Please visit our website, PATTCh.org, and from there go to our Facebook page for helpful exchanges of ideas.

I hope you find this book as useful as I have in understanding and alleviating postpartum mood disorders!

Penny Simkin, PT, CD DONA, CCE
Co-founder of PATTCh (Prevention and Treatment of Traumatic Childbirth),
and author (with Phyllis Klaus) of *When Survivors Give Birth:*
Understanding and Healing the Effects of Early Sexual Abuse on a
Woman's Later Childbearing

Reference

Larsen, V., Evans, T., & Martin, L. 1967. Differences between new mothers: psychiatric admissions vs. normals. *Journal of the American Medical Women's Association*, 22(12), 995–998.

Preface

I wrote my first book on postpartum depression 26 years ago.[1] Armed with a brand new PhD in developmental psychology, and a growing conviction that postpartum depression was not simply a matter of "hormones," I summarized the existing research, and tried to explain why some women got depressed after having a baby. The general depression literature clearly demonstrated that factors such as abuse, trauma, pain, low socioeconomic status (SES), lack of support, or sleep deprivation increased women's risk of depression. However, there were few studies at the time that demonstrated that these factors increased depression risk in perinatal women. While the rest of the depression field was making tremendous strides, in the perinatal depression world, we were all still talking about hormones.

So much has changed. Hundreds of new studies from around the world have now confirmed that all of the factors listed above contribute to depression in perinatal women. This book summarizes and gives you access to these studies.

One of the concepts I introduced in the second edition of this book was the role of systemic inflammation in perinatal depression. This has been a critical shift in how we understand depression. Inflammation is not simply *a* risk factor for depression; it is *the* risk factor, the one that underlies all the others (Kendall-Tackett, 2007). Individual risk factors are still relevant, but psychoneuroimmunology (PNI) research provides a unifying framework for understanding why we see what we see. PNI researchers have also found that all effective treatments for depression are also anti-inflammatory. By lowering inflammation, we can both prevent and treat depression in new mothers.

In addition, we now know much more about the complex role of breastfeeding and sleep in the etiology of postpartum depression. When I first started in this field, postpartum depression experts pretty much ignored breastfeeding, and mothers were routinely told to wean. The situation has improved—somewhat. Mothers are often still pressured to wean, which can be quite counterproductive. PNI researchers have found that breastfeeding actually protects maternal mental health because it turns off the inflammatory response system. On a related topic, mothers are also given a lot of advice about infant sleep that, if followed, actually increases their risk of depression. As you will see, it's impossible to talk about infant sleep in the first 6 months without considering how a baby is fed. If advice interferes with how babies are fed, it becomes counterproductive.

Another recent development is the large number of studies on trauma as a risk factor for perinatal depression. We now have a large literature on birth trauma. In addition, recent studies also focus on partner violence, childhood abuse, and even natural disasters. These studies are welcome additions to the field.

Mothers now have more treatment choices than ever before. Psychotherapy is still the front-line treatment, particularly interpersonal psychotherapy (IPT). We also have more studies on complementary and integrative treatments for depression. Antidepressants are still the most common form of treatment, but some confusion remains about whether antidepressants are safe for pregnant and lactating women. I will address that topic in much detail in Chapter 18.

These newer findings have changed the way we think about depression, and have given us a truer picture of it. Unfortunately, the need is critical. Many experts still say that incidence of postpartum depression is 10–15 percent. I believe the percentage is much higher, especially once we consider women of color, low-income women, women in developing countries, immigrants, and other high-risk populations. Ten percent to 15 percent is what you see in studies of affluent, white women. Once we broaden our scope, a very different picture emerges. We need to find ways to reach out to these high-risk mothers as well.

You have before you an opportunity to make a real difference in the lives of mothers and babies. Pediatrician Dr. Ray Helfer once described the perinatal period as a "window of opportunity" in our work with families. At no other time are they as interested and willing to learn. If you can identify postpartum depression, and help mothers get the treatment they need, you can save them, and their families, years of suffering. It's a worthy goal. My goal is to equip you to do just that.

Note

1 I wrote the first book in 1992. The original title was *Postpartum Depression: A Comprehensive Approach for Nurses*. I changed the title *Depression in New Mothers* with the 2005 edition because I felt it more accurately represented the content. Depression can occur well outside the 6-week postpartum window.

Part I

Symptoms, incidence, and consequences

Chapter 1

Depression in new mothers
Myth vs. reality

> Depression is among the most disabling disorders for women in their childbearing years. For women aged 15 to 44 years around the world it is second only to HIV/AIDS in terms of total disability. Moreover, in the United States, depression is the leading cause of non-obstetric hospitalization among women aged 18 to 44 years.
>
> (Michael O'Hara, 2009, p. 1258)

Depression is one of the most common complications of childbirth, and one of the most disabling. Yet people often do not recognize it when they see it. Postpartum depression isolates mothers when they most need the help of others. Mothers may be ashamed to admit that life with a new baby is not always bliss. They may assume that everyone has made a smoother transition to motherhood than they have. They may be truly embarrassed that they are not able to "cope" better, as Beck (2006) describes:

> Postpartum depression is a serious mood disorder that can cripple a woman's first months as a new mother. I have described it as "a thief that steals motherhood." Without appropriate clinical intervention, postpartum depression can have long-ranging implications for both mother and child.
>
> (p. 40)

Myths about postpartum depression

Misperceptions abound regarding depression in new mothers. Unfortunately, myths and misperceptions can keep mothers from receiving the attention they need. Here are some of the most common.

Myth #1: Depression in new mothers is not serious

Some people still trivialize depression in new mothers. What they fail to understand is that depression can cause serious, if not life-threatening, consequences for mothers and babies.

Myth #2: Postpartum depression is caused by shifts in estrogen and progesterone

This description of depression still exists despite the fact that many studies contradict it. Unfortunately, this hypothesis can distract us from the real underlying causes of depression, and can also lead to ineffective, and even harmful, treatment practices.

Myth #3: Postpartum depression is more common in white middle-class women

Revelations of postpartum depression by such well-known women as Brooke Shields, Marie Osmond, and the late Princess Diana, have been undeniably helpful in that they have increased awareness. The downside, however, is that they have inadvertently reinforced the notion that postpartum depression is a condition of privilege. The reality is that postpartum depression affects women in many different cultures, and across all income levels. In fact, lower-income and racial/ethnic-minority women are often at higher risk.

Myth #4: We don't really know what causes postpartum depression

Yes, we do. The causes of depression vary from woman to woman. But we have identified the major risk factors for depression.

Myth #5: Postpartum depression will go away on its own

Unfortunately, untreated postpartum depression can last for months—or longer. Zelkowitz and Milet (2001) identified 48 couples where one or both partners had postpartum mental illness. Four months later, 54 percent of the mothers, and 60 percent of their partners, still had psychiatric diagnoses. In another study, mothers were assessed at 2, 3, 6, and 12 months postpartum. Mothers who were depressed at 2 months continued to be depressed at each subsequent assessment point throughout the first year (Beeghly et al., 2002).

Myth #6: Women with postpartum depression cannot breastfeed

Sadly, when women seek help for depression, many are told to wean. For some mothers, weaning is no problem. But for others, weaning is experienced as a significant loss. The good news is that exclusive breastfeeding actually protects mothers' mental health. Supporting breastfeeding can help her recover, and almost all treatment options are compatible with breastfeeding.

Myth #7: Women should avoid nighttime breastfeeding to prevent depression

There is no evidence that supports this myth, and the advice that follows is totally impractical, and may actually undermine mothers' mental health. Several recent, large research studies have demonstrated that exclusively breastfeeding mothers get more sleep than their mixed- or formula-feeding counterparts. Once mothers start supplementing, they actually get less sleep. I will describe these studies in Chapter 7.

Symptoms of depression

Postpartum depression can manifest in a wide variety of symptoms. These include moods of sadness, anhedonia (the inability to experience pleasure), low self-esteem, apathy and social withdrawal, excessive emotional sensitivity, pessimistic thinking, irritability, sleep disturbance, appetite disturbance, impaired concentration, and agitation (Preston

& Johnson, 2009). They may feel mentally foggy, anxious, angry, or guilty. They may believe that their lives will never be normal again (Beck, 2002). For some women, it may be more acceptable to talk about physical ailments, rather than depression, so they may present with pain, fatigue, and sleep and appetite disturbances (Alexander, 2007). Missing their postpartum appointment may also indicate possible depression. A study from Brazil of 516 postpartum women found that 22 percent of women who came to their postpartum appointment screened positive for depression compared to 33 percent of women who missed or rescheduled their appointment (Lobato, Brunner, Dias, Moraes, & Reichenheim, 2012).

Donna describes how her symptoms came on suddenly after the birth of her daughter.

> I never really went into labor. They did three inductions ... I knew I was going to have a C-section ... When they said it was a girl, I just went numb. I just didn't feel like I had a given birth. I felt disconnected from my body. I was up for 24 hours. I was crying hysterically. She wanted to eat a lot. I never was able to breastfeed. I was in the hospital crying. I didn't feel like her mother. I was very disconnected. I was freaking out. My friends kept telling me that it was the baby blues.

Women in non-Western cultures may describe the symptoms of postpartum depression in quite different terms. For example, in a qualitative study of 12 women from Ghana, the predominant symptom of depression was described as "thinking too much" (Scorza, Owusu-Agyei, Asampong, & Wainberg, 2015). The thoughts these women describe could be rumination, a classic symptom of depression. They could also be related to posttraumatic stress disorder (PTSD).

> I don't sleep at night or in the day because the eyes cannot close while the mind is still thinking.
>
> You sleep small, and when those thoughts come into your mind, you cannot sleep anymore.

Mothers, and their partners and mothers (serving as key informants), described the mothers' symptoms including body pain, trouble eating and sleeping, low milk supply, intrusive thoughts, social withdrawal, sadness, and tearfulness (Scorza et al., 2015). Seven of the 12 women believed that their condition would kill either them or their babies, and 5 of the 12 had suicidal thoughts. Contributing factors included financial problems, family stress and lack of support, and problems between women and their partners.

Diagnostic criteria for major depressive disorder

While many mothers may exhibit symptoms of depression, major depression is a more serious manifestation of depressive symptoms that has specific diagnostic criteria in the *Diagnostic and Statistical Manual-5* (DSM-5). For a diagnosis of major depression, patients must have at least five of the following symptoms during the same two-week period:

(1) Depressed mood
(2) Markedly diminished interest or pleasure in all or almost all activities

(3) Significant (> 5 percent body weight) weight loss or gain
(4) Decrease or increase in appetite
(5) Insomnia or hypersomnia
(6) Psychomotor agitation or retardation
(7) Fatigue or loss of energy
(8) Feelings of worthlessness or inappropriate guilt
(9) Diminished concentration or indecisiveness
(10) Recurrent thoughts of death or suicide.

The above symptoms should not be due to psychosis, and the woman should never have had a manic or hypomanic episode. Further, the woman's symptoms should not be due to physical illness, alcohol, medication or illegal drugs, or normal bereavement. In addition, these symptoms must represent a change in previous functioning, and must include at least depressed mood and anhedonia. These symptoms can be by subjective report or observation of others, and must occur nearly every day (American Psychiatric Association, 2013).

Is postpartum depression a distinct condition?

Professionals frequently raise the question of whether postpartum depression is distinct from depression that occurs outside the puerperium. Some have argued that puerperal and non-puerperal mental illnesses are similar in terms of their symptomatology and factors predicting onset, and that the *only* distinguishing characteristic of puerperal mental illness is onset and triggers that are specific to new motherhood (e.g. infant characteristics, sleep deprivation, and birth experience).

At the present time, there is no specific diagnostic category for postpartum illness in the DSM-5. The specifier "with peripartum onset" can be added to a current or recent depressive, manic, or hypomanic episode in major depressive disorder, bipolar disorder I or II if the episode happens during pregnancy and up to 4 weeks postpartum (American Psychiatric Association, 2013; Sharma & Mazmanian, 2014).

Critics of this new diagnostic category note that they are unable to include anxiety disorders, obsessive–compulsive disorder (OCD), or PTSD under the peripartum specifier, even though the DSM acknowledges that anxiety and panic attacks can co-occur with perinatal depression. In addition, 4 weeks postpartum is far too short a time period for this diagnosis in that depression can happen any time in the first year (Sharma & Mazmanian, 2014). The DSM-5 also cites the incidence of depression as 3–6 percent—far below the actual number of even the most conservative estimate.

MRI studies of depression

Beginning in the 1990s, the number of studies that compared anatomical brain variations between depressed and non-depressed people dramatically increased. The brains of depressed people had reduced volume of structures that process emotions including the prefrontal cortex, orbitofrontal cortex, cingulum, hippocampus, and striatum. The white matter also had notable abnormalities in depressed people. Perhaps the most important contribution to magnetic resonance imaging (MRI) research of depression is "blood oxygen level dependent" (BOLD), which shows levels of hemodynamic response to stimuli. In functional MRI studies, people with depression often show significant decrease in activation of key structures, such as the medial prefrontal cortex and amygdala (Fiorelli et al., 2015).

To consider the issue of whether postpartum depression was a distinct condition, Fiorelli and colleagues (2015) reviewed the literature on postpartum/postnatal depression and MRI/neuroimaging. They identified 11 studies. These studies examined women's reactions to threatening words or negative facial expressions. Depressed women had reduced activation in the amygdala and dorsomedial prefrontal cortex. Another study found that the depressed women did not show a difference in activation when hearing their own infants' cries vs. those of other infants. Fiorelli et al. noted that the MRI studies of postpartum depression replicated those of major depressive disorder, and concluded that the data did not support a distinct neurobiological profile for postpartum depression. They did also note, however, the relative dearth of MRI studies on perinatal depression (11 studies) compared to studies of major depressive disorder (over 1,000). With an increase in MRI studies, a distinct profile may still be identified.

Incidence and prevalence of depression in new mothers

Incidence of postpartum depression ranges quite a bit depending on the population studied and how depression is defined. The typical range is 12–25 percent of new mothers, with rates in some high-risk groups being as high as 40 percent or more. A study of 86,957 mothers and fathers in the US found that they are at highest risk for depression in the first year postpartum (Dave, Petersen, Sherr, & Nazareth, 2010). By the time their children are 12 years old, 39 percent of mothers and 21 percent of fathers have been depressed.

Studies that report higher percentages of depressed mothers may have included both major depression and depressive symptoms in their totals. Similarly, the percentage will be higher if major and minor depression are included in the "depressed" group. Below is a summary of studies from around the world.

US studies of postpartum depression

The Childbirth Connections' Listening to Mothers' Survey II included a nationally representative sample of 1,573 mothers in the US found that one in three mothers reported depressive symptoms in the past two weeks: 34 percent reported feeling down, depressed, or hopeless, and 36 percent reported anhedonia (little interest or pleasure in doing things) (Declercq, Sakala, Corry, & Applebaum, 2008). In a large US population study, 14,093 women, ages 18–50, were interviewed about past pregnancy status (Vesga-Lopez et al., 2008). Women who were currently pregnant women had the lowest risk of mood disorders. Postpartum women had significantly higher rates of major depression compared with non-postpartum women. Risk factors for psychiatric disorders in pregnant and postpartum women included age, marital status, health status, stressful live events, and history of trauma.

The Centers for Disease Control published prevalence data on postpartum depressive symptoms in 17 US states (Centers for Disease Control and Prevention, 2008). The prevalence ranged from 12 percent in Maine to 20 percent in New Mexico. In this sample, women at highest risk for depressive symptoms were younger, had lower levels of education, and received Medicaid benefits. In addition, smoking during the last trimester of pregnancy, and partner-related, traumatic, or financial stress during pregnancy were related to higher depressive symptoms. In a smaller number of states, NICU admission and having a low birthweight baby were associated with depressive symptoms. Depressive symptoms were assessed with the Patient Health Questionnaire-2 (PHQ-2).[1]

In a sample drawn from a national evaluation of the Healthy Steps for Young Children program, 4,874 mothers completed interviews at 2–4 months postpartum (McLearn, Minkovitz, Strobion, Marks, & Hou, 2006b). Using the Center for Epidemiologic Studies Depression Scale (CES-D), they found that 18 percent of mothers had depressive symptoms. Depressed mothers were less likely to continue breastfeeding, show their infants a book at least once a day, play with their infant at least once a day, talk to their infants while working, or follow two or more routines. The authors concluded that depression is common in the early postpartum period and can lead to unfavorable parenting practices.

US ethnic group differences

Several recent studies have found that incidence of depression varies by ethnicity within the US. A study from North Carolina compared rates of depression in new mothers (N = 586) among four American ethnic groups: Hispanics, Native Americans, African Americans, and Whites (Wei et al., 2008). Hispanic women had by far the lowest rates of depression: 2.5 percent. In contrast, Native Americans had the highest rates of major depression (19 percent), and an average rate of minor depression (11 percent). White women had the second-highest rates of major depression (18 percent), and the highest rate of minor depression (20 percent). The rate for African Americans was 15 percent, and 10 percent for major and minor depression, respectively. Breastfeeding was associated with lower depressive symptoms; Hispanic women had the highest breastfeeding rate, which the authors thought explained their low rate of depression. Women's history of or treatment for depression were related to higher depressive symptoms.

In contrast, 23 percent of low-income Hispanic mothers (N = 218) were depressed (EPDS ≥10),[2] with only half of the women indicating that they needed help for sadness or depression since their child's birth (Chaudron et al., 2005). Using the more stringent cutoff (EPDS ≥13), the rate of depression was 13 percent. In this sample, adolescents had higher rates of depression.

In a prospective of 1,735 women, Mora and colleagues (2009) described the trajectories of depressive symptoms in a sample of low-income, multiethnic, inner-city women. Seventy percent of the women were African American, 17 percent were Latina, and the remaining 13 percent were White or other ethnicities. The women were recruited during pregnancy and interviewed once during pregnancy, and at three times postpartum interviews up to two years later. Based on their analyses, they grouped the women into five distinct groups: chronically depressed (7 percent); antenatal depression only (6 percent); postpartum only—resolves in the first year postpartum (9 percent); late, present at 25 months postpartum (7 percent); and never having been depressed (71 percent). The authors thought it remarkable that 71 percent of the women were not depressed at any assessment, and that a further 15 percent had transient symptoms. Depression across the three classes shared some risk factors: high stress and fair to poor self-rated emotional health. Women were more likely to have chronic depression if they had a high number of pregnancies. If they were ambivalent about being pregnant, they were more likely to be depressed during pregnancy and have chronic depression.

Unfortunately, racial/ethnic minority women are at higher risk for depression, and were less likely to be diagnosed and treated than their White counterparts. Another recent study also found that younger women, African Americans, Hispanics, other non-White women were least likely to be diagnosed with depression (Centers for Disease Control and Prevention, 2015).

International incidence of postpartum depression

Studies from the European Union

Researchers in Norway found that rates of depression ranged from 11 percent in the second and third trimesters of pregnancy to 7 percent at 12 months postpartum using the EPDS ≥ 10. Depression prevalence did not significantly vary from the second and third trimesters of pregnancy to 12 months postpartum (Eberhard-Gran, Tambs, Opjordsmoen, Skrondal, & Eskild, 2004).

A study from Spain screened 1,453 women for depression and other psychiatric disorders, and found that 18 percent had at least one psychiatric disorder, with mood disorders being the most common (Navarro et al., 2008). When mothers experienced more than one psychiatric condition, the combination of depression and anxiety was the most common. Eating disorders and depression was another common combination.

Postpartum depression occurred in comparable rates in mothers from Turkey (Danaci, Dinc, Deveci, Sen, & Icelli, 2002). In this study, 14 percent of 257 mothers were depressed at 6 months postpartum. Risk factors for depression included a higher number of living children, living in a shanty, being an immigrant, having a baby with a serious health problem, the mother's or her husband's previous history of psychiatric illness, and poor relationships with her spouse or his family.

Another Turkish study of 479 pregnant women found a similar rate using the EPDS, cutoff 12/13: 18 percent in the first week postpartum and 14 percent at 6 weeks (Kirpinar, Gozum, & Pasinlioglu, 2010). The strongest predictors of postpartum depression were a history of depression or anxiety during pregnancy, poor marital relationships in early postpartum, lack of health insurance, and lack of contraceptive use.

A third study from Turkey had results consistent with the previous two (Turkcapar et al., 2015). In this study, 15 percent ($n = 83$) had an EPDS score >13. Women who had suicidal thoughts during pregnancy were seven times more likely to have postpartum depression. Other risk factors included previous psychiatric history or postpartum depression, depressive symptoms during pregnancy, and physical violence during pregnancy or postpartum. Depression was assessed via EPDS and Hospital and Anxiety and Depression Scale (HADS) (Kirpinar et al., 2010; Turkcapar et al., 2015).

Studies from Australia

A recent study from Australia found that mothers had the highest rates of depression at 4 years postpartum, much later than we typically think of as a high-risk period (Woolhouse, Gartland, Mensah, & Brown, 2015). In this study, 1,507 women were recruited during pregnancy from six Melbourne public hospitals. The mothers were assessed at 3, 6, 12, and 18 months postpartum, and at 4 years postpartum. Depression was defined as ≥13 on the EPDS. The study revealed that 31 percent of women had depressive symptoms at some time in the first 4 years postpartum. Women with one child at 4 years postpartum had significantly higher rates of depression (23 percent) than women with more than one child (11 percent). The strongest predictors of depression at 4 years were depression in early pregnancy and in the first 12 months postpartum, young maternal age at baseline, stressful life events, social adversity, intimate partner violence, and low income.

Another study from Australia looked at hospital admissions for depressive disorders for first-time mothers before and after birth (Xu, Austin, Reilly, Hilder, & Sullivan, 2012). The sample included 728 women with first admissions for depressive disorder. Fewer women were admitted during pregnancy, but that the rate increased dramatically in the first 3 months postpartum. The highest rate was in month 2. Rate of admissions remained high throughout the second year postpartum, but was significantly elevated across the entire first year. Those admitted to the hospital were likely to be older mothers, those who smoked, had an elective cesarean, and had babies admitted to the NICU or special care nursery. Women with lower SES and immigrants were also more likely to be admitted.

Studies from Asia

In Korea, 49 percent of 148 women at 2–6 weeks postpartum were identified as being depressed on the Beck Depression Inventory. The majority had mild depression. Risk factors included smoking before pregnancy, low marital satisfaction and support, "bad mood" during and after pregnancy, and lack of sleep postpartum. Interestingly, they also investigated an entire list of activities that Korean traditional postpartum care dictates. They found that none of the traditional care practices were related to a lower depression score. These activities included keeping the windows sealed, heating the floor, avoiding hard or tough foods, lifting heavy things, and covering their whole body with a blanket (Lee & Hwang, 2015).

Another study from Korea found similarly high percentages of depressed mothers (Park, Karmaus, & Zhang, 2015). In this study, 153 women were recruited from maternity clinics, and evaluated during the first, second, and third trimesters of pregnancy, and at 4 weeks postpartum using the EPDS-Korean version. The prevalence of depression ranged from 41 percent to 61 percent. Depression in the second and third trimesters predicted postpartum depression, and unemployment and household income predicted prenatal depression.

Mothers in India ($N = 252$) also suffered from postpartum depression. They were interviewed during their third trimester, at 6–8 weeks and 6 months postpartum. Twenty-three percent were depressed, and 78 percent of these women had "substantial" clinical morbidity. Their risk factors for depression included economic deprivation, poor marital relationships, and gender of the infant. The factor unique to this culture was gender of the infant; mothers were more likely to become depressed if they had a girl (Patel, Rodrigues, & DeSouza, 2002).

Murray and colleagues (2015) compared urban ($n = 216$) and rural ($n = 215$) samples from Central Vietnam. They examined son preference and traditional confinement practices, as well as poverty, parity, infant health, partner violence, and infant health in its relationship to postpartum depression. Using an EPDS cutoff of 12/13, they found that 20 percent of the urban women and 16 percent of the rural women had depressive symptoms. Infant gender was not related to depression, but poverty, food insecurity, breastfeeding difficulties, being frightened of family members, mother-in-law reacting negatively to the baby, and recent partner violence were. Regarding traditional confinement practices, some were significantly related to lower EPDS scores if they were *not* practiced. Mothers had lower depression scores if they did not avoid watching TV, bathing for 1–3 months, washing their hair, reading, and if they avoided eating special foods. Other traditional practices had no impact on depression. Only using traditional medicine resulted in lower EPDS scores.

Mothers in Nepal had surprisingly low rates of depression (Regmi, Sligl, Carter, Grut, & Seear, 2002): 12 percent at 2–3 months postpartum. The authors were surprised at this low rate, and pointed out that Nepal is one of the poorest countries in the world, with an infant mortality rate of 75 per 1000. So although these women suffer from many adversities, they also display amazing resilience.

A recent longitudinal study of Han Chinese women examined whether a history of major depression was related to previous postpartum depression (Yang et al., 2015). In the sample of women who had had recurrent major depression, 18 percent experienced postpartum depression, 59 percent of which were first-onset major depression ($N = 5,391$). Mothers with a history of both depression and postpartum depression had more comorbid symptoms including generalized anxiety disorder (GAD), dysthymia, agoraphobia, animal phobia, and situational phobia. Risk factors for major depression for women with a history of postpartum depression included childhood sexual abuse (reported by 16 percent), stressful life events, lack of social support from husbands and friends, severe premenstrual syndrome (PMS), a higher number of births, and a stronger family history of major depression.

Studies from South America

In a study of mothers from Costa Rica and Chile, one-third of the mothers were dysphoric after childbirth, and 35–50 percent had had at least one episode of major depressive disorder (MDD) in their lifetimes. All the mothers were low-income and had at least one child under the age of three (Wolf, De Andraca, & Lozoff, 2002).

A study of 892 women from nine countries found that the rates of depression were highest in non-Whites from Asia and South America (Affonso, De, Horowitz, & Mayberry, 2000). Europeans and Australians had the lowest rates. The rate for American mothers was somewhere in between. The countries included were the US, Guyana, Italy, Sweden, Finland, Korea, Taiwan, India, and Australia.

Studies from the Middle East

In a prospective study of 137 women from the United Arab Emirates (UAE), 16.8 percent had a score ≥10 on the EPDS, and 10.1 percent were formally diagnosed with depression via MINI[3] at 2 months postpartum (Hamdan & Tamim, 2011). Non-Arabic women were excluded. The factors that predicted postpartum depression were depression in pregnancy for both second and third trimesters, number of children, non-Muslim religion, and formula feeding. (Non-Muslims were religious minorities in the UAE.)

Another study compared women in two rural communities in Pakistan ($n = 1,727$) and Malawi ($n = 1,732$) (Zafar, Jean-Baptiste, Rahman, Neilson, & van den Broek, 2015). The researchers found marked differences in "postpartum psychological morbidity" (defined as an EPDS score ≥9): 27 percent in Pakistan and 3 percent in Malawi. The authors hypothesized that some of this difference could be attributable to where data were collected (in the home setting in Pakistan vs. a busy clinic in Malawi). They also noted that women in Malawi were more likely to be involved in agricultural or other work, and not confined to home. In Malawi (and other African cultures), admitting to anxiety or worry may be associated with "wishing it upon yourself," so disclosure rates are likely to be lower. Finally, mothers in Malawi may experience more support that actually acts to prevent depression and anxiety from occurring. Risk factors for psychological morbidity included complications during a previous pregnancy, and intrapartum or postpartum hemorrhage.

Studies from Africa

In the Sudan, a sample of 300 pregnant women were identified and enrolled in a study, and 238 participated at 3 months postpartum (Khalifa, Glavin, Bjertness, & Lien, 2015).Women were screened for depression at 3 months postpartum using the EPDS. Using a cutoff of ≥12, 9 percent were identified as having postpartum depression. Depression was confirmed using the MINI. The authors indicated that EPDS was a valid tool for screening Sudanese women, but suggested a shorter screening test would be helpful due to the limited resources in the Sudan. The percentage is surprisingly low in this country given the ongoing civil war and major social disruptions. The authors are applying a more stringent definition of depression, which tends to result in lower percentages. Surprisingly, the authors say little about this low percent. However, they recommended that screening for depression take place after 6 weeks postpartum due to the intense level of social support families provide for mothers in the first 6 weeks. Could this level of support be the factor that leads to these low levels of depression?

Depression in new fathers

A new area of study in the postpartum depression field is depression in new fathers. Many of the risk factors for depression in fathers are similar to those in mothers. A recent study from Canada compared fathers with and without depression (deMontigny, Girard, Lacharite, Dubeau, & Devault, 2013). The infants of all the fathers in the study were exclusively breastfeeding. Risk factors for depression included previous perinatal loss, decreased marital adjustment, a child with a difficult temperament, and perceived low parental efficacy.

A longitudinal study of 200 couples from Hong Kong showed that high levels of depressive symptoms during pregnancy, and partner's depressive symptoms, significantly increased fathers' depressive symptoms at 6 months postpartum (Ngai & Ngu, 2015). The prevalence rate for fathers was 7 percent during pregnancy, and 11 percent at 6 months postpartum. The prevalence rate for mothers was 16 percent during pregnancy, and 13 percent at 6 months postpartum. Lack of social support was related to depression for mothers, but not for fathers. Depression was measured using the General Health Questionnaire.

A survey from Japan of 837 new parents found that 14 percent of fathers, and 10 percent of mothers, were depressed based on their score on the EPDS (Nishimura, Fujita, Katsuta, Ishihara, & Ohashi, 2015). Depression in fathers was positively associated with depression in mothers, and negatively associated with marital satisfaction. For fathers, the risk factors for depression included a history of infertility treatment, going to a medical facility for treatment of a mental disorder, and economic anxiety.

Summary

The above-cited studies indicate that postpartum depression occurs in many different countries, in fathers, and in all racial/ethnic groups in the US. The pattern is not entirely clear from these studies which ethnic group is most at risk, but what we do know is that postpartum depression can affect mothers and fathers from a broad range of backgrounds, ethnicities, and nationalities.

Notes

1 The Patient Health Questionnaire (PHQ-2) will be described in more detail in Chapter 5.
2 EPDS = Edinburgh Postnatal Depression Scale. This scale will be described in more detail in Chapter 5.
3 MINI = Mini International Neuropsychiatric Interview, a structured, diagnostic interview for depression.

Chapter 2   Conditions comorbid with postpartum depression

Depression is often a highly comorbid condition. A woman with depression may also have anxiety disorders, OCD, PTSD, and possibly bipolar disorder. A recent study of 245 in Brazil found that 18 percent of mothers ($n = 45$) met the criteria for depression (EPDS $\geq$ 13 and positive MINI PLUS) (Figueira, Malloy-Diniz, Romano-Silva, Neves, & Correa, 2009). Of the 45 women with depression, 42 had at least one other psychiatric disorder, and 34 had at least two other psychiatric disorders. The most common comorbid symptoms include anxiety disorder, OCD, social phobia, and agoraphobia. The most common co-occurring conditions are described below.

Postpartum anxiety disorders

Postpartum anxiety disorders include panic disorders, GAD, social phobia, OCD, and PTSD. Several factors appear to contribute to postpartum anxiety disorders including additional responsibilities, and changing social, family, and professional roles (Rapkin, Mikacich, Moatakef-Imani, & Rasgon, 2002).

A study from Australia assessed 139 women during pregnancy, and 105 at a follow-up appointment at 4–6 months postpartum (Clout & Brown, 2015). The authors examined a number of possible predictors of postpartum depression, anxiety, and stress. They found that cesarean delivery was associated with all three. Child and maternal sleep problems were related to depression. Child health problems were related to anxiety. However, these results were no longer significant once antenatal stress, anxiety, and depression were controlled for.

Another study of 207 mothers in Australia examined the relationship between depression and anxiety in pregnancy and postpartum, noting that this relationship is often bidirectional (Skouteris, Wertheim, Rallis, Milgrom, & Paxton, 2009). In their study, depressive symptoms in early pregnancy predicted anxiety symptoms in later pregnancy. Anxiety in later pregnancy predicted depressive symptoms postpartum. These relationships were present even after controlling for social support, prior depression, and sleep quality. Anxiety scores were more stable than depression scores across the multiple assessment points, and the authors suggested that clinicians screen for both depression and anxiety.

In contrast, 159 Australian women participated in a study of depression and anxiety from late pregnancy to 12 months postpartum. The researchers were interested in the cycle of comorbidity of depression and anxiety in perinatal women (Moss, Skouteris, Wertheim, Paxton, & Milgrom, 2009). They controlled for social support, prior depression, and sleep quality. Depression was measured with the short form of the Beck

Depression Inventory, and anxiety was measured with the State–Trait Anxiety Inventory. Moss et al. found that depression did not predict anxiety symptoms at any time point, and anxiety only predicted depression from late pregnancy to early to mid postpartum, but not when social support was controlled for. They recommended screening for both depression and anxiety. Non-depressed women may have other psychiatric conditions. Clinicians should not assume that a non-depressed woman has no other conditions.

A study from Japan included 99 pregnant women, and assessed them during late pregnancy, and at 5 days and 12 months postpartum (Kokubu, Okano, & Sugiyama, 2012). The researchers found that anxiety during pregnancy predicted postpartum depression and bonding failure. Depression in pregnancy did not predict depression postpartum, in contrast to previous studies. "Bonding failure" included positive responses to items such as "I resent my child" or "I feel nothing for my child," and negative responses to items such as "I feel loving towards my child" or "I enjoy doing things with my child."

Panic disorder

Panic disorder is characterized by sudden, recurrent, and unpredictable panic attacks. Symptoms include palpitations, shortness of breath, chest pain, dizziness, fear of losing control, and fear of dying. In a review, Ross and MacLean (2006) noted that 50 percent of individuals with panic disorder also have major depression. A more recent pregnancy cohort study from Australia of 1,507 women found that 9 percent reported intense anxiety or panic attacks that occurred from occasionally to often, and 10 percent reported depressed mood between 6 and 9 months postpartum (Woolhouse, Brown, Krastev, Perlen, & Gunn, 2009). The authors used only a single item to assess anxiety/panic attacks, not a standardized measure. In addition, because anxiety and panic attacks were both included in this item, these data do not provide an accurate measure of incidence of panic disorder. However, these data do suggest that anxiety is a common problem in the postpartum period. Their findings also revealed that mothers were significantly more likely to seek assistance for depressive symptoms vs. anxiety. However, they were most likely to seek assistance if they experienced both.

Panic disorder was assessed retrospectively in 128 women from Germany, 93 of whom had 195 pregnancies (Bandelow et al., 2006). Women had fewer panic attacks during pregnancy. They were more frequent in the postpartum period compared with the control period. Breastfeeding and miscarriages were not significantly related to panic attacks. For 3 percent of the pregnancies, mothers reported that their panic attacks improved. For 79 percent of pregnancies, mothers reported no difference. For 18 percent of pregnancies, mothers reported that they increased.

A sample recruited from an urban healthcare center in Philadelphia included 188 mothers of infants who were assessed for mood and anxiety disorders (Cerulli, Talbot, Tang, & Chaudron, 2011). Twenty-eight percent had been assaulted by their current or ex-intimate partner, and 20 percent reported intimate partner violence (IPV) within the past year. Not surprisingly, women reporting IPV were more likely to have mood and anxiety disorders, including depression and panic disorder. The authors suggested that when women have perinatal mood disorders, practitioners consider a possible contributory role of IPV. The authors note the following:

> The findings reveal a portrait of a patient that may appear in a pediatrician's office for a well-baby visit—exhausted, overwhelmed, and anxious. Without

inquiry into the mother's experiences, it is easy for one to jump to a conclusion that she is only a nervous, sleep-deprived new mother. The findings suggest that the clinical picture may be more complex, however, and that careful assessment of the possible co-occurrence of IPV and mood and/or anxiety disorder is warranted.

(p. 1801)

Obsessive–compulsive disorder

Obsessive–compulsive disorder (OCD) is another anxiety disorder that often co-occurs with postpartum depression. It is characterized by recurrent, unwelcome thoughts, ideas, or doubts that give rise to anxiety and distress (obsessions). These obsessions lead to excessive behavioral or mental acts (Abramowitz et al., 2002; Ross & McLean, 2006). Although data are limited, the postpartum prevalence of OCD is approximately 3–4 percent (Ross & McLean, 2006).

A study of 60 mothers seeking treatment for perinatal mood disorders measured depression, anxiety, and OCD symptoms (Abramowitz et al., 2010). The researchers found that the majority of the sample (52 of 60) had both obsessive-like thoughts and compulsive behaviors (neutralizing strategies). The majority had mild symptoms, but 23 had clinically significant OCD symptoms. Both depression and anxiety were associated with obsessive–compulsive symptoms. Women who had EPDS scores ≥11 had significantly higher scores on the measure of obsessive–compulsive symptoms.

A prospective cohort study of 461 postpartum women found that 11 percent screened positive for OCD, while another 38 percent had subclinical obsessions and compulsions (Miller, Hoxha, Wisner, & Gossett, 2015). Subclinical OCD was associated with both depression (24 percent) and state–trait anxiety (8 percent). The obsessions included fear of doing something embarrassing, harming others because they're not careful enough, being responsible for something terrible happening, dirt and germs, not saying just the right thing, or losing things, and being obsessive about symmetry or exactness, feeling like they need to know or remember certain things. The compulsions included being bothered by certain sounds or noise or mental images, having superstitious fears, washing hands excessively or in a ritualized way, checking that they did not make a mistake, and needing to reread or rewrite things. The authors noted that nearly half of all women experience obsessions and compulsions postpartum, and that the majority of these do not represent overt OCD. They recommended that clinicians offer reassurance if these obsessions and compulsions are not disruptive in a woman's life.

Karin describes how she developed symptoms of OCD and panic disorder after a previous stillbirth and high-risk pregnancy. Her symptoms started about 6 months after her baby was born.

> I was nervous about everything. About germs, development, baby care, all of it. I started having these thoughts about Zeke's safety. The scariest part were these weird thoughts about harming him myself. I was afraid to say anything to anybody. They terrified me. I kept hoping it would go away. It didn't.
>
> My whole life up to that point had been defined by my successes at school and work. I was an over-achiever. Someone else had cared for my baby at birth and done a better job than me. And now I was just a glorified babysitter. I loved my son, but I always felt disconnected from him.

I went back to school when Zeke was 10 months old and it was such a relief for me. He weaned almost as soon as I went back. I didn't know what a nursing strike was. I just assumed he didn't want me anymore. But at school I was finally being recognized for what I knew how to do. My husband, Jared, was working full-time on swing shift and going to school full-time. I didn't see him much. We had moved into my parents' basement during my pregnancy, and I was spending a lot of time with my parents. My mother and sister helped with some of Zeke's care. After 1 year of classes, I was exhausted. Cleaning up the same mess over and over from a toddler was sheer drudgery. Then one night, I had a panic attack just as Jared was getting home from work. I didn't know what was happening. I was terrified. But I knew something was wrong.

My husband had an Employee Assistance Program that was also available to spouses. I didn't know where else to go, but I called them the next day when nobody else was there. I used a quiet voice and felt huge shame. They gave a name to my "incident" the night before. It could have been a panic attack. They got me set up with a counselor in my area who diagnosed me with post-partum depression. Since the EAP only provided 3 sessions, the counselor gave me a few CBT techniques and said I was "ready to go," and discharged me from care.

By that time, it was getting very difficult to even get out of bed. I couldn't sleep without prescription sleep medication, and I knew I was not "ready to go." I found out about the student counseling center on campus and made an appointment there. My first appointment was a disaster. I don't remember what was said, but the counselor said I sounded great. Just as part of policy, they had to administer a depression questionnaire. She looked at my paper, raised her eyebrows, and left the room. When she came back, she graciously said, "I thought you were OK, but this questionnaire shows me you clearly need further help, so I am going to transfer your care to my colleague."

That next counselor was a godsend. She talked to me about my expectations, reassured me that I wouldn't actually hurt my baby, and helped me know when it was time for antidepressants. I slowly got better.

I have since discovered after several counselors, that I actually had postpartum OCD that was left untreated for far too long. I have experienced differing severity of postpartum OCD with every child since then (I now have 7 living children).

Obsessions about infant harm

In postpartum women, obsessive thoughts are often focused on infant harm. Even when there is depression, but no OCD, approximately 40 percent of mothers report also having these thoughts (Ross & McLean, 2006). Some concern fears of hurting the baby with knives, or throwing the baby down stairs or out a window (Abramowitz et al., 2002). Other types of obsessive thoughts concerned their babies dying in their sleep, that they would sexually misuse their babies, or physically misplace them. Not surprisingly, obsessive thoughts can be very troubling to mothers, as DeeDee describes.

My postpartum depression was basically weird thoughts toward the baby, and he was a wonderful baby. The perfect baby. One time I had him on the bathroom floor with me. All of the sudden, I had this thought to kick the baby. This was the first weird thought I had toward him. My pediatrician told me that this was very normal. "You had a traumatic delivery" … I would have weird thoughts when I was breastfeeding. I was constantly worried that the baby would hit his head on the table. I was also scared to walk through the doorway, that he would hit his head. These thoughts would become obsessive. I was afraid if I told anyone, they'd take the baby away. I finally told my mom. She said it was normal and not to worry. This lasted around five months … If I was ironing, I'd be terrified that the baby would be burned. Even if he was upstairs asleep in his bed. Then I would start to analyze my thoughts. "Am I thinking he'd be burned because I wanted him to be burned?" I was also scared of knives … I didn't want to do these things. I couldn't understand why I was thinking this way … These thoughts happened every day, all the time. Slowly, I had fewer thoughts. I'd think "there's no way he can hit his head when I'm holding him" … The hardest thing was I couldn't find anyone who had this experience. I knew about it, but I couldn't seem to find anyone who had been through it. [DeeDee]

A study of four men revealed that they too experienced postpartum OCD that coincided with their partners' deliveries. These obsessions were very similar in content to the obsessional thoughts of new mothers. The men responded with feelings of shame and guilt (Abramowitz, Moore, Carmin, Wiegartz, & Purdon, 2001).

Beck (2002) identified anxiety, relentless obsessive thinking, anger, guilt, and contemplating self-harm as part of her "spiraling down" dimension of postpartum depression. This dimension was part of a meta-synthesis of 18 qualitative studies of postpartum depression. Obsessive thoughts were so intrusive for the women in Beck's (2002) study that they often became intolerable. Women tended to ruminate over feelings of failure as a mother, fearing that they or their babies might be harmed, wondering if they would ever feel normal again, and constantly worrying about the baby. These mothers tended to self-silence and isolate themselves because they were sure no one would understand what they were going through.

Responding to concerns about infant harm

Descriptions of thoughts about harming the baby must also be handled with care. Women I've spoken with indicated that professionals either reacted with great alarm, or assured them that the thoughts were "normal." The women who were troubled by these thoughts indicated that one of the worst reactions people had was to express concern that they would kill their babies. This reaction did not stop the thoughts, but actually fed into them and made them more intense.

Speisman, Storch, & Abramowitz (2011) distinguished obsessive thoughts of infant harm from psychosis. Psychotic symptoms are not present in OCD. In psychosis, thoughts of harm are consistent with a person's delusional thinking. A person acts out aggressive behavior because she believes she has to do it. In contrast, obsessive thoughts do not increase risk of infant harm. These thoughts are unwanted and inconsistent with a person's normal behavior, and so distressing that people suffering from OCD will go to great lengths to keep these bad things from happening.

When speaking to a mother, say something like this: "it must be very distressing to you to have such thoughts. Many other women have these thoughts, and they do not mean that you are a bad mother or will harm your baby. These thoughts usually mean that you are under some type of stress, and it may help to talk with someone about it." Then you can offer some names of people who can help. This type of approach validates her experience while taking the problem seriously.

In more serious cases, you may need to take additional action. If the mother refuses help, or if you fear that the baby is in danger, you may be legally obligated to make a report to the department of social services or your local child protective agency.

Posttraumatic stress disorder

Another co-occurring disorder is posttraumatic stress disorder (PTSD). Women may come into the postpartum period with pre-existing PTSD that could be due to prior trauma, such as previous abuse or sexual assault, or could be caused by the birth itself. Depression and PTSD share several diagnostic features including diminished interest in significant activities, restricted range of affect, difficulty falling and staying asleep, difficulty with concentration, and restricted range of affect. Therefore, we should not be surprised by depression being highly comorbid with PTSD (Kendall-Tackett, 2014a).

Even if women do not meet full criteria for PTSD, they may have troubling posttraumatic stress symptoms. The diagnostic criteria for PTSD have recently changed, and are now described in the Diagnostic and Statistical Manual-5 (American Psychiatric Association, 2013; Friedman, Resick, Bryant, & Brewin, 2011). PTSD will be described in more detail in Chapters 8 and 12, but below is a brief overview of how it intersects with postpartum depression.

A recent review of 78 studies estimated that postpartum PTSD ranges from 3 percent in community samples to 16 percent in at-risk samples (Grekin & O'Hara, 2014). Risk factors for community samples include current depression, birth events, and a history of affective disorders. For at-risk samples, risk factors include current depression and infant complications. The strongest relationship was between postpartum PTSD and postpartum depression. Maternal and infant complications also had a large effect size. This included infants in the NICU. History of trauma and single marital status both had moderate effect sizes, and there was a stronger relationship between trauma history and postpartum PTSD for racial/ethnic minority women.

In a study of Vietnamese and Hmong women living in the US, Foss (2001) found that PTSD was highly correlated with depression. Similarly, a study of 54 Caucasian, Asian, and Pacific Islander women with PTSD found that PTSD during the postpartum period was highly comorbid with depression (73 percent), anxiety (64 percent), and moderate to high life stress (73 percent) (Onoye, Goebert, Morland, & Matsu, 2009). Although there were no significant differences in rates of PTSD based on ethnicity (possibly due to the small N), Pacific Islanders had the highest rates of behavioral health problems related to the condition.

A study from England found that obstetric complications and admission to the ICU were related to maternal PTSD at 6–8 weeks postpartum (Furuta, Sandall, Cooper, & Bick, 2014). This sample was recruited from an inner-city hospital over 6 months (N = 1,825). Eight percent (n = 147) experienced severe maternal morbidity. The complications included hemorrhage, eclampsia, severe hypertension, HELLP syndrome, and admission to intensive care. A total of 6 percent had clinically significant intrusion and 8 percent had clinically significant avoidance. In addition, 14 percent of these mothers had an EPDS score ≥13, but there was no significant difference based on complication status. Women experienced fewer, and less severe, symptoms if they had a higher level of perceived control during their labors. The authors suggested that future studies focus on interventions that can increase mothers' sense of control even when there is an emergency, such as explaining treatments, and involving them in the decisions about their care. Hall (2014/2015) offers a number of specific suggestions on how to help these mothers, and what healthcare providers should say—and not say.

PTSD can also occur during pregnancy. Seng and colleagues (2009) found that rates of lifetime, and current, PTSD were high in a sample of 1,581 pregnant women from diverse backgrounds. The lifetime rate was 20 percent: 17 percent for those with private insurance, and 23 percent had public-payer insurance. The current prevalence of PTSD was 8 percent, but was 14 percent for those who had public-payer insurance. Women with PTSD were more likely to be African American, pregnant as a teen, living in poverty, with a high school education or less, and living in a high-crime neighborhood. Eighty-six percent of women in the PTSD group were experiencing partner violence. The overall rate of major depressive disorder was 12 percent; 85 percent of depression cases were comorbid with either full or partial PTSD. Childhood physical and sexual abuse were major risk factors for both groups. They found that 50 percent of mothers with depression in this study also had comorbid PTSD. The authors argued that screening for depression alone would likely miss the comorbid PTSD.

In data from this same sample as cited above, African American women had the highest rate of trauma exposure and PTSD ($n = 709$) (Seng, Kohn-Wood, McPherson, & Sperlich, 2011a). The rate of lifetime PTSD for African Americans was 24 percent, with current prevalence of 13 percent (compared to 3.5 percent for the predominantly White comparison group). In other words, the current prevalence of PTSD for African Americans was more than four times the rate for Whites and other ethnicities.

Similarly, women with hypertension during pregnancy can also develop PTSD. In a sample recruited from the Preeclampsia Foundation website, 1,076 mothers who experienced hypertension, and 372 with no history of hypertension, completed a survey (Porcel et al., 2013). The conditions related to hypertension included preeclampsia, eclampsia, and HELLP syndrome. Women who had hypertension in pregnancy were 4.46 times more likely to have PTSD.

A qualitative study of 27 pregnant and postpartum living in extreme poverty in Vancouver, Canada found that these women had experienced multiple types of trauma as children and adults (Torchalla, Linden, Strehlau, Neilson, & Krausz, 2015). Many had addictions, been involved in the sex trade, and experienced gender-based violence. The themes that emerged from these women were that trauma and adversities were common, and happened in a variety of contexts, from a variety of perpetrators. The women had experienced partner violence; physical, sexual, and emotional abuse; and child neglect. All of them had been maltreated as children, and 77 percent reported past sexual abuse. The women worried that what they experienced could be passed on to the next generation.

A recent longitudinal study of 119 women in Hawai'i examined the change in symptoms of PTSD, depression, anxiety, and maternal stress during pregnancy and postpartum (Onoye et al., 2013). PTSD symptoms declined over the course of the pregnancy, with a spike in symptoms in the last weeks of pregnancy. Anxiety did not change over time, however, and there was a wide range of individual variability. For depression and stress, there was also a declining trend. This is consistent with studies showing higher rates of depression in pregnancy than postpartum.

PTSD in postpartum women will be described more fully in Chapters 8 and 12.

Eating disorders

Eating disorders can also co-occur with depression during pregnancy and the postpartum period. In one study, active bulimia nervosa also increased the risk of postpartum depression, miscarriage, and preterm birth (Morgan, Lacey, & Chung, 2006). In this study, a cohort of 122 pregnant women with active bulimia were compared with 82 pregnant women with quiescent bulimia. The risk of depression (OR 2.8, CI = 1.2–2.6), miscarriage (OR = 2.6, CI = 1.2–5.6), and preterm birth (OR = 3.3, CI = 1.3–8.8) were all increased among women with active bulimia. These effects were not explained by the confounding factors of laxative misuse, demographic differences, alcohol/substance abuse, cigarette use, or absolute weight difference.

The rate of postpartum depression was 35 percent in a sample of 49 newly postpartum women with eating disorders (Franko et al., 2001). The majority of these women had had normal pregnancies, but three women had babies with birth defects. Among the women in the study, those who had active symptoms of either anorexia or bulimia during pregnancy were at increased risk for postpartum depression. The authors recommended close monitoring of women with past or current eating disorders during pregnancy and in the postpartum period.

Binge eating and vomiting before pregnancy predicted postpartum depression in another study of 181 women. Mothers whose eating disorders were active during pregnancy were the most distressed in this sample, particularly those with a binge or purge type of eating disorder. However, low-intensity exercise was associated with less distress (Abraham, Taylor, & Conti, 2001).

Substance abuse

Finally, substance abuse can also co-occur with postpartum depression. In a review of 17 studies, Ross and Dennis (2009) found that women who were actively abusing substances were at increased risk for postpartum depression. Regarding substances, alcohol, cocaine, and illegal drugs were the substances specifically considered.

In another study (Pajulo, Savonlahti, Sourander, Helenius, & Piha, 2001b), 8 percent of 391 pregnant women were depressed. Substance abuse and life stress both predicted depression in pregnancy, as did difficulties with their social networks (friends, partners, and the women's own mothers). A second study by these same authors (Pajulo et al., 2001a) compared 12 mothers who abused substances, and 12 control mothers in their emotional health and interactions with their babies at 3 and 6 months postpartum. Not surprisingly, the substance-abusing mothers were significantly more depressed, had less social support, and more life stress than the control mothers. They also had less positive interactions with their babies.

Substance abuse is obviously a serious problem for both mothers and babies. If women abuse substances during pregnancy, the state may intervene and remove the baby from the mother's care after delivery. For substance-abusing mothers, intervention for depression alone would be incomplete. Mothers who abuse substances also need referrals to programs that can directly address their substance abuse.

Postpartum psychosis

Postpartum psychosis is the most serious form of postpartum mental illness. Although postpartum psychosis is not the focus of this book, it is important to mention because of its severity, and its co-occurrence with depression. It occurs in 0.1–0.2 percent of all new mothers, and most episodes begin abruptly between days 3 and 14 postpartum (Rapkin et al., 2002).

Miller (2002) noted that the most common differential diagnoses for postpartum psychosis include major depression with psychotic features, bipolar disorder, schizoaffective disorder, schizophrenia, and brief reactive psychosis. Some medical conditions can be related to postpartum psychosis, and should be ruled out before diagnosing these symptoms as due to mood disorders. These other conditions include thyroiditis, hypothyroidism, B12 deficiency, and adult GM_2 gangliosidosis. Substances that can trigger a psychotic episode include bromocriptine, metronidazole, and addictive substances, including LSD, PCP, and ecstasy.

Bipolar disorder

Bipolar disorder is a common type of postpartum psychosis. It is often misdiagnosed because it usually manifests in the puerperium as major depression without psychosis (Beck, 2006). With this disorder, women may experience hypomanic episodes that include inflated self-esteem, increased talkativeness, decreased sleep, racing thoughts, and increased goal orientation. Unlike the mania that occurs in bipolar I disorder, hypomania is not socially disabling. Differentiating major depression from bipolar disorder, particularly bipolar disorder II, can be challenging. But bipolar disorder is associated with a significantly earlier age of onset, more recurrences, atypical and mixed depressions, and a family history of bipolar disorder or completed suicide compared with major depression (Beck, 2006; Yatham et al., 2009). The Canadian Network for Mood and Anxiety Disorder's (CANMAT) guidelines noted that postpartum is a time when rates of hypomania may be at their highest levels (Yatham et al., 2009).

In a study of 30 women with bipolar disorders who had children, 66 percent had a postpartum mood episode (Freeman et al., 2002). Most of these episodes were exclusively depressive. Of the women who became depressed after their first child, all were depressed after subsequent births. Depression during pregnancy also increased the risk of postpartum depression.

A recent study from Italy of 276 women with bipolar disorder tracked their progress through the postpartum period (Maina, Rosso, Aguglia, & Bogetto, 2014). All of these women had been medication-free throughout their pregnancies. Seventy-five percent of them had a history of postpartum mood disorders. The majority of these postpartum mood disorders were depressive (80 percent), but 14 percent had had manic episodes, and 4 percent had mixed episodes. Thirteen patients had psychotic disorder. The authors noted that there was a significant association between postpartum manic and mixed episodes with type I disorder and with psychosis. Their findings indicated that women with bipolar disorder, who are not medicated during pregnancy, are at high risk for mood disorders and psychosis postpartum.

Birth can also trigger episodes of psychosis in bipolar women with a family history of postpartum psychosis (Jones & Craddock, 2001). One study examined 313 deliveries of 152 women with bipolar disorder. Twenty-six percent of the deliveries were followed by an episode of puerperal psychosis, and 38 percent of the women had at least one puerperal psychotic episode. Family history also increased risk. There were 27 women with bipolar disorder who had a family history of postpartum psychosis. Seventy-four percent of these women developed postpartum psychosis. In contrast, only 30 percent of the women with bipolar disorder, but without a family history of postpartum psychosis, had a postpartum psychotic episode.

Although bipolar has a strong genetic component, recent studies have also found a link between bipolar disorder and childhood trauma (Etain, Henry, Bellivier, Mathieu, & Leboyer, 2008). In Etain et al.'s review article, they noted that people with bipolar have often experienced severe and frequent childhood trauma. Trauma in childhood may increase susceptibility, modulate the clinical expression of the disease, and is associated with more severe symptoms. Childhood trauma may affect the age of onset and suicidal behavior, and comorbid depression, panic disorder, and substance abuse. It can also affect patients between episodes. There is a growing body of literature that childhood trauma can dramatically increase women's risk of depression, PTSD, and anxiety disorders. Given this, a link between childhood trauma and bipolar disorder is plausible.

Antidepressants should be used cautiously in women with postpartum depression due to the risk of inducing postpartum psychosis, mania, and rapid cycling (Freeman et al., 2002; Moses-Kolko & Roth, 2004). In published case reports, induction of mania happened with a family history of bipolar disorder (Yatham et al., 2009). For these women, the anticonvulsant medications may be more appropriate in that they have both mood-stabilizing and antidepressant effects (Leibenluft, 2000).

Sleep deprivation and psychosis

Sleep deprivation has been related to delusional thinking and other psychotic symptoms in men and non-postpartum women. Should it surprise us that it could have this same effect on women who have recently given birth? Personal accounts of postpartum psychosis, and accounts given by women interviewed for this book, indicated that women who developed psychosis had been unable to sleep for two to three days before the onset of their illness. *Inability to sleep is a red-flag symptom that requires immediate medical attention.* Charlotte describes her experience.

> My second postpartum experience was a nightmare. I was exhausted … I decided to wean my baby at 2 months because I was so exhausted and depressed … I thought about suicide, institutionalization, and separation from my family constantly … That postpartum psychosis exists was such a revelation to me because in April I had experienced a week of near-total insomnia. During these truly sleepless nights, I had no control over my thoughts, as if my brain had been put in a food processor. The first half of a thought would be rational and the second half would be totally unrelated, nonsensical.

The exact mechanism for the sleep-deprivation/psychosis link is unclear at this time. Psychosis could be the result of biochemical changes resulting from lack of sleep. Or the lack of sleep may have been due to an underlying condition, such as bipolar disorder.

Summary

Mothers who are depressed during pregnancy or postpartum have a high likelihood of having comorbid conditions. These recent studies indicate that screening for depression alone will likely lead to treatment that is only partially effective. However, these studies have also provided a reasonable idea of what types of symptoms and co-occurring conditions they need to look for.

Chapter 3　Why depression is harmful for mothers

Depression is not benign

Depression is harmful for those who experience it. Studies on the Global Burden of Disease indicate that depression, and other mental disorders, more than double all-cause mortality (Walker, McGee, & Druss, 2015). These findings were related to an analysis of 148 studies. Based on 24 studies, the median potential lost life was 10 years. The researchers estimated that 14 percent of deaths worldwide, or 8 million deaths per year, were attributable to mental disorders.

Not surprisingly, depression increases healthcare costs. A study from Canada found that depressed mothers had healthcare costs that were twice those of non-depressed mothers. Mothers who were very depressed had costs that were five times higher (Roberts et al., 2001).

In adults, depression increases the risk of a number of serious diseases including coronary heart disease, myocardial infarction, chronic pain syndromes, premature aging, impaired wound healing, and even Alzheimer's disease (Kiecolt-Glaser et al., 2005). According to the US Center for Disease Control and Prevention, depression and anxiety are common among childbearing women and affects women's lives in many ways including their family relationships, their ability to function at home or at work, and their future risk of chronic disease, including diabetes and heart disease (Centers for Disease Control and Prevention, 2015). Unfortunately, in one US study conducted by the Centers for Disease Control and Prevention, 66 percent of women who were depressed during pregnancy were not diagnosed (Centers for Disease Control and Prevention, 2015).

These findings indicate that depression is far too serious to ignore and hope that symptoms will improve. Below is a summary of findings describing the specific ways depression harms mothers.

Decreased health behaviors

Depressed women are less likely to use contraception, or to use less-effective forms, and are more likely to smoke, have high BMIs, and use emergency medical services (Centers for Disease Control and Prevention, 2015). They are also more likely to binge drink or drink heavily. In a review article, depression was related to poor eating habits, use of tobacco, and abuse of alcohol and drugs. Depressed people even ate more chocolate (Salovey, Rothman, Detweiler, & Steward, 2000).

Postpartum depression is also related to prenatal health behaviors. A prospective cohort study recruited 664 new mothers on a postpartum floor of a US hospital and interviewed them at 8 weeks postpartum (Dagher & Shenassa, 2012). Smoking cigarettes at any time during pregnancy, and not taking prenatal vitamins in the first trimester, were related to significantly higher scores on the EPDS.

Depressed people are more likely to smoke, and smokers are more likely to be depressed. In a prospective study of 236 new mothers, non-smokers were the least likely to be depressed on the EPDS (Mbah, Salihu, Dagne, Wilson, & Bruder, 2013). Interestingly, there appeared to be a dose–response effect between depression and smoking: the more a mother smoked, the higher her depression score. Pregnant women exposed to second-hand smoke were also at increased risk of depression.

In a sample of 71 women with gestational diabetes, cesarean delivery and higher gestational weight gain were associated with depressive symptoms on the EPDS >9 at 6 weeks postpartum (Nicklas et al., 2013). Thirty-four percent of these mothers had an EPDS score >9. The authors concluded that it was important to identify women with depression as it might interfere with health changes that might be necessary in the postpartum period.

Another large, epidemiological study (N = 18,109) found that women with gestational diabetes mellitus (GDM) had significantly higher risk for depression and anxiety postpartum (Walmer et al., 2015). Socioeconomic status attenuated this relationship. Hispanic women with gestational diabetes were at higher risk, but Asian and Black women had lower rates compared to White women. Black women with GDM had higher rates of depression compared to Black women without GDM.

Postpartum depression also predicted maternal sexual dysfunction in an Australian sample of 325 women at 12 months postpartum (Khajehei, Doherty, Tilley, & Sauer, 2015). In this study, depression predicted sexual dysfunction, infrequent sexual activity, not being the initiator, and relationship dissatisfaction. Nineteen percent were depressed in this sample.

Increased risk of chronic disease

Depression is a risk factor for a number of chronic diseases, including cardiovascular disease. This link is important because it gives us insight into the physiological processes involved in depression (Frasure-Smith & Lesperance, 2005). Patients who become depressed after a myocardial infarction are 2–3 times more likely to have another one. They are also 3–4 times more likely to die (de Jonge, van den Brink, Spijkerman, & Ormel, 2006). The risk was not only for those suffering from major depression, but for milder forms as well.

A study of 586 women investigated the link between short sleep duration to 6 months and 1 year postpartum, and adiposity and cardiovascular status at 3 years postpartum (Taveras et al., 2011a). After the researchers adjusted for age, race/ethnicity, education, parity, pre-pregnancy BMI, and excessive weight gain during pregnancy, they found that when mothers slept less than 5 hours/day, they were more likely to have a higher postpartum BMI and higher waist circumference at 3 years postpartum. Short sleep duration was related to somewhat higher leptin levels at 3 years postpartum. They did not find a relation between short sleep duration and other cardiovascular symptoms, such as LDL, HDL, trigylcerides, and insulin resistance.

Impact on relationships

Depression can also impair women's relationships. Posmontier (2008a) found that women with postpartum depression were significantly impaired on personal, household, and social functioning in a study of 23 women with postpartum depression, and a matched group of 23 non-depressed women. Depression was identified via the MINI, SCID,[1] and PDSS.[2] Posmontier controlled for infant gender, number of nighttime awakenings, and income, and found that depressed women were 12 times less likely to achieve pre-pregnancy levels of functioning.

Depressed women reported more communication problems with their partners, and have marital dysfunction that persists long after the depression has resolved in another study (Roux, Anderson, & Roan, 2002). A study of 80 women in Iran found that depressed women were more likely to report marital dissatisfaction than their non-depressed counterparts (Kargar Jahromi, Zare, Taghizadeganzadeh, & Rahmanian Koshkaki, 2014). Another study compared women who were currently depressed, those with a history of depression, and those with no history of depression. The depressed and formerly depressed women were impaired on every measure of interpersonal behavior, had less stable marriages, and reported lower levels of marital satisfaction than women with no history of depression (Hammen & Brennan, 2002).

Suicidal ideations

As with thoughts of harming the baby, it is difficult to know the percentage of women who think about suicide, but research suggests it is fairly common. For example, in a sample of hospitalized women in Australia (Fisher, Feekery, Amir, & Sneedon, 2002), 5 percent reported suicidal ideations. Similarly, in a study of 831 low-income pregnant women in Sao Paulo, Brazil, 6 percent reported suicidal ideation (Huang et al., 2012). Risk factors included past or current psychiatric disorders, single partner status, and smoking. A study of 147 Canadian women found that 17 percent reported thoughts of self-harm, and 6 percent reported suicidal ideation, in the first year postpartum (Pope, Xie, Sharma, & Campbell, 2013). The sample included women with major depression and bipolar disorder II. Self-harm was assessed via the EPDS item 10, and suicidal ideation was assessed using the Hamilton Depression Rating Scale item 3. Women with higher levels of depression were more likely to have suicidal ideations, and those with hypomanic symptoms were at highest risk.

A study from Bangladesh found that 33 percent of a sample of 361 women were depressed (Gausia, Fisher, Ali, & Oosthuizen, 2009). Depression was assessed via the EPDS and structured questionnaires. The strongest risk factors included being beaten by a husband before or during their pregnancies, having an unsupportive mother-in-law or husband, and preferring a male child. Of the women with antenatal depression, 14 percent had thoughts of self-harm. The mothers often felt that they had no way out of their current situation. Twenty percent could not read and had never been to school, and another 25 percent had only been to school for 1–5 years. Most were not employed, and they could not return to their families of origin because of the shame that it would bring on their families.

Suicidality was measured using two measures during pregnancy and at 12 months postpartum in a study from Italy (Mauri, Oppo, Borri, & Banti, 2012). The researchers defined "suicidality" as "thoughts of death or self-harm and suicide attempts." They used the EPDS and the Mood Spectrum Self-Report (MOODS-SR). The sample was 1,066 women recruited in the third month of their pregnancies. Five hundred women completed the assessment at 12 months postpartum. Their findings revealed that the point prevalence for suicidality was 7 percent during pregnancy, and 4 percent postpartum for the whole sample assessed with the MOODS; and 12 percent during pregnancy, and 9 percent postpartum using the EPDS. If women had major or minor depressive episodes, the suicidality rate ranged from 26 percent by MOODS, and 34 percent via EPDS during pregnancy, to 18 percent via MOODS, and 31 percent EPDS postpartum.

In some mothers, suicidal ideations co-occur with obsessive thoughts of infant harm. Valerie first developed thoughts about the baby being hurt, and then thoughts about her actually hurting the baby. She also thought about ending her own life. She had a family history of severe depression, and a history of miscarriage and infertility. Her thoughts became severe enough that she finally talked to her midwife about postpartum depression.

> My family has a history of depression. During my growing-up years, my father spent years in bed because of it. So I was no stranger to what it can do to a person.
>
> My husband and I tried for four years to get pregnant. During that time we had two miscarriages: one at 6 weeks and one at 10 weeks in. When we finally did get pregnant, I stifled my excitement till about the third trimester because I was sure something was going to happen and my son was going to die.
>
> I hadn't even had a problem with depression myself, so I was not prepared for it when it hit me after the baby was born. I didn't think it would happen to me because I wanted to have a baby so badly. About a week after my son was born, I started having horrible images pop into my head of me hurting my son. They started out as images of accidents happening: me dropping him accidentally on the pavement. But by the time he was a month and a half old, they turned into images of me doing things on purpose to him, like walking into the corner of the wall and hitting his head on the corner until he was unconscious. I specifically remember one night, in particular, I had nursed my son to sleep, and then laid him on my chest and rocked him. I was in a little nook area right next to my kitchen, and I went from enjoying my baby to suddenly having the urge to grab a knife and put it through my baby's back and into my heart. It took everything I had in me to stop myself from doing it. Once I was able to dismiss the desire to end both of our precious lives, I got up away from the knives and found my husband. I didn't have the courage to tell him why, but I told him I was going to talk to the midwife about postpartum depression at my 6-week appointment that week.
>
> My wonderful midwife talked to me about my depression. She didn't ask for specifics, bless her soul, because I wasn't ready to talk about them just yet. I felt so guilty for the thoughts I had that I thought it would be better for the baby if I just left him and his dad. I didn't know what I would do once I left, but I didn't think I should have the privilege of being in my baby's life.
>
> My midwife put me on Prozac, and sent me to a psychiatrist (who was amazing). She helped me realize that all of these thoughts of harming myself and my baby were the depression talking, and that it wasn't my fault. It just happens to some women.
>
> I had, and still have, lots of people rooting for me, and I am very grateful for all their support and love.

Sleep and suicidal ideations

A recent study from the PTSD literature indicates that sleep problems can indicate possible suicidal ideation. In this study of 311 military personnel, self-reported insomnia was related to suicidal ideation even after controlling for depression, hopelessness, PTSD, anxiety symptoms, and substance abuse (Ribeiro et al., 2012).

Along these same lines, in a study of 628 depressed mothers, sleep problems predicted suicidal ideation (Sit et al., 2015). In this sample, 5 percent said that they "sometimes" or "quite often" had thoughts of self-harm. Using logistic regression, childhood physical abuse increased frequent thoughts of self-harm. If mothers had not been physically abused, frequent thoughts of self-harm were related to sleep disturbance and anxiety symptoms. Interestingly, anxiety and sleep disorders did not predict self-harm in mothers with a history of childhood abuse.

Four mothers I've interviewed indicated that they too had suicidal ideations.

- "I'm still dealing with the sexual abuse [her own past history]. I hadn't dealt with it before the birth. I told my husband for the first time in the hospital. I was hysterical … I was afraid of being alone, so my husband stayed the night. If I could've opened the window, I would have jumped out" [Val].
- "I had breastfeeding problems. He was colicky. I was afraid I wouldn't be able to comfort him. I didn't have thoughts of hurting him, but I thought of suicide. That's how depressed I was" [Elizabeth].
- "The severe depression would come on and go away. One time I was sorting through all our medicines, sorting the ones that were very lethal into a pile. The severe episodes only lasted about 1/2 minutes, but the moderate depression stayed. I couldn't be left alone" [Melissa].
- "My husband and sister thought they would take care of me. I started having visions of my own funeral. I was having all kinds of scary thoughts. At that point, they decided I needed to go into the hospital … The week after my daughter's birthday, I was acutely suicidal. I packed some clothes and my pills. I was going to go to New York City, rent a hotel room, and kill myself. My husband said I was rambling and saying, 'Please take care of her.' As I was getting on the train, my husband was at the train station because they found my car" [Donna].

Mothers' suicidality can also affect their interactions with their babies. In a clinical study of 32 mother–infant dyads, suicidality was examined as a possible influence on mother–infant interaction (Paris, Bolton, & Weinberg, 2009). These mothers were participating in a study of a home-based intervention for treatment of postpartum depression. The researchers noted that suicidality can lead to cognitive distortions in which a small stressor can turn into a lethal one. These mothers may view themselves as the "worst mothers in the world," and truly believe that their babies would be better off without them. The mothers with high suicidality had more mood disturbances, lower maternal self-esteem, and more parenting stress. They were less sensitive to their infants' cues and aware of their babies' social signals, and were limited in their ability to respond consistently. The infants demonstrated less positive affect and involvement with their mothers, and were more passive and less engaged in the interactions. The authors speculated that the mothers might feel that they were "toxic" for their babies, and were attempting to distance themselves from their babies in order to protect them.

The authors indicated that these beliefs could be addressed in therapy, and that mothers could establish a more functional interaction pattern.

Maternal suicide

Suicide is another frightening response to postpartum depression, and is the leading cause of death in postpartum women (Sit et al., 2015). Fortunately, it is relatively rare, but suicide attempts appear to be more common. In a sample from Liverpool, UK, of 73 mothers referred to a perinatal mental health clinic, 24 percent had made a definite suicide attempt, and 25 percent had made a possible suicide attempt. The remaining 52 percent were referred with no suicide attempt, or for a non-postpartum-related attempt (Healey et al., 2013).

When postpartum depression leads to suicide, it leaves behind a heartbroken family. Depression activist Joan Mudd writes, "In 2001 my dear daughter, Jennifer Mudd Houghtaling, lost her battle with postpartum depression." A tribute to Jennifer described her as follows.

> No one would be more stunned by the turn of events that created the Jennifer Mudd Houghtaling Postpartum Depression Foundation than Jennifer. Her ebullient joy, and laser beam of personal interest and insight, were her gifts to everyone she knew and loved. Carefree, energetic, devoted, and nonjudgmental, Jennifer would want to know what she could do to help this cause, how does this terrible disease occur, and most of all, what needs to be done to solve it.
>
> It was her generosity of spirit that was so special.
>
> Be it being an active member of the "Big Sister" program, teaching adults to read, keeping in touch with an aged friend who had become blind, or trying to convert her dog (unsuccessfully) to being a vegetarian, Jennifer made all those around her feel like they mattered.
>
> That light should have shone brightly on her much desired and cherished baby boy, Brandon. More than anything, Jennifer wanted Brandon. When she found out that she was carrying a baby boy, she named him immediately, and changed the password on her computer to Brandon so she could see his name and say it every day.

In 2004, Joan and her husband founded the Jennifer Mudd Houghtaling Foundation to increase awareness of postpartum depression among healthcare providers, increase screening for new mothers, and save other women from Jennifer's fate.

In Chapter 5, I describe some general screening questions for suicide risk and need for hospitalization. Sleep is also important in assessing suicidal risk. In Chapter 7, I describe what we know about the sleep of perinatal women, and what are the characteristics of disturbed sleep. Practitioners must also use caution with regard to medication choice for mothers at risk for suicide. Safer choices for potentially suicidal mothers are described in Chapter 5.

Suicide is a tragedy with wide-ranging implications for everyone who is left behind. Fortunately, if warning signs are heeded, the risk of maternal suicide can be greatly reduced.

Summary

The studies summarized in this chapter indicate that mothers suffer when they are depressed. There are serious long-term implications for them. These effects may not manifest immediately, but they mean that practitioners must learn to ask mothers how they are doing, and be prepared to act once they identify depression. It's too serious to ignore.

Notes

1 SCID = Structured Clinical Interview for Depression.
2 PDSS = Postpartum Depression Screening Scale. See Chapter 5.

Chapter 4   **Why maternal depression harms babies and children**

Mothers are not the only ones who are harmed by depression. Over the past 30 years, researchers have thoroughly documented the harmful effects of maternal depression on children, from the neonates to young adults. Many things modify these negative effects, such as chronicity and severity of the mother's depression, her education level, other adults in the infant's life, and other types of adversity. Nevertheless, without intervention, maternal depression can have serious and long-lasting negative consequences for infants and children. Not treating depression should never be an option. Below is a brief summary of these findings, starting with the *in utero* effects of untreated depression.

The impact of untreated depression on fetal development

The impact of maternal depression on infants begins during pregnancy. A number of studies have demonstrated that depression during pregnancy is a strong risk factor for preterm birth and low birthweight. Depressed mothers are also at increased risk for having babies who are small for gestational age.

In a prospective cohort study of 681 women from France, the rate of spontaneous preterm birth for depressed women was more than double that of non-depressed women (10 percent vs. 4 percent) (Dayan et al., 2006). A study in Goa, India ($N = 270$) found that mothers who were depressed during their third trimester were significantly more likely to have low birthweight babies than their non-depressed counterparts. The most-depressed mothers were at highest risk. This was true even after controlling for other factors that influence birthweight, such as maternal age, maternal and paternal education, and paternal income (Patel & Prince, 2006).

Another study specifically examined the impact of depression in pregnancy in a sample of 261 African American women (Kim et al., 2013). The women who were screened during pregnancy. Those with an EPDS score ≥10 had increased risk for preeclampsia, preterm birth, and low birthweight. Approximately 35 percent screened positive for depression, and the rate of preterm birth was 11 percent. An EPDS score ≥10 was also associated with increased intrauterine growth retardation, but this was not significant after behavioral risk factors were controlled for. Thyroid disease during pregnancy and history of preterm birth also increased the risk of preterm birth.

A review of 29 studies pooled data and calculated relative risk with regard to depression, low birthweight, and preterm birth (Grote et al., 2010). The researchers found that preterm birth and low birthweight were both associated with antenatal depression.

The risk is especially great for women in developing countries compared with women in North America or Europe. To put their findings into context, they noted that antenatal depression was comparable in risk to smoking ten or more cigarettes a day, but less than the risk associated with Black race and abusing substances. The researchers also noted that there was an effect of cumulative adversities, such as depression, living in poverty, facing discrimination, and experiencing food insecurity.

Not every study has found a relationship between depression and low birthweight or prematurity, however. In a large cohort study of 10,967 women, investigators found that women depressed during pregnancy were significantly more likely to have low birthweight babies (Evans, Heron, Patel, & Wiles, 2007). However, once the investigators controlled for confounding factors, such as smoking, this relationship disappeared. The authors concluded that there was no independent effect of depression on low birthweight. However, given that depressed women are more likely to smoke, and that depression may mediate smoking, the authors' statement about lack of a relationship may be premature.

Anxiety disorders and preterm birth

Anxiety can also increase the risk of preterm birth. A study of 1,820 women from Baltimore found that women with high levels of anxiety about their pregnancies were significantly more likely to have preterm babies (Orr, Reiter, Blazer, & James, 2007). Indeed, women with the highest levels of pregnancy-related anxiety had three times the risk of preterm birth compared to women with low anxiety. These findings were significant even after controlling for traditional risk factors for preterm birth including race/ethnicity, first- or second-trimester bleeding, drug use, unemployment, previous preterm or still birth, smoking, and low BMI, maternal education, and age.

Another study of 415 pregnant women from Los Angeles had similar results (Glynn, Schetter, Hobel, & Sandman, 2008). In this study, pregnant women were assessed at 18–20 and 30–32 weeks gestation. The sample was 23 percent Hispanic, 48 percent White, 14 percent African American, and 15 percent women from other ethnic groups. Higher stress and anxiety increased the risk of preterm birth. These findings persisted even after controlling for obstetric risk, pregnancy-related anxiety, race/ethnicity, parity, and prenatal life events. The authors concluded that prenatal stress and anxiety are important predictors of preterm birth.

Women with panic disorder also had a higher rate of preterm birth, and shorter gestation, than women without panic disorder in a large population study of 38,151 pregnant women in Hungary (Banhidy, Acs, Puho, & Czeizel, 2006). In this sample, diagnoses of panic disorders were rare (0.5 percent), but the proportion of preterm births was significantly larger than in mothers without panic disorder (17 percent vs. 9 percent). Anemia was also more common, as was having a male infant. Women with panic disorder were also more likely to be low-income.

Trauma, posttraumatic stress disorder, and preterm birth

A study of 2,654 pregnant women in Massachusetts and Connecticut examined the link between depression, PTSD, use of benzodiazepines and SSRIs, and preterm birth (Yonkers et al., 2014). The women were part of a longitudinal, prospective, multisite trial. Using logistic regression, the authors were able to consider the independent contribution of each. They found that PTSD was independently related to preterm birth. However, risk increased by four times if a mother has both PTSD and depression, independent of use of medications. The researchers also found that a history of child sexual abuse increased the risk for adverse birth outcomes, and one prior preterm birth quadrupled the risk. The researchers posited a relationship with trauma's link to increased levels of the stress hormone corticotropin-releasing hormone (CRH), which serves as a "placental clock." Severe or traumatic stress can disrupt this clock, promoting preterm birth.

A mother's history of adverse childhood experiences may also contribute to many of the physiologic changes that can increase her risk of preterm birth. Abuse history also increases the likelihood that the mother will participate in harmful behaviors, which also increases risk. A Swiss study compared 85 women with histories of childhood sexual abuse (CSA) to 170 matched unexposed women (Leeners, Rath, Block, Gorres, & Tshudin, 2014). During pregnancy, women with CSA histories were significantly more likely to smoke and have a partner who was abusing substances. Women with a CSA history were also more likely to experience physical, sexual, and emotional abuse, and to report depression and suicidal ideation than women without a CSA history, and were at increased risk for preterm delivery.

Similarly, a study of 148 women who had had a baby in the past five years found that intimate partner violence (IPV), PTSD, and depression were related to low birthweight, as was the combination of IPV and PTSD/depression (Rosen, Seng, Tolman, & Mallinger, 2007). The rates of all three were high: 24 percent were depressed, 26 percent had PTSD, and 21 percent reported IPV in the past year. Fifty-four percent of these mothers were African American, and 73 percent were living below the poverty line. Food insufficiency was the most common form of economic deprivation, with 60 percent reporting that they did not have enough food in their house to eat. This was also associated with low birthweight.

In a study comparing three groups of pregnant women—trauma-exposed, PTSD+ ($n = 255$); trauma-exposed, resilient ($n = 307$); and non-exposed ($n = 277$)—current PTSD was related to low birthweight (Seng, Low, Sperlich, Ronis, & Liberzon, 2011b). Women who were PTSD+ had infants who weighed, on average, 283 g less at birth compared with trauma-exposed, PTSD− women, and their babies weighed 221 g less than non-exposed women. PTSD related to CSA was also associated with shorter gestation, and was a stronger predictor of gestation length than African American race. The authors proposed that abuse-related PTSD may be a better predictor of adverse perinatal outcomes generally associated with low SES and African American race in the US. For the PTSD+ group, the rate of preterm birth was 22 percent, with 13 percent being low birthweight.

Possible underlying mechanisms for preterm birth and other effects

Some of the increased risk of preterm birth may be due to elevated levels of stress hormones. A recent study examined cortisol levels and pro- and anti-inflammatory cytokines during the third trimester of pregnancy for 96 pregnant women. The researchers hypothesized that without the system of cytokine–cortisol feedback, a pregnant woman's ability to regulate inflammation is impaired, which can potentially contribute to adverse effects for mother and baby. The study compared cortisol and cytokine levels for low-income, minority women, and affluent, Caucasian women (Corwin et al., 2013). They found higher cortisol in the low SES, racial/ethnic-minority women. In addition, the negative-feedback system that would normally turn off the inflammatory response was active in the affluent,

White women, but not in the low-SES, minority women. Chronic stress in the low-SES/minority women led to cortisol resistance, which limited their bodies' ability to control inflammation.

Cortisol and preterm birth

Prenatal exposure to cortisol is also hypothesized to influence the connectivity between the brainstem, limbic system, and cortex, which are thought to influence behavior. In another study, mothers' plasma cortisol was assessed at 15, 19, 25, 31, and 36 weeks gestation, and mothers' stress, anxiety, and depression was assessed at each time point (Davis, Glynn, Waffarn, & Sandman, 2011). The infants were tested via heel-stick procedure in the first 24 hours, and their cortisol was measured via saliva. The study results indicated that mothers with higher cortisol levels during pregnancy had infants who had an exaggerated cortisol response to the heel stick. The infants also took longer to recover behaviorally. The strongest relationship between maternal cortisol and infant behavioral response was with maternal cortisol measured at 25 weeks gestation. The authors concluded that exposure to prenatal stress may have programmed infants with an exaggerated stress response.

Mothers with high levels of urinary cortisol were significantly more likely to have premature babies in a study of 300 women in their last trimester of pregnancy (Field et al., 2006b). These infants also had lower habituation and high reflex scores on the Behavioral Neonatal Assessment Scale. Using discriminate function analysis, the researchers found that cortisol levels more accurately predicted short gestation and low birthweight than did scores on the depression inventory.

Cortisol changes the placental environment directly across the placenta. CRH, a precursor hormone to cortisol, induces vasodilatation, causing the uterine artery to constrict, reducing blood flow to the fetus. This may restrict oxygen and nutrient delivery, and has been associated with preterm birth. The placenta also produces CRH, which increases over pregnancy and triggers parturition. Researchers have hypothesized that stress-related CRH may induce preterm labor because it is a normal signal for labor to begin (Coussons-Read et al., 2012).

Catecholamines

Norepinephrine can affect fetal growth via its effects on the cardiovascular system. It is related to uterine-artery resistance, and indirectly to blood flow and fetal growth in animal studies, but it does not cross the placenta (Dayan et al., 2006; Field, Diego, & Hernandez-Reif, 2006a). These hormone levels can also be influenced by other mood states that are often comorbid with depression, such as stress and anxiety.

Inflammatory response

Another possible pathway by which depression increases the risk of preterm birth involves the immune system (see Chapter 6). Depression activates the proinflammatory cytokines, such as IL-6 and TNF-α, and prostaglandin E2, which is secreted in response to cortisol and proinflammatory cytokines. Prostaglandin E2 plays a major role in uterine contractions (Dayan et al., 2006). IL-6 and TNF-α are elevated in depressed mothers and also ripen the cervix before delivery.

In a study of 30 pregnant women, Coussons-Read and colleagues (2005) found that TNF-α and IL-6 levels were significantly higher, and the anti-inflammatory cytokine

IL-10 was significantly lower in mothers who were stressed compared with mothers who were not. The authors hypothesized that inflammation was the likely mechanism to explain the relationship between maternal stress and preterm birth. They noted that high levels of inflammation (particularly IL-6 and TNF-α) were associated with preeclampsia and premature labor. Infection also increases the risk of preterm delivery, and TNF-α is released in response to both viral and bacterial infections. They concluded that high levels of proinflammatory cytokines may, in fact, endanger human pregnancies.

In a more recent study, Cousson-Read and colleagues (2012) followed 173 women through the second trimester of pregnancy and found that women who delivered preterm had higher overall and pregnancy-related stress levels, and higher IL-6, and TNF-α, compared with women who delivered at term. The population was 66 percent Latina, and 81 percent were either White or Latina. The overall rate of preterm birth was 11 percent. The researchers noted that prenatal stress, as marked by the increase in proinflammatory cytokines, shortens gestation by altering the circulating cytokines.

PTSD and inflammation

Posttraumatic stress disorder also appears to have an inflammatory basis. In a recent review, Baker and colleagues (2012) noted a plausible link between inflammation and PTSD, especially when there is comorbid depression. A study of 3,049 adults found that people with PTSD were 2.27 times more likely to have high inflammation as indicated by elevated C-reactive protein (Spitzer et al., 2010).

Similarly, in a meta-analysis of 25 studies that included C-reactive protein (CRP), IL-6, and TNF-α found that those exposed to childhood trauma had significantly higher levels of all three (Baumeister, Akhtar, Ciufolini, Pariante, & Mondelli, 2016). The authors noted that those inflammatory molecules are a potential pathway by which early trauma can translate into adult psychiatric conditions. TNF-α and IL-6 were related to childhood physical and sexual abuse, but not CRP. CRP was most strongly associated with parental absence in early childhood. Another recent study found that childhood social adversity was related to elevated CRP in older adults in Canada, but not in their Latin American counterparts (Li et al., 2015). Social adversity included parental alcohol or drug abuse, witnessing parental partner violence, and childhood physical abuse.

Cognitive beliefs, such as shame, could mediate the relationship between trauma and inflammation. Shame is common in trauma survivors. In a study of 56 young women, trait shame was related to sympathetic nervous system activity, but it was not related to activity of the hypothalamic–pituitary–adrenal (HPA) axis (Rohleder, Chen, Wolf, & Miller, 2008). Chronic shame was associated with inflammation and glucocorticoid resistance.

In another study of 139 women in an urban health clinic, researchers examined the link between IPV, psychological stress, and inflammation (CRP) (Heath et al., 2013). Participants who had clinical levels of PTSD had higher CRP, and this was true even after controlling for comorbid depression. Their analysis revealed that the re-experiencing symptoms may explain the link between PTSD and elevated CRP. IPV predicted both depression and PTSD.

This finding is not surprising in light of recent research in older adults showing that couples with high levels of trait hostility also have high levels of CRP (Smith, Uchino, Bosch, & Kent, 2014). The link between hostility and inflammation was true for both partners. On a related note, pessimism increased inflammation in a study of 6,814 adults with no cardiovascular disease (Roy, Janal, & Roy, 2010). Pessimism was related to significantly elevated IL-6, CRP, fibrinogen, and homocysteine. The effects were attenuated, but still significant, when depression, mistrust, and health behaviors were accounted for.

In a review, Baker and colleagues (2012) described pathways by which PTSD is related to inflammation. They noted that the combination of PTSD and major depression is related to the highest amount of IL-6. Interestingly, they also noted that suicide is related to high inflammation levels: IL-6 levels were elevated in suicide attempters, and highest in the violent attempters.

Sleep disorders, depression, and inflammation

Pregnancy could also increase the risk of disordered breathing during sleep, which increases depression, which increases both cortisol and inflammation. One study of 166 pregnant women found that sleep quality was related to preterm birth (Okun, Schetter, & Glynn, 2011). The researchers administered the Pittsburg Sleep Quality Index (PSQI) and found that sleep quality was related to preterm birth. The strongest effects were for sleep problems early in pregnancy, with more modest effects in later pregnancy. For every point increase on the PSQI, the risk of preterm birth increased 25 percent for early pregnancy, and 18 percent in later pregnancy. The researchers hypothesized a possible inflammatory link between sleep-disordered breathing, preeclampsia, and preterm birth.

In a study of 189 pregnant women from Australia, mothers were assessed during pregnancy with the EPDS, PSQI, and the Berlin Questionnaire for Sleep-Disordered Breathing (Mellor, Chua, & Boyce, 2014). PSQI-assessed poor sleep quality was significantly related to higher EPDS scores, as was the Berlin score. The participants also perceived that sleep problems were related to their depressive symptoms. The authors proposed a number of possible mechanisms that include increased proinflammatory cytokines, IL-6, and CRP, as these are associated with depression as well as preterm birth. Another possible mechanism is the upregulation of the HPA axis and sympathetic nervous system.

The anti-inflammatory impact of social support

Interestingly, social support can modify these effects. In a study from Los Angeles, 1,027 preterm birth were compared with 1,282 full-term birth in a retrospective case-control study (Ghosh, Wilhelm, Dunkel-Schetter, Lombardi, & Ritz, 2010). Sixty-five percent of the mothers were Hispanic. The researchers examined whether chronic stress in mothers increased the risk of preterm birth, and whether social support lessened the risk. Social support downregulates the stress system by increasing oxytocin, so there are sound physiological reasons for why it might help. Thirty-seven percent of the women reported moderate stress, and 14 percent reported high chronic stress. Women reporting low support and/or high chronic stress were more likely to be young, with low levels of education, Black or US-born Latina, single, and low SES. The results indicated that social support did decrease the risk of preterm birth. Chronic stress, low confidence in normal birth, and fear for the baby's health increased the risk. Support from fathers lowered the risk. However, mothers who had low support and moderate to high stress had more than double the risk of preterm birth. The authors suggested that future studies could examine more types and sources of support, particularly in diverse populations.

Effects of maternal depression on infants

After babies are born, mothers' depression can still affect them. A number of physiological indicators are more common in infants of depressed mothers. For example, abnormalities in electroencephalograms (EEGs) have been observed in infants of depressed mothers at 3–6 months. Babies of depressed mothers had depressed affect and right frontal EEG asymmetry as early as 3 months. Right frontal asymmetry is an abnormal pattern found in chronically depressed adults, and is a physiologic marker of depression in babies (Field, Diego, & Hernandez-Reif, 2006a). A study of 48 neonates (Field, Diego, Hernandez-Reif, Schanberg, & Kuhn, 2002) found that babies with greater relative right-frontal EEG activation had elevated cortisol levels, showed more variability in state changes during sleep/wake observations, and had less than optimum performance on the Brazelton Neonatal Behavioral Assessment Scale. Their mothers also had lower pre- and postnatal serotonin levels, and higher levels of cortisol (both consistent with depression). The authors concluded that greater relative right-frontal activation may place these infants at increased risk for developmental problems.

Emotional regulation and reactivity

Infants of depressed mothers often exhibit an exaggerated stress response. A study of 91 Portuguese women assessed them at 3 months before birth and 3 months after (Figueiredo & Costa, 2009). In the third trimester of pregnancy, 25 percent had STAI[1] scores >45 or an EPDS ≥10. At 3 months postpartum, 15 percent had STAI >45 and 27 percent an EPDS ≥10. Mothers' depression predicted poorer prenatal attachment, but had no impact on their postpartum interaction with their infants. Conversely, mothers' anxiety was not related to prenatal attachment, but predicted worse involvement with their babies postpartum. They did note that even with depression and anxiety, the majority of mothers were emotionally involved with their infants.

A prospective study of 88 women and their 7-month-old infants examined the link between prenatal anxiety disorder, and mothers' caregiving sensitivity, on infants' salivary cortisol (Grant et al., 2009). Maternal anxiety was assessed in the last 6 months of pregnancy. At 7 months, the infants' cortisol levels were measured 15, 25, and 40 minutes after exposure to the still-face mother procedure, a condition where mothers do not respond to their babies' cues. It raises babies' cortisol levels. Mothers' caregiving was measured during the play times of the still-face procedure (2 minutes each). Mothers were classified as high- or low-sensitive based on analysis of video play sessions. The findings indicated that maternal prenatal anxiety, and postpartum caregiving sensitivity, impacted the stress response of 7-month-old infants to the still-face procedure. Mothers rated as low-sensitive, and who had prenatal anxiety, had infants with a more reactive stress response following the still-face paradigm. This was independent of the effects of pre- or postpartum depression and anxiety. Interestingly, the infants of more-sensitive mothers had lower cortisol levels when they arrived at the laboratory than infants of less-sensitive mothers. The authors hypothesized that sensitive caregiving could buffer against elevated cortisol in novel and stressful situations.

Chronicity and severity of depression also influences the amount of its negative impact. Diego and colleagues (2005) recruited four groups of mothers (N = 80) in their second trimester of pregnancy: non-depressed women, women only depressed during pregnancy, women only depressed postpartum, and women who were depressed during both pregnancy and postpartum. They found that babies of mothers with prenatal depression spent more time fussing and crying, and showed more stress behaviors than babies whose mothers were not depressed, or who were only depressed postpartum. The authors concluded that infants are influenced by the timing and duration of depression, not simply its mere presence.

A study of mothers' PTSD showed similar results. In this study of 52 low-income, ethnic-minority mother–infant dyads, women completed questionnaires about their trauma exposure, and that of their infants (Enlow et al., 2011). The mothers were exposed to an average of 2.62 traumatic events, with 25 percent being exposed to 4 or more events. Infants were assessed using the still-face paradigm at 6 months of age, and mothers completed a measure of infant temperament at 13 months. Consistent with previous studies, mothers' report of PTSD symptoms predicted more infant internalizing, externalizing, and dysregulation at 13 months. The authors concluded that maternal PTSD is related to infant difficulties with emotional regulation.

Emotional and social development

A study of mother–infant dyads up to age 9 months found that infants of depressed mothers had the poorest scores on measures of social engagement, maturity of regulatory behaviors, and negative emotionality (Feldman et al., 2009). Consistent with previous studies, infants of depressed mothers also had the highest cortisol reactivity. The study compared 22 dyads with maternal depression, 19 with maternal anxiety, and a group of matched controls. The infants of anxious mothers were suboptimal on the measures compared to the control mothers on maternal sensitivity and infant social engagement. Maternal sensitivity moderated the effect of maternal depression on social engagement.

In a study from Finland of 520 mothers, data were collected in the second trimester of pregnancy, and at 2 and 12 months postpartum (Punamaki et al., 2006). Mothers' prenatal depression and anxiety predicted infant's developmental problems at 12 months. Postpartum depression at 2 months was related to infant developmental problems, and difficult child temperament characteristics at 12 months.

Mother–infant bonding

A mother's ability to bond with her baby (i.e., develop a warm, affectionate relationship) may also be impaired if she is depressed. A study from Michigan examined the trajectory of mother–infant bonding over the first year postpartum (Muzik et al., 2013). The researchers were interested in bonding in the context of risk factors, such as the mother's history of child abuse and postpartum depression. They compared 97 women with a history of child abuse with 53 women with no abuse history, and assessed them at 6 weeks, and 4 and 6 months postpartum. They also examined positive parenting behaviors, such as engagement, flexibility, sensitivity, and warmth. They found that all women increased in bonding over the 6 months, but that women with postpartum depression or PTSD were impaired in their bonding at each time point. Women's perceptions of their relationships with their babies also influenced their behavior during playtime. If they perceived that they had not bonded with their babies, they had fewer positive parenting behaviors. The author concluded that early detection of both depression and PTSD was needed in order to prevent these problematic parenting behaviors and disturbed mother–infant relationships.

Another longitudinal study from London also examined the effects of postpartum depression over the first year (O'Higgins, St. James Roberts, Glover, & Taylor, 2013). Women who had an EPDS score ≥13 at 1–4 weeks postpartum were scored on the Mother–Infant Bonding Scale at 1–4, 9, and 16 weeks, and 1 year postpartum. There were 50 depressed mothers and 29 non-depressed mothers. The authors concluded that women who are depressed in the first 4 weeks postpartum fail to bond well with their babies at all time points. The authors recommended early intervention.

A study of 180 women participating in a partial hospitalization program demonstrated that not all women with depression, or other psychiatric problems, have impaired bonding (Sockol, Battle, Howard, & Davis, 2014). In this study, women completed self-report measures of depression and mother–infant bonding. Additional data were collected from their charts. After controlling for demographic variables, EPDS score was the only significant predictor of impaired bonding and risk of abuse. Women having cesareans reported more rejection and pathological anger. They noted that the majority of women in the study had depression in the clinical range (>11 EPDS). However, even compared to other depressed women, women with severe depression were at higher risk of bonding problems.

A German study included 78 mother–infant dyads: 30 mothers with anxiety disorders and 48 healthy mothers (Tietz, Zietlow, & Reck, 2014). Mothers with anxiety disorders reported significantly less bonding with their babies than mothers without anxiety. However, some of this effect could also be explained by co-occurring depression.

Finally, a meta-analysis on 28 published and unpublished studies found that depression in fathers also affected parenting (Wilson & Durbin, 2010). The effect size was small, but depressed fathers engaged in fewer positive, and more negative, parenting behaviors. The effect sizes found were comparable to studies on mothers. Positive behaviors included warm, sensitive, engaged, accepting, and supportive interactions. Negative behaviors included hostile, coercive, intrusive, restrictive, controlling, critical, and dysfunctional behaviors or interactions. The analysis revealed that mothers and fathers had comparable negative parenting behaviors, but that the effect of depression on positive behaviors is actually larger for fathers than it is for mothers.

Sudden Infant Death Syndrome (SIDS)

A truly frightening finding has to do with postpartum depression in the neonatal period, and increased risk of SIDS (Sanderson et al., 2002). In this cohort study of 32,984 births in Sheffield, UK from 1988 to 1993, there were 42 infant deaths attributed to SIDS. Multivariate analyses identified three significant risk factors for SIDS: smoking, a high EPDS score, and living in a poor area. The authors concluded that a high EPDS score, and by implication, high depressive symptoms, was possibly implicated in SIDS.

Effects of maternal depression on toddlers and preschoolers

In a study of 17 depressed and 19 non-depressed adolescent mothers, toddlers were observed in a cleanup task in order to observe parenting styles (Pelaez, Field, Pickens, & Hart, 2008). The parenting styles were classified as: (1) Authoritative, mother provides firm control and sets limits in a warm, respectful manner; (2) Authoritarian, mother shows verbal or physical rejection, or control, or lacks positive encouragement; (3) Permissive, mother provides positive verbal communication, but sets no limits or provides no instructions; and (4) Disengaged, mother is uninvolved, unresponsive or avoidant, and has flat affect. Depressed mothers were more likely to be classified as authoritarian or disengaged. Mothers' depression also appeared to affect their children's behaviors. The toddlers of depressed mothers spent less time following instructions, displayed aggressive play for a greater percentage of time, and had less time on-task than toddlers of non-depressed mothers.

In a secondary analysis of data from the Healthy Steps National Evaluation with 3,412 mothers, McLearn et al. (2006a; 2006b) found that mothers with depressive symptoms at 2–4 months were less likely than non-depressed mothers to participate in infant safety activities, and were also less likely to play with their children at 30–33 months. Mothers who were currently depressed were significantly less likely to use electric-outlet covers and safety latches, talk with their children, limit TV or video watching, follow daily routines, and be nurturing. In addition, currently depressed mothers were more likely to slap their children's face or spank them with an object.

In a study of 112 mother–infant dyads, researchers found that brief maternal depression did not negatively impact infant performance at either 12 or 15 months (Cornish et al., 2005). However, chronic maternal depression was related to lower infant cognitive and psychomotor development, with similar effects for boys and girls. Twenty-five percent of infants with chronically depressed mothers were delayed in psychomotor development, and were less likely to be walking competently by 15 months. Chronic maternal depression was not related to delays in infant language development.

A study of mother–child dyads ($N = 838$) assessed depression during mid-pregnancy, and child outcomes at age 3, including BMI and overall adiposity (Ertel, Koenen, Rich-Edwards, & Gillman, 2010). The mothers were predominantly White and affluent. Eight percent were depressed during pregnancy, and 7 percent were depressed postpartum. Antenatal depression was associated with smaller infant size, and more central adiposity in children at age 3. Postpartum depression was associated with higher overall adiposity. Postpartum depression was hypothesized to impact adiposity through negative impact on breastfeeding, unhealthy maternal diet, and lower physical activity levels. Mother–infant interactions could also influence child weight gain.

A recent study from 791 mothers in Canada found that 3-year-old girls of depressed mothers were almost 5 times more likely to wheeze or have chronic breathing problems (Alton, Zeng, Tough, Mandhane, & Kozyrskyj, 2016). This relationship was not true for boys.

Black and colleagues (2002) found that maternal depression, and the mother's perceptions of her partner, were related to children's behavior problems at 4–5 years. In this sample, 42 percent of the children had been maltreated, 36 percent had externalizing scores in the clinical range, and 11 percent had internalizing scores in the clinical range. When mothers were depressed, they perceived the quality of their relationship with their partner more negatively, and their children showed more symptoms.

Unfortunately, children who were premature may be more susceptible to the negative effects of maternal depression. In a series of two studies, researchers measured children's cortisol levels after interacting with their mothers (Bugental, Beaulieu, & Schwartz, 2008). The children were 14–16 months old. Infants who had been preterm were more reactive to their mothers' depression than infants who were full term. The preterm infants had higher cortisol levels when interacting with their depressed mothers, and lower cortisol levels when interacting with a non-depressed mother, than full-term infants. The authors concluded that premature infants were more sensitive to the emotional environment of their homes, including their mothers' depression.

Effects on school-age children

The negative impact of maternal depression has also been documented in elementary- and school-aged children. In an American study of 5,000 mother–infant pairs, children of depressed mothers had more behavior problems and lower vocabulary scores at age 5 (Brennan et al., 2000). The researchers assessed mothers for depression during pregnancy, immediately postpartum, and at 6 months and 5 years old. Severe and chronic depression was related to more behavior problems, as were more recent episodes of maternal depression.

In a longitudinal study of 14,000 infants born in 2001, maternal depression, based on the CES-D[2] score, increased the risk of childhood obesity at age 5 (Vericker, 2015). Low-income mothers were more likely than high-income mothers to be depressed, and 38 percent had recently been depressed. Maternal depression was associated with poor eating habits. Children of depressed mothers ate vegetables and milk less often, and were more likely to drink sweetened beverages and eat sweet snacks.

Murray and colleagues (2001) found that children of depressed mothers were more likely, at age 5, to have depressive cognitions, such as hopelessness, pessimism, and low self-worth, especially when exposed to a mild stressor. The authors noted, however, that current maternal hostility towards the child accounted for much of this relationship. In another study, maternal depression during the child's first two years of life was the best predictor of elevated baseline cortisol in response to a mild stressor at age 7 (Ashman, Dawson, Panagiotides, Yamada, & Wilkins, 2002).

In a prospective study of 65 healthy mother–infant dyads, high maternal cortisol in early pregnancy was related to amygdala and hippocampal volume at 7 years of age (Buss et al., 2012). This study found that higher cortisol levels in early pregnancy were associated with greater volume of the right amygdala volume in girls, but not in boys. This increased volume was related to girls' behavioral problems at age 7, as indicated on the Child Behavior Checklist. There was no impact on the hippocampus.

Chronicity and severity of symptoms makes a difference in terms of child outcomes. In a study of 3,332 mothers and children from Brazil, psychiatric disorders were identified in the children at age 6. Mothers had been evaluated for depression via EPDS at 3, 12, 24, and 48 months, and at age 6 (Matijasevich et al., 2015). The researchers identified five trajectories of maternal depression, ranging from low to high chronic. Thirteen percent of the children had a DSM-IV psychiatric disorder. The probability of child psychiatric disorders, as well as internalizing and externalizing behaviors, increased as mothers' symptoms became more severe and chronic.

Children of mothers who had postpartum depression had lower social competence scores at ages 8–9 in a study from Finland (Luoma et al., 2001). Social competence included parents' reports of children's activities, hobbies, tasks and chores; functioning in social relationships; and school achievements. Mothers were assessed for depression pre- and postnatally, and when their children were 8–9 years old. Mothers' current depression was also associated with children's low social competence and adaptive functioning.

Ten-year-olds exposed to maternal depression since birth ($n = 17$) were compared with children with non-depressed mothers ($n = 21$) on cortisol levels, hippocampal, and amygdala volumes (Lupien et al., 2011). Changes in these brain structures are often associated with poor maternal care in both animal and human studies. The results revealed no differences in hippocampal volumes, but right and left amygdala volumes were higher, and there were increased levels of glucocorticoids in the children of depressed mothers. The amygdala is related to CRH. The authors noted that their findings suggest that amygdala volume is a marker of biological sensitivity to quality of maternal care, and that duration of exposure may be the key variable related to amygdala volume.

Negative findings also appear at age 11 in a study of 132 children (Hay et al., 2001). Women were assessed for depression at 3 months postpartum ($N = 149$), and the children were tested at age 11. If mothers were depressed at 3 months postpartum, their children had significantly lower IQ scores, and more problems in school, including attentional and mathematical-reasoning difficulties at 11. The children of depressed mothers were more likely be in special education, and the effects were particularly pronounced for boys. Neither social disadvantage nor mothers' subsequent mental health problems accounted for the link between postpartum depression and IQ.

Effects on young adults

The impact of mothers' depression can last into early adulthood. Depression in either mothers or fathers increased the risk of depression in their offspring in a study of 2,427 young adults (Lieb, Isensee, Hofler, Pfister, & Wittchen, 2002). Interestingly, paternal depression was associated with an earlier onset, and severity, impairment, and recurrence of their children's depression.

Panic disorder was related to parenting behavior in a study of 86 Swiss mothers and their children, ages 13–23. Mothers with panic disorder showed more verbal control, were more criticizing, and less sensitive during mother–child interactions than mothers without panic disorder (Schneider et al., 2009). These mothers were observed in a structured-play situation, and there were more conflicts between mother and child if the mothers had panic disorder. There were no differences in parenting behaviors based on the children's anxiety levels. Parental overcontrol appears to undermine their children's self-efficacy.

A study of 150 pregnant women found that antenatal and postpartum depression predicted smoking in adolescent offspring (Hay, Pawlby, Water, & Sharp, 2008). In this study, 31 percent of the mothers were depressed during pregnancy, and 22 percent were depressed at 3 months postpartum. Mothers who were depressed at either of these time points were more likely to be depressed at subsequent assessment points. The authors concluded that mothers' lifelong symptoms of depression created a risky environment before birth, and in the postpartum period. Depression in the perinatal period was a robust predictor of child behavior problems. The exact causal chain of events is unknown, but perinatal depression predicted cumulative stress for families, which promoted adolescent disorder, including teen smoking.

A 20-year follow-up of children of depressed parents compared them with a matched group of children whose parents had no psychiatric illness. The adult children of depressed mothers and fathers had three times the rate of major depression, anxiety disorders, and substance abuse compared with children of non-depressed parents. In addition, children of depressed parents had higher rates of medical problems and premature mortality (Weissman et al., 2006).

A 22-year longitudinal study of adult children of mothers with postpartum depression found that the children of depressed mothers had an increased biological response to stress (Barry et al., 2015). This study from Belgium measured cortisol response to a social-evaluative threat, comparing children of depressed mothers ($n = 38$) with children of non-depressed mothers ($n = 38$). Children whose mothers had postpartum depression demonstrated greater cortisol reactivity in response to a perceived threat (a 5-minute speech followed by a 5-minute spoken mental-math test), even when controlling for subsequent maternal depression.

The interaction styles of depressed mothers

As described in the previous section, mothers' depression can lead to long-lasting and serious effects in their babies. The next logical question to ask is why this occurs. To understand why, it's instructive to look at the interaction styles of depressed mothers. Depressed mothers tend to have one of two basic interaction styles: avoidant and angry/intrusive (Field, 2010). Depressed mothers touch their infants less and are less physically affectionate. Their vocalizations also differ from those of non-depressed

---

Interaction styles of depressed mothers

There are two basic styles of interaction that depressed mothers have with their infants: avoidant and angry/intrusive. Avoidant is the most common, but mothers can manifest both, and both are stressful for babies.

In the avoidant style, mothers spend most of their time disengaged from their babies, ignoring their cues. Mothers with this style are unresponsive, have flat affect, and do not support their infants' activities; they only respond to infant distress. Babies react to this style by trying to engage their mothers in interaction. Unfortunately, they are generally not successful. Lack of maternal responsiveness is highly stressful for babies, as demonstrated by elevated cortisol levels and abnormal EEG patterns. The babies disengaged, or engaged in self-comforting, self-regulatory behaviors, such as thumb-sucking, looking away, being passive, and withdrawing to help them cope with their state. When they cannot engage their mothers, they often respond by "shutting down."

In the angry/intrusive style, mothers are more engaged with their babies, but the interactions are characterized by hostility and intrusiveness. In this style, mothers expressed anger and irritation, and roughly handled their babies. These mothers also ignore their babies' cues. Mothers with the angry/intrusive style speak in an angry tone, poked at their babies, and interfered with their babies' activities. Rather than interacting in a give-and-take fashion, these mothers dominated the relationship. Babies react to this style by trying to disengage from their mothers. These infants are often angry, and show frustration easily in anticipation of their mothers' intrusiveness. Mothers may interpret this behavior as rejection.

---

mothers. They have a more negative effect, they explain things less, and make fewer references to their infants' behavior. Depression reduces the synchrony between mothers and infants, and has less infant-directed speech. All of these interaction activities are important for infants' later cognitive, social, and emotional development.

Intervention for the interaction style of depressed mothers

Does mother–baby interaction improve when depression resolves? Conversely, does depression remit when the mother–infant interaction improves? These questions have important clinical implications, and the findings so far have been mixed. In a study of 117 postpartum women with depressive symptoms (Horowitz et al., 2001), half of the women were assigned to a treatment group where they were coached to improve their responsiveness to their infants. At the end of the interven-

---

The Still-Faced Mothers studies

The Still-Faced Mother paradigm was developed by Dr. Edward Tronick to provide an analog, under laboratory conditions, to the effects of maternal depression. Tronick and colleagues asked mothers to pretend that they were depressed when interacting with their 3-month-old babies. These mothers spoke in a monotone, had little or no facial affect, and seldom touched their infants. It only took about 3 minutes before the infants became distressed at the way their mothers were acting. The infants became wary, and tried to engage their mothers in normal interactions. The infants continued to be wary even when mothers returned to their normal affect. These studies demonstrate that it is highly stressful for infants when their mothers do not respond to them, as evidenced by their elevated levels of cortisol (Buss et al., 2012).

---

tion, mothers in the intervention group did show significantly higher levels of maternal responsiveness, but the intervention had no effect on their depressive symptoms.

Two studies from the UK have found that infant massage can help with maternal depression, and the effects may be due to improved mother–infant interactions. The first was a small pilot study with 12 mothers in the massage group, and 13 in the control group (Glover, Onozawa, & Hodgkinson, 2002). All the mothers had scored over 13 on the EPDS. At the end of the trial, depressive symptoms improved more for the mothers in the massage group than for mothers in the control group (although both improved). In addition, mothers' interactions with their babies improved. The authors highlighted that massage relaxed mother and baby, increased maternal confidence, increased mothers' understanding of babies' cues, and released oxytocin, which promoted bonding.

The second study assigned 34 depressed mothers to infant-massage or support-group conditions (Onozawa, Glover, Adams, Modi, & Kumar, 2001). There were five weekly sessions. The EPDS scores fell in both groups by the end of 5 weeks, with a larger effect in the infant-massage group. There was also significant improvement in mother–infant interaction in the massage group. The mothers in the massage condition were specifically taught how to read their babies' cues.

A study of 151 mother–infant pairs examined the impact of antidepressants on mother and child psychopathology (Weissman et al., 2006). They found that remission of maternal depression was associated with a reduction of child symptoms and diagnoses. A maternal response of at least 50 percent was required to see an improvement in the child.

In another study, researchers taped mother–infant interaction for 27 women and their infants (Logsdon, Wisner, & Hanusa, 2009b). The women completed a measure of maternal-role gratification, and the Infant Care Survey. The results indicated that antidepressants did improve maternal gratification and overall functioning, but did not have an effect on maternal self-efficacy or maternal–infant interaction. The percentage of positive infant affect did improve over time. Self-efficacy increased for the mother when the infant demonstrated a higher percentage of positive affect, but the correlation was not significant. McLennan and Offord's (2002) review raised similar concerns about whether targeting postpartum depression alone was sufficient to ameliorate negative child outcomes. Depression and negative interaction style may need to be addressed separately.

Another study examined the impact of breastfeeding on infants of depressed mothers (Jones, McFall, & Diego, 2004). This study compared four groups of postpartum women: depressed women who were either breast- or bottle-feeding, and non-depressed women who were either breast- or bottle-feeding. The outcome was babies' EEG patterns. In this study, babies of depressed, breastfeeding mothers had *normal* EEG patterns. In contrast, babies of depressed, non-breastfeeding women did not. In other words, breastfeeding protected babies from the harmful effects of maternal depression. The authors observed that depressed, breastfeeding mothers touched, stroked, and made eye contact with their babies more than depressed, non-breastfeeding women because these behaviors are built into the breastfeeding relationship. This is one more reason to encourage and support breastfeeding in depressed mothers. Research on breastfeeding and depression will be described in more detail in Chapter 6.

Summary

What these above-cited studies indicate is that it is possible to reverse the harmful effects of maternal depression on infants and children. However, particularly when symptoms are long-lasting, both the depression and the dysfunctional interaction may need to be addressed.

Infanticide

One of the most serious manifestations of maternal depression is when a mother takes the life of her baby. Fortunately, the incidence of infanticide is rare. As I described in Chapter 2, thoughts of infant harm can be fairly common among depressed mothers, but most do not involve the mother thinking of actually harming her baby. Rather, these thoughts are obsessive concerns for infant safety, and what may happen to the baby. Even when women have thoughts about harming their babies, most never act on them.

A qualitative study of 15 women with non-psychotic depression in Brisbane, Australia explored the themes that mothers presented regarding their thoughts of infanticide (Barr & Beck, 2008). Mothers with non-psychotic depression are at lower risk of harming their infants, yet we know little about what and how often they think about infanticide. All of the women in this study had babies 0–12 months old. The authors found specific themes regarding their thoughts.

Experience of horror: Women experienced horror when they thought about harming their babies.
Distorted sense of responsibility: Women felt despondent and that their situation was hopeless. Infanticidal thoughts occurred alongside suicidal thoughts.
Consuming negativity: They hated and were angry with their babies when they thought about infanticide.

Keeping secrets: They were ashamed of their thoughts, and kept them from family and healthcare providers.

Managing the crisis: They developed plans to keep their babies safe at times when they might harm them (e.g., scheduling help at high-stress times of day).

Barr and Beck (2008) noted that depressed mothers often thought about harming their infants. Mothers with non-psychotic depression may not be at increased risk for actually harming their infants. However, Barr and Beck urged healthcare providers to assess women for psychotic or delusional symptoms and/or behavior that puts the infants at risk, and concluded that women thinking about infanticide need to seek out help and support.

Chandra and colleagues (2002) studied 50 women from India who had been admitted to a psychiatric hospital postpartum. They collected data from three sources: the mother's partner, nursing observations made during the first week in the hospital, and the psychiatric assessment within the first week of admission. In this sample, 43 percent reported infanticidal thoughts, 36 percent reported infanticidal behavior, and 34 percent reported both infanticidal thoughts and behavior. Infanticidal ideas and behavior tended to co-occur. In a logistic regression, depression and psychotic ideations predicted infanticidal ideations. Psychotic ideations also predicted infanticidal behavior.

A study from Korea included 45 women who either killed, or attempted to kill, their infants. Women were included in the sample if they had diagnoses of either major depression or bipolar disorder (Kim, Choi, & Ha, 2008). The data were collected via chart review, and the researchers were interested in whether depressive symptoms at admission that could predict later diagnoses of bipolar disorder. They found that while only 24 percent of the patients had a diagnosis of bipolar disorder at admission, 73 percent had this diagnosis at discharge. Among women admitted with a diagnosis of major depression, 65 percent were later reclassified based on the appearance of hypomanic or manic episodes. Thirty-six percent of their sample attempted suicide immediately after committing filicide. The researchers suggested that healthcare providers consider the diagnosis of bipolar disorder when examining filicidal depressive mothers. They also noted that treating bipolar women with antidepressants could be detrimental for patients. Indeed, 77 percent of their subjects had been treated with unopposed antidepressants, with or without antipsychotics.

Meyer and Oberman (2001), in their book on mothers who kill their children, noted that in the case of infanticide, it is often difficult to distinguish "mad" from "bad." There are often elements of both. In some cases, there are clear indications of postpartum psychosis, such as delusional thinking. In other cases, there are often pre-existing life stresses, such as past or current abuse, substance abuse, or some other impairing factor.

Conclusion

Depression causes more harm to mother and baby than people generally realize. These effects provide ample reason to take depression seriously, and encourage mothers to seek treatment. In working with mothers, however, you must be careful with the information, particularly about infant harm. While helping mothers see that seeking help for depression is good for them and their babies, we must never communicate to mothers that their depression has somehow "ruined" their babies or children. Many times, mothers fear this, and this belief has been a motivating factor in some cases of infanticide. Providers can, however, use this information to gently encourage mothers to get help because when they get better, it will also be good for their babies.

Notes

1 STAI = State–Trait Anxiety Inventory.
2 CES-D = Center for Epidemiologic Studies-Depression.

Chapter 5   Assessment of postpartum depression

> Postpartum depression is often suffered privately. Because clinicians identify fewer than half of the women with this mood disorder, routine, periodic screening for one year after delivery is imperative.
>
> (Beck, 2006, p. 47)

Healthcare providers often fail to detect depression in new mothers because they are not familiar with it, or do not know what to look for. In addition, mothers themselves may hide their depression (Beck, 2006). Because of its serious consequences for mothers and babies, clinicians should routinely screen for depression in pregnant and postpartum women (American Colleage of Obstetricians and Gynecologists, 2015; Siu & US Preventive Services Task Force (USPSTF), 2016). Depression is much more common than conditions that occur during pregnancy that are routinely screened for (Beck, 2006). For example, in one study, 15 percent of women had depressive symptoms. In contrast, 2.4 percent had gestational diabetes, 5.5 percent had pregnancy-associated hypertension, and 10 percent had a preterm birth (McGarry, Kim, Sheng, Egger, & Baksh, 2009).

Challenges to assessing postpartum depression

Postpartum depression is often missed because mothers do not seek care for it. In fact, they may actively conceal it. Sixty percent of women with depressive symptoms in the Utah PRAMS[1] study did not seek help (McGarry et al., 2009). Women's inability to disclose their feelings was a common help-seeking barrier, in a review of 40 studies (Dennis & Chung-Lee, 2006). The authors noted that women did not proactively seek help, and family members and health professionals often reinforced this lack of care-seeking. Other women viewed depression as a normal part of becoming a mother. Mothers also feared losing their babies, or did not want to bear the stigma and shame of depression. Another barrier was when care providers offered medications as the only treatment alternative. The combination of a lack of knowledge of postpartum depression, and acceptance of myths, were significant barriers to seeking help.

In a qualitative study of 18 women's barriers to seeking care at 8 weeks postpartum, Sword and colleagues (2008) examined individual-, social network-, and health system-related factors that facilitated or hindered care-seeking. Factors that facilitated mothers seeking care included being aware that they were depressed and not feeling like themselves. In addition, supportive relationships, outreach and follow-up, legitimization of postpartum depression, and timeliness of care, facilitated care-seeking.

Hindering factors included women's beliefs that depressive symptoms were just a normal part of motherhood and their limited understanding of postpartum depression. Mothers waited for symptoms to improve on their own, were uncomfortable discussing mental health concerns, and feared being judged or having their children taken away. Friends, family, and healthcare providers sometimes hindered care because they told mothers that their symptoms were normal. Healthcare providers hindered care when they offered treatments that the women found unacceptable (Sword et al., 2008).

In a survey of 94 mental health providers in Rochester, New York, Springate and Chaudron (2006) found that 80 percent were not experienced with perinatal mood disorders. These clinicians offered several types of psychotherapy including interpersonal (90 percent), supportive (86 percent), and cognitive-behavioral (76 percent). Only 16 percent offered direct medication management. While most providers accepted private insurance, only a small percentage took government insurance (e.g., only 12 percent accepted Medicaid). These findings highlight several barriers for women receiving perinatal mental healthcare, such as limited access to care for women on government insurance, and a long waiting period to see a psychiatrist.

Increased healthcare use

High rate of healthcare use is one possible indication of depression. In an Australian study (Webster et al., 2001), depressed mothers made more visits to pediatricians or their primary care providers. They were also significantly more likely to visit a psychiatrist or social worker, seek the assistance from a postpartum depression support group, and contact the Nursing Mothers' Association of Australia. They were also significantly less satisfied with those services than non-depressed mothers. The depressed women felt that their providers did not listen, and that they received poor quality information. Webster et al. speculated that the mothers could be unhappy because depression—the real reason for their visit—was not identified. The women rarely raised the issue of depression themselves, but provided "hints" to their providers about the way they were feeling. The authors recommended using screening questions to help identify mothers with depression.

A Canadian study also found that women with postpartum depression used more healthcare services (Dennis, 2004b). A cohort of 594 women in British Columbia completed questionnaires at 1, 4, and 8 weeks postpartum. At 4 weeks, women with depressive symptoms had seen family practice physicians and public health nurses more times, and were twice as likely to be classified as high utilizers of healthcare services at both 4 and 8 weeks. In addition, depressed women were more likely to perceive their health as poor. The author emphasized that family care physicians were important in identifying and treating depression in new mothers. They also recommended that women who use a lot of healthcare services be screened for possible depression.

Increased use of healthcare services come at a substantial cost. In the Ontario Mother and Infant Survey (Roberts et al., 2001), mothers who were depressed, and mothers who made less than $20,000 per year, had the highest healthcare costs. The total health and social service costs were almost double for both groups (calculated separately) compared to the rest of the sample. Other variables that predicted higher healthcare costs included mothers' perception of their own health as poor, perception of inadequate help and support at home, and a postpartum hospital stay of less than 48 hours.

Not every study has found an increase in healthcare utilization among depressed mothers. A study of 665 Canadian mothers of infants 2–12 months found no increase in use of any type of healthcare services for mothers with either depression or anxiety (Anderson, Campbell, daSilva, Freeman, & Xie, 2008). The main outcome variable was use of services over a six-month period including visits to the primary care provider, Emergency Department, and walk-in clinics for the baby. Eleven percent had postpartum depressive symptoms and 9 percent had postpartum anxiety.

Screening for depression

As indicated above, women may provide hints that they are depressed, but may not actually say it unless asked. Active screening, with a standardized instrument, is much more likely to identify mothers who are depressed.

One way to screen is to ask mothers if they have any of the known risk factors for depression. An Australian study screened 2,118 women during pregnancy (Webster, Linnane, Dibley, & Pritchard, 2000b). Of these women, 33 percent had one or more risk factors for depression during pregnancy. At 4 months, 26 percent of women with one or more risk factors were depressed, compared with 11 percent of women with no risk factors. The risk of depression increased with the number of risk factors; 48 percent percent of the women with five risk factors were depressed. The authors felt they could have improved predictions by adding questions about infant behavior, severe blues, and a history of childhood abuse. They acknowledged that many of the women in their local postpartum support group were sexual abuse survivors, and adding this variable, in particular, would have improved detection rates.

Another study found that depression at 1 week postpartum predicted depression at 4 and 8 weeks (Dennis, 2004a). This study included 594 women from British Columbia. Using an EPDS cutoff score of >9, Dennis found that 30 percent of mothers had depressive symptoms at week 1, and rates of 23 percent and 21 percent at 4 and 8 weeks, respectively. Mothers with a score >9 at week 1 were 30 times more likely at 4 weeks, and 19 times more likely at 8 weeks, to have postpartum symptoms.

Non-response can also indicate depression. In a study of obsessive-compulsive disorder during pregnancy, George and Elliot (2004) found that failure to respond to the antenatal questionnaire predicted higher rates of postpartum depression than the screening questionnaire itself. They concluded that non-response to a questionnaire conveys as much information as actually completing one, and urged clinicians to follow up on non-response.

A study of 211 pregnant women examined whether women would be more likely to report depression on an anonymous questionnaire vs. a questionnaire where they needed to use their name (Matthey, White, & Rice, 2010). Seventy-seven percent of health professionals ($N = 44$) assumed that mothers would be more likely to report depression on the anonymous questionnaire. However, there were no significant differences between the two groups, so anonymous assessment tools may not be necessary, and that mothers seem willing to reveal their depression when asked specifically about it.

Screening in obstetric settings

Morris-Rush and Bernstein (2002) indicated that screening for depression during the postpartum visit is often helpful and is standard of care. The current guidelines from the American College of Obstetricians and Gynecologists (2015) and the US Preventive

Services Task Force (Siu & US Preventive Services Task Force (USPSTF), 2016) recommends that all perinatal women be screened at least once during the perinatal period for depression and anxiety using a standardized instrument. Unfortunately, this guideline to screen "at least once" may be too conservative to accurately detect depression and anxiety in the perinatal period. Once depression is identified, the healthcare provider is urged to refer women for follow-up care. They recommend using the EPDS, PHQ-9, Beck Depression Inventory, and CES-D as screening tools.

In a survey and chart-review study, obstetric providers charted EPDS score in 39 percent of the visits, and counseled their patients in 35 percent of the visits (Delatte, Cao, Meltzer-Brody, & Menard, 2009). All respondents to the survey of 47 providers agreed that they are responsible to screening for depression, and 94 percent were confident that they could diagnose it. Far fewer were actually doing it. There was a significant difference in referral rates depending on the provider type. Residents had the lowest rates (17 percent), followed by attendings (42 percent), certified nurse midwives (67 percent) and nurse practitioners (94 percent). This study was designed to evaluate the effectiveness of a policy of universal screening at a local medical center. The researchers noted that their results highlight the gap between what providers know should be done, and what is actually being done at postpartum visits.

Another study of 19 obstetricians and 3 midwives also found that most respondents indicated that it was important to screen, but that few were consistently doing it (Kim et al., 2009). The EPDS was used as a screening instrument. Ninety-five percent of the providers overestimated their rates of screening, and 67 percent thought they had achieved universal screening. If providers did not directly participate in the process, only 37 percent were screening. If they were involved, 59 percent actively screened. Some indicated that there was no office prompt to remind them to screen. Others were concerned about giving the PPD screen to everyone ("not everyone needs this"), that there was no time to do it, or that they lacked expertise to handle mental health issues. Higher screening rates appear to depend on more active provider commitment.

Screening in pediatric settings

The American Academy of Pediatrics' statement indicates that perinatal and postpartum depression is within the purview of pediatricians (Earls & Health, 2010). They noted that perinatal depression leads to increased medical costs and inappropriate care, child maltreatment, discontinuation of breastfeeding, family dysfunction, and adversely affects infant brain development. They stated that screening and referral to resources in the community are key to supporting healthy attachment and parent–child relationships.

Many consider pediatric visits to be the perfect time to screen for maternal depression (Currie & Rademacher, 2004; Freeman et al., 2005; Heneghan et al., 2007). Depressed mothers, particularly those with severe depression, may neglect self-care and not go to the doctor for themselves. Therefore, screening in a pediatric setting is even more important. Heneghan and colleagues (2007) noted that pediatricians see infants approximately seven times in the first year for well-baby checks, making it quite feasible to identify maternal depression. They surveyed 662 pediatricians with the goal of exploring characteristics of pediatricians associated with identifying and managing maternal depression. They found that 77 percent reported that they had "ever" identified maternal depression, and 82 percent of these referred the mother to services. Pediatricians were more likely to identify depression if they practiced in the Midwest, used more than one method to address maternal depression, worked in a practice that provides child mental health services, thought that maternal mental health has a substantial impact on child health, and had attitudes that inclined them to identify and manage maternal depression.

Head and colleagues (2008) also found that pediatricians were in an ideal position to detect maternal depression, and they surveyed 1,600 members of the American Academy of Pediatrics regarding perceived barriers to addressing maternal depression. There were three groups of pediatricians in the study: those in practice for five or more years, those in practice less than five years, and pediatric residents. Residents were more likely to have attended a course on maternal depression in the past two years, although only approximately 20 percent had done so. Pediatricians in practice for five or more years reported more barriers to addressing maternal depression than did pediatric residents. Some of these barriers included lack of training in adult mental health, and lack of interest in maternal depression. Even with residency reforms, 81 percent of current residents reported no training in adult mental health issues. The authors concluded that education for pediatricians during their residency appears to be helpful when it is present, but a large percentage still haven't had training on the topic.

A study of screening in Arizona well-baby clinics included 96 mothers at 8 weeks postpartum (Freeman et al., 2005). Of the mothers screened, 15 percent had a score of ≥12 on the EPDS. Higher scores were associated with smoking, and a family history of psychiatric disorders or substance abuse. Interestingly, a number of traditional risk factors for postpartum depression did not predict it. These included mother's age and ethnicity, marital status, employment, lifestyle habits, medical complications during pregnancy, labor or delivery, reproductive history, and perceived help with the baby.

Researchers in Turkey screened for depression at well-child visits (Orhon, Ulukol, & Soykan, 2007). They found that 34 percent of mothers were in the clinical range on the EPDS. Eighty percent of these mothers were identified at the one-month visit. Mothers with depressive symptoms had more negative perceptions of their infants, and reported more fussing, crying, sleep, and temperament problems. When depression was treated, these symptoms improved, especially poor quality of mothers' sleep, infant cry-fuss problems, and mothers' perceptions of infant temperament. However, there was a 59 percent dropout rate for treatment. Depressed mothers were more likely to complain of insufficient milk supply during the first 2 months, but infant feeding pattern was not associated with depressive symptoms. Further, the rate of breastfeeding initiation was 100 percent, with high continuation rates among the depressed mothers.

Barriers to screening

A focus group of 27 new mothers with a history of perinatal depression identified women's barriers to care in pediatric settings (Byatt, Biebel, Friedman, Debordes-Jackson, & Ziedonis, 2013). These barriers included stigma and fear of coming forward. The women didn't want their pediatricians to judge them or think they would kill their babies. Mothers also indicated that the providers were not knowledgeable and that they minimized the mothers' concerns. In contrast, mothers reported that they felt empowered when their pediatricians listened empathically, and offered tangible referrals and resources.

Pediatricians' attitudes about maternal depression were also measured in another study (Park et al., 2007). In a survey of 651 practicing, non-trainee pediatricians, the authors used an exploratory principal components analysis to examine interrelationships among the measures of pediatricians' attitudes. The analysis indicated three subscales:

acknowledging maternal depression (confidence in their ability to identify and treat depression; belief that advice from a pediatrician is the best way to help mothers seek treatment for depression), perception of mothers' beliefs (that mothers don't want pediatricians to investigate their depression; mothers are fearful of losing their children if they disclose depression; pediatricians feel that they are invading mothers' privacy); and treating maternal depression (confidently treat maternal depression with medications or brief counseling; pediatricians can be effective in treating maternal depression; mothers want pediatricians to treat their depression). Only 25 percent felt confident that they could identify depression. Most relied on observation, rather than using screening instruments, which tends to result in lower rates of detection.

Screening by telephone may be problematic in well-baby settings (Tam, Newton, Dern, & Parry, 2002). After being screened, women in the study were asked to pick up packets that contained depression assessment screening scales. Out of 160 packets distributed, only seven were completed. The author concluded that women were reluctant to participate in the study. Five of these women were in the clinical range. All refused to participate in phase 2 of the study, a clinical interview, but they all accepted referrals to a psychiatrist. Provider barriers included lack of confidence in their ability to handle a situation, such as a crying mother or a mother with suicidal thoughts. The pediatricians indicated that asking about depression would be like "opening Pandora's box." However, Tam and colleagues reiterated that pediatricians were the ideal professionals to screen for depression, and they recommended that pediatricians find a way to screen in a non-threatening way. Tam et al. also suggested offering a range of treatment options for patients.

With this in mind, Wisner, Logsdon, & Shanahan (2008) described a web-based education program for physicians and other primary-care healthcare providers, as these providers have the most ongoing contact with postpartum women: the website www.MedEdPPD.com. This site was designed to provide tools: CME modules, current literature and classic papers, a comprehensive slide library, and other resources. Nurses were the largest percentage of visitors (34 percent), followed by mothers (27 percent), and social workers (18 percent). Clinical psychologists (7 percent) and physicians (5 percent) were still represented in small numbers. Wisner et al. concluded that the site provides numerous training opportunities, is flexible and cost-effective, and meets the needs of healthcare providers.

Pediatricians should use a screening tool to assess depression rather than relying solely on observation, as observation misses a substantial number of cases. Hilt (2015) points out that if pediatricians do not ask mothers about depression, chances are no one else will either. The American Academy of Pediatrics recommends using either the EPDS with a cutoff of ≥10 or the PHQ-2 (Earls & Health, 2010), two scales I describe in the next section.

Screening and assessment scales

There are a number of screening scales for depression, including two designed specifically for postpartum women. The most widely used are described below.

Patient Health Questionnaire-9 (PHQ-9)

The PHQ-9 is a multiple-choice inventory that is used as a screening and diagnostic tool for depression. It is designed for primary care settings to detect major depression in adults. It is both sensitive and specific, and is widely used. It has been validated to use with perinatal patients (Walker, Gao, & Xie, 2015). Its major limitation is the lack of an item about suicidal ideation. It is based on the diagnostic criteria for major depression in the DSM-IV. A shorter version of the PHQ-9 is the PHQ-2 (see below).

A recent study compared two measures for detecting postpartum depression: Patient Health Questionnaire-9 (PHQ-9) and the Pregnancy Risk Assessment Questions (PRAMS-6), which were divided into the PRAMS questions for depression and PRAMS questions for anxiety (Davis, Pearlstein, Stuart, O'Hara, & Zlotnick, 2013). These measures were compared to the Structured Clinical Interview for Depression (SCID) and the Hamilton Rating Scale for Depression. The PRAMS-6 and PHQ-9 were both effective for screening for postpartum depression when compared with the Hamilton Rating Scale for Depression, and had moderate accuracy when compared with the SCID. The PHQ-9 had slightly better accuracy that the PRAMS-6.

A study of 745 pregnant women suggests that the PHQ-9 may be helpful in identifying depression in pregnancy as well (Sidebottom, Harrison, Godecker, & Kim, 2012). Patients received an assessment pack that included the PHQ-9. At a later appointment during their pregnancy, they were assessed via the SCID. The researchers noted that the PHQ-9 had good sensitivity (85 percent) and specificity (84 percent) for a diagnosis of depression, and the prevalence of major depression was 4 percent and 7 percent for the mild, subdiagnostic category. The researchers concluded that the PHQ-9 effectively identified depression in pregnant women.

Patient Health Questionnaire-2 (PHQ-2)

The 2-item Patient Health Questionnaire (PHQ-2) is a reliable initial health screening that can be used in all healthcare settings. Like the PHQ-9, it was designed to be used with adults in primary care settings, but it has been validated for use in perinatal women (Walker et al., 2015). Both the American Academy of Pediatrics and the American College of Obstetricians and Gynecologists recommend its use as a screening tool (Earls & Health, 2010).

The PHQ-2 includes the following two questions, and assesses frequency of anhedonia ("little interest or pleasure in doing things") and depressed mood ("feeling down, depressed or hopeless") during the past two weeks.

Over the past two weeks, how often have you been bothered by any of the following problems?

- Little interest or pleasure in doing things
- Feeling down, depressed, or hopeless

The response categories include Not at All, Several Days, More than Half the Days, and Nearly Every Day and are scored from 0 to 3. The higher the number, the higher the depressive symptoms.

One study found that it was highly sensitive for identifying postpartum depression during well-child visits (Gjerdingen, Crow, McGovern, Miner, & Center, 2009). A study examined the accuracy of the Patient Health Questionnaire-2 (PHQ-2) particularly for identifying depression in low-income women (Cutler et al., 2007). Ninety-four women participated in this study from an inner-city well-child clinic. The children ranged in age from 3 days to 5 years. The agreement between the PHQ-2 and EPDS was moderate. The sensitivity of the PHQ-2 was 44 percent and the specificity 93 percent. The sensitivity was higher for mothers with more education. The authors concluded that the PHQ-2 is not an effective screen with low-income, ethnically diverse women.

The PHQ-2 is designed to screen for depression in general, and can be used as a quick screen. However, results are likely to be more accurate with one of the two measures designed specifically for new mothers.

Edinburgh Postnatal Depression Scale (EPDS)

The EPDS continues to be the most widely used screening tool for postpartum depression in the world. The EPDS is a 10-item self-report questionnaire that can be completed in 5 minutes (Cox, Holden, & Sagovsky, 1987). It was designed to give primary-care providers, and other healthcare workers, a simple tool for screening in the postpartum period. There are also shortened versions available of this scale, including a 2-, 3-, and 7-item version (Walker et al., 2015).

Women are asked to report how they have felt in the past week, and the items are scored from 0 to 3. The standard cutoff is 12, but higher and lower cutoffs have been used. EPDS has been used in numerous research studies in populations all over the world. The authors have granted use of their questionnaire without charge or permission as long as the source of the scale is listed, and the copyright is respected.

Scale cutoffs

The cutoff used on the EPDS can vary depending on the intended on its purpose, and whether it is used for broad screening, or to more specifically identify only women with more serious depressions. Dennis (2004a, 2004b) used ≥9 as the cutoff for depressive symptomatology, which increases its sensitivity and makes it more appropriate for community screening (Dennis, 2004a). Dennis argued that a lower cutoff, with higher sensitivity, leads to fewer false-negatives. In contrast, a higher cutoff has more specificity, but might miss some depressed women. In her sample with 594 women, a cutoff of 12/13 at week 1 failed to detect depression in 43 percent of mothers at 4 weeks, and 53 percent of mothers at 8 weeks.

In a sample of 137 women from the United Arab Emirates, a cutoff of 9 resulted in 9 false-positive cases when the mothers were also assessed using the MINI (Hamdan & Tamim, 2011). Further, none of the mothers with scores under 10 qualified as cases when the MINI was used, so there were no false-negatives. When the cutoff was raised to 12, there were 4 false-positive and 3 false-negatives. The authors noted that while a score of 12 had better accuracy compared to the MINI, it also results in more false-negatives.

Moses-Kolko and Roth (2004) recommend the following: if a woman scores above 9, she is likely depressed, and they recommend a full psychiatric evaluation. This evaluation includes assessment of whether she is thinking of harming herself or her baby. The full assessment includes a psychiatric history of herself and her family members, gravid history, psychosocial history, routine lab results (including TSH), and screening for bipolar disorder. If symptoms have persisted for more than two weeks, she should be referred for treatment that can include psychotherapy, support, and possibly medications. If a woman scores between 5 and 9 on the EPDS, she may be at risk for depression within the next 6–12 months. Clinicians can give women copies of the EPDS and instruct them to seek care if they score >9. If she indicates that she intends harm to herself or her baby, she should be seen immediately (Moses-Kolko & Roth, 2004). A woman with an EPDS score <5 is unlikely to be depressed and needs no further follow-up.

Logsdon and colleagues (2009a) noted that the EPDS has been validated with a sample of adult women around the world. However, it has not been used with teen mothers. In their sample of 149 adolescent mothers, they found that the EPDS was a valid screening tool to use with teens. It had an internal consistency reliability of 0.88. The CES-D was used as the measure of criterion validity. In this sample of teen mothers, 26 percent had an EPDS score ≥12. With the CES-D, 44 percent had significant symptoms of depression. The analyses also indicated that the EPDS was measuring both depression and anxiety symptoms. They concluded that the EPDS was a valid instrument to use with adolescent mothers.

Previous studies have noted that the EPDS measures not only depression but also other disorders, such as anxiety. One way to determine if there are other conditions that the EPDS measures is to run confirmatory factor analyses on the various models presented in these previous studies. One recent study used the EPDS as a screening tool for 169 low-income African American women, a group typically underrepresented in postpartum depression studies (King, 2012). King used confirmatory factor analysis to determine which model of factors in the EPDS fit best with this particular sample. She found high rates of depression with her sample. When the cutoff was ≥10, 30 percent screened positive for depression, and 19 percent did when the cutoff was ≥13. With confirmatory factor analysis, she found that the three-factor model with depression, anxiety, and anhedonia was the best fit for this sample of low-income African American women. These findings suggest that anxiety and anhedonia factors are distinct from depression, and are relevant for this sample.

A study from Western Australia had a large sample of mothers, both antenatal (N = 4,706) and postnatal (N = 3,853), and demonstrated the validity of using the EPDS to measure anxiety (Swalm, Brooks, Doherty, Nathan, & Jacques, 2010). They demonstrated the concurrent validity of the anxiety subscale by its significant relationship to the items on a psychosocial risk factor questionnaire that were anxiety-related. The items related to anxiety are numbers 3, 4, and 5 ("I have blamed myself unnecessarily when things went wrong," "I have been anxious or worried for no good reason," and "I have felt scared and panicky for no very good reason"). A score of 4 or more on those three items captures the top quartile of mothers at possible high risk for perinatal anxiety disorders.

EPDS-Partners and EPDS-Lifetime

A recent version of this has also been developed for screening for depression in partners (EPDS-P) (Fisher, Kopelman, & O'Hara, 2012), which detects partners' depression through mothers' report. This instrument demonstrated reliability and validity in detecting fathers' depression in a sample of 810 couples. They compared mothers' reports on fathers, and the fathers' self-reports. Both types of reports were accurate, but fathers' self-reports were somewhat more accurate than mothers' reports about fathers.

Another recent variant on the EPDS is the EPDS-Lifetime. The EPDS was modified to include questions about lifetime incidence of postpartum depression, the worst episode, and the timing of symptoms onset. A study using data from the Netherlands Study of Depression and Anxiety sought to assess the EPSD-Lifetime (Meltzer-Brody, Boschloo, Jones, Sullivan, & Penninx, 2013). This study assessed the prevalence of lifetime postpartum depression in women who had histories of prior major depression, and to evaluate the risk factors for postpartum depression. Fifty-four percent of the women had had an episode of major depression before their first episode of postpartum depression. They found that women with a lifetime history of depression and a live birth, 40 percent had an EPDS score ≥12. Regarding timing of onset, 57 percent happened during postpartum, and 43 percent occurred during pregnancy. They found that 2 out of 5 parous women with a history of major depression had lifetime postpartum depression. The episodes of postpartum depression were more severe than major depression that happened outside the perinatal period.

Advantages and disadvantages of the EPDS

The EPDS offers a number of advantages. It is easy to complete and score. Mothers can answer all the questions in a few minutes. It is specifically written for new mothers. Indeed, the EPDS was developed to address the limitations of more generic depression measures.

Although widely used, there are some disadvantages to the EPDS. The scale is written in British, rather than American English. American mothers sometimes find the wording of some of the questions confusing, or a little odd. Lappin (2001) cautions that the EPDS is designed to be used in the early postpartum period, and has only been validated for that use. It should not be used for screening for depression in pregnancy, or to diagnose depression beyond the postpartum period; however, it is often used in both of these situations. Lappin (2001) also cautions against interpreting one-to-two point differences as indicating increased severity. This instrument is best at predicting depression with a cutoff of 12. Similarly, Elliot and Leverton (2000) noted that the EPDS is a reliable and valid screening tool, but it has been misused. They emphasized the importance of ongoing training and quality control to ensure that it is used properly.

Guedeney and colleagues (2000) raise another caution. They provided a case report of three false-negatives on the EPDS with women with major depressive disorder (according to the Research Diagnostic Criteria). They noted that the EPDS seems better able to identify depressed postpartum women with anhedonic and anxious symptoms than depressed women with psychomotor retardation.

Scoring difficulties with the EPDS

The EPDS contains several items with reverse scoring that may increase the likelihood that scores may be miscalculated. Matthey et al. (2013) collected 496 EPDSs from client files, and examined them for scoring errors from six practices in Australia. They also surveyed 22 clinicians and asked them to estimate the rate of errors. The error rate was far above what the clinicians estimated. Matthey et al. found that 17 percent of the forms had at least one error. Most were from clinicians scoring them incorrectly. Most were incorrect by only one point, and this difference generally did not seem clinically relevant. However, there was some concern because being off by one point could make the different between a positive and negative screen for depression. The authors noted that the EPDS is not easy to manually score despite claims in the literature that it is.

Variations of the EPDS with better predictability

A sample of 299 women completed the EPDS at 2–3 days, and 4–6 weeks postpartum (Chabrol & Teissedre, 2004). The authors used exploratory factor analysis to predict EPDS scores at 4–6 weeks. The three factors they extracted were anxiety, depressive mood, and anhedonia. Of these, anxiety was the best predictor of higher EPDS scores at 4–6 weeks, and was the only significant predictor of postpartum depression. The items included under anxiety were self-blame (item 3), anxiety (item 4), scared or panicked (item 5), inability to cope (item 6), and difficulty sleeping (item 7).

Another study specifically used three items of the EPDS, the anxiety subscale, and compared them with the accuracy of the full 10-item scale, and the ultrabrief 2-item screener (Kabir, Sheeder, & Kelly, 2008). Their sample was 199 14- to 26-year-old participants in an adolescent-oriented maternity program. A total of 21 percent of the mothers met the criteria for depression (EPDS >10). The EPDS-3 had the best performance, with 95 percent sensitivity and 98 percent negative predictive value. It identified 16 percent more mothers as depressed than the full EPDS did. The EPDS 2-item scale was markedly inferior, and did not identify mothers who were depressed as well as the other versions. The three-item screener included the following questions:

> I have blamed myself unnecessarily when things went wrong
> I have felt scared and panicky for no very good reason
> I have been anxious or worried for no good reason

In contrast, the two-item screen resembles the PHQ-2, and was much less effective, with a sensitivity of 48 percent, and a negative predictive value of 80 percent. These items included the following:

> I have looked forward with enjoyment to things
> I have felt sad or miserable

They suggested that the EPDS-3 is brief enough to be incorporated into well-baby checks, and it identified a higher percentage of women as possibly depressed than the full EPDS.

A more detailed study of 1,549 women in Australia found that adding a simple interval question to the EPDS increased its accuracy using the Composite International Diagnostic Interview (CIDI) (Austin et al., 2010). This question asked if they had experienced any depressive symptoms since the last EPDS ("During the last 2 months, has there been any period of one week or more when you felt so miserable or sad that it interfered with your ability to get things done, or with your relationships with friends/family?"). Mothers who scored >12, and/or were positive on the interval question, were then administered the CIDI. The interval question increased the ability to identify caseness on the CIDI by 1.7 times. The authors concluded that using the EPDS alone, and only one time, likely underestimates CIDI caseness.

Postpartum Depression Screening Scale (PDSS)

Another tool designed specifically for new mothers is the PDSS. The PDSS is a 35-item, Likert-scale, self-report instrument. It measures functioning on seven dimensions: sleeping/eating disturbances, anxiety/insecurity, emotional lability, cognitive impairment, loss of self, guilt/shame, and contemplating harming oneself. It takes 5–10 minutes to complete, and is available for a small fee from Western Psychological Services (www.wpspublish.com). A shorter version of this scale has been validated for use with postpartum women (Walker et al., 2015).

Like the EPDS, the PDSS is useful for screening new mothers for depression. In addition, the subscales can provide information for clinicians in treating mothers by highlighting specific areas of difficulty. In developing this scale, Beck and Gable (2000) attempted to address the limitations of the EPDS. For example, they noted that the EPDS did not measure postpartum feelings, such as loss of control, loneliness, irritability, fear of going crazy, obsessive thinking, concentration difficulty, and loss of self. In a study of 525 new mothers, confirmatory factor analysis supported the seven dimensions of the PDSS. The internal consistencies on the seven dimensions ranged from 0.83 (sleeping/eating disturbances) to 0.94 (loss of self). A panel of experts also established the content validity of the scale, and item-response theory techniques provided further construct validity (Beck & Gable, 2000).

In another study (Beck & Gable, 2000, 2001a, 2001b), 150 mothers who were 12 weeks postpartum completed the PDSS, EPDS, and the Beck Depression Inventory-II (BDI-II). Following completion of these questionnaires, a nurse/psychotherapist interviewed each woman using the Structural Clinical Interview for DSM-IV Axis I disorders. The results of the PDSS correlated with the EPDS ($r = 0.79$), and the BDI-II ($r = 0.81$). The authors then performed a hierarchical regression to ascertain the level of variance that the PDSS accounted for above and beyond the other two measures. The results indicated that the PDSS accounted for an additional 9 percent of the variance in the diagnosis of depression. A cut-off score of 80 for major depression has a sensitivity of 94 percent, and a specificity of 98 percent. A cutoff of 60 can be used for both major and minor depression, has a sensitivity of 91 percent, and a specificity of 72 percent. The PDSS was superior in this sample in identifying major depression partly because it included items on sleep and cognitive impairment (Beck & Gable, 2001b).

A more recent study used both the EPDS and PDSS with a sample of 842 Chinese pregnant women with complications (Zhao et al., 2015). They found that the EPDS and PDSS scores were strongly correlated, and that each scale did well in detecting both major and minor depression, but they found that the PDSS had better psychometric performance than the EPDS. Ten percent of women had an EPDS score ≥13, and 31 percent had an EPDS of 9–12. When both scales were used together, the authors recommended a cutoff of 8/9 on the EPDS, with 72 percent sensitivity and 88 percent specificity. The cutoff recommended on the PDSS was 79/80 for major depression, with sensitivity of 86 percent and specificity of 100 percent. However, although the PDSS was, overall, a better tool, it did miss some cases of depression. The authors noted that both tools were reliable assessments for Chinese pregnant women with complications, and recommended using lower cutoffs to reduce misdiagnosis, and improve validity of screening. They also recommended using both screening tools to decrease rates of false-positives and -negatives. They also feel that the optimal time to screen pregnant women is at the first prenatal appointment.

Other measures specifically for postpartum women

There are some other measures that may prove useful for both practitioners and researchers. These are listed below.

Postpartum Social Support Questionnaire (PSSQ)

The PSSQ is a 50-item self-administered questionnaire designed to measure social support that new mothers receive. It identifies mothers who have little support as this can be a substantial risk factor for postpartum depression (Miller, Hogue, Knight, Stowe, & Newport, 2012).

Postpartum Depression Predictors Inventory-Revised (PDPI-R)

The PDPI-R is a 13-item self-report measure used to identify risk factors for postpartum depression. It accurately identifies mothers at risk for depression during pregnancy and the postpartum period (Oppo et al., 2009).

Perinatal Anxiety Screening Scale (PASS)

The PASS screens for a wide variety of anxiety symptoms that may present in the perinatal period. It is useful in a number of different settings including antenatal clinics, in- and out-patient facilities, and in mental health treatment settings. It addresses acute anxiety and adjustment; general work and specific fears; perfectionism; control and trauma; and social anxiety. It is a 38-item self-report questionnaire (Somerville et al., 2014).

Childbirth Perception Scale (CPS)

The CPS is a 12-item scale that measures women's perceptions of their births. There are two parts to this questionnaire: women's perception of their deliveries, and perception of the first week postpartum. It was initially designed to compare home and hospital births, taking into account women's mental health, and how it can color perceptions of birth. It correlates highly with the EPDS (Truijens, Wijnen, Pommer, Guid Oei, & Pop, 2014).

Additional factors to assess

Once you have determined a mother is depressed, you may want to make some additional assessments to guide her to the right level of help and support. These additional factors include the severity of the current episode, and whether she is abusing substances, at risk for suicide, or requires hospitalization.

Unfortunately, simply identifying mothers who are depressed is not enough. In a study of 2,199 pregnant women, 19 percent had a cutoff >9, and 5 percent had an EPDS ≥14. None of the women pursued follow-up referrals. Similarly, of the 2,199 women, only 569 were available for assessment at 6 weeks postpartum, 28 women screened positive for depression, and only 5 followed-up with behavioral healthcare referrals (Rowan, Greisinger, Brehm, Smith, & McReynolds, 2012). If depressed women do not seek care, there is little impact to be gained from screening.

Severity of current episode

When evaluating the severity of the current depressive episode, consider three factors: duration and intensity of symptoms, and level of impairment. Symptoms must be present for at least 2 weeks for a diagnosis of major depression. Intensity of the symptoms and level of impairment can also indicate whether aggressive treatment is warranted. Indications of severe impairment can include when patients suddenly stop paying attention to personal grooming, cannot manage their households, or have days when they cannot get out of bed. If serious enough, hospitalization might be necessary.

If mothers are hospitalized while still breastfeeding, and they want to continue, make arrangements to protect their milk supply, or to help them wean gradually, as sudden weaning increases their risk of infection. These mothers need access to a hospital-grade electric pump. For mothers who choose to continue, a regular schedule of pumping can ensure that their milk supply is maintained. It also gives mothers a vision of life beyond the hospital.

> **When to make an emergency referral to a mental-health specialist**
>
> - Suicidal thoughts or plans, concerns about patient's safety
> - Plans that include assaulting or killing others, concerns about safety of other people
> - Recent episode of psychosis
> - Inability to care for self or others
> (Mitchell et al., 2013)

Suicide risk

Suicide risk is always an important consideration when working with depressed mothers. Although rare, the consequences are so serious that it is useful to screen all mothers who are depressed. The Institute for Clinical Systems Improvement (Nicolson, Judd, Thomson-Salo, & Mitchell, 2013) lists some specific risk factors for suicide. Even with these signs, it is still difficult to predict all potential suicides, but screening will detect many mothers who are at risk. Be sure to chart your assessment of suicide risk.

- Previous history of suicide attempts
- Suicidal ideation, particularly with specific suicide plans
- Substance abuse or dependency
- Personality disorder or physical illness
- Family history of suicide
- Single status
- Recent death of a loved one
- Recent divorce or separation
- Insomnia
- Panic attacks
- Diminished concentration
- Severe anhedonia or hopelessness
- Comorbid PTSD

If even one of these risk factors is present, a more specialized consult may be in order. Potentially suicidal patients should be closely monitored through frequent visits, encouraging the mother to reside with family or friends, or by being hospitalized. Contact your local suicide-prevention hotline for information about how best to proceed, and for referrals of people who can help.

Conclusion

Mothers are often not forthcoming about their depression. They may not even realize that they are depressed, but they often know that *something* is wrong, which may prompt them to seek healthcare often for themselves and their babies.

You can screen for depression by using some general questions about their level of fatigue and stress. You can also use one of the standardized screening measures for depression. Screening can also help you determine whether a mother is suicidal, needs to be hospitalized, or needs a referral for other assistance.

Once depression has been identified, mothers need to be treated. There are a wide range of treatments available for depressed new mothers. These are described in detail in Part III.

Note

1   PRAMS = Pregnancy-Risk Assessment Monitoring Study.

Part II

Risk factors

Chapter 6

Physiology of postpartum depression I

Inflammation and psychoneuroimmunology

The field of psychoneuroimmunology (PNI) has brought about some of the major developments in postpartum depression research. PNI research examines the role of the immune system in stress and depression. Of particular interest is the role of proinflammatory cytokines and the HPA axis in the etiology of depression (Corwin & Pajer, 2008; Kendall-Tackett, 2007; Leonard, 2010). Proinflammatory cytokines are messenger molecules of the immune system. They have the adaptive function of fighting infection and healing wounds, but when these molecules are systemic and chronically elevated, they increase the risk of depression and a number of serious diseases. Cytokines increase the risk of depression by dysregulating neurotransmitter metabolism, impairing neuronal health, and altering activity in parts of the brain related to mood (Kiecolt-Glaser, Derry, & Fagundes, 2015).

Maes and colleagues (2000b) were the first to document that women with postpartum depression and anxiety had elevated levels of proinflammatory cytokines. When describing the relationship between depression and inflammation, Maes and Smith (1998) noted that there are a number of plausible explanations for why inflammation might increase the risk for depression. First, when inflammation levels are high, people experience classic symptoms of depression, such as fatigue, lethargy, and social withdrawal. Researchers discovered this connection when using inflammatory cytokines as treatments for conditions such as cancer or hepatitis. When patients are treated with cytokines, depression increases in a predictable and dose–response way: the greater the dosage of cytokines, the more depressed the patients. When the dose is tapered, depression drops (Baumeister et al., 2016; Kiecolt-Glaser et al., 2015). Second, inflammation activates the hypothalamic–pituitary–adrenal (HPA) axis, dysregulating levels of cortisol. Cortisol generally keeps inflammation in check. However, depression dysregulates cortisol, which then fails to restrain the inflammatory response. Finally, inflammation decreases serotonin by lowering levels of its precursor, tryptophan.

To further understand the role of inflammation in depression, it's helpful to first review the human stress response—the normal physiologic response to a perceived threat. Inflammation is part of the three-part stress response.

How humans respond to a perceived threat

When faced with a threat, human bodies have a number of interdependent mechanisms designed to preserve our lives. This physiologic response is the same for both physical and psychological threats (Kim & Ahn, 2015).

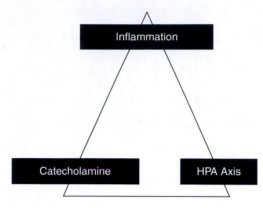

FIGURE 6.1 The three-part stress response

Catecholamine response

The sympathetic nervous system responds first by releasing catecholamines (norepinephrine, epinephrine, and dopamine). This is the fight-or-flight response, and it occurs instantly.

With regard to postpartum depression, the HPA axis and immune response are of most interest.

HPA axis

The HPA axis also responds to threat with a cascade of stress hormones within 15–20 minutes after threat exposure. The hypothalamus releases corticotrophin-releasing hormone (CRH), which causes the pituitary to release adrenocorticotropin hormone (ACTH), which causes the adrenal cortex to release cortisol, a glucocorticoid. The HPA axis has far-reaching effects on immunity, metabolism, and reproduction. This system returns to baseline a few hours after stress exposure. If stress continues, however, it becomes dysregulated, and patterns of either hyperactivity or hypoactivity appear (Brummelte & Galea, 2016; Corwin & Pajer, 2008; Kim & Ahn, 2015).

The regulation of the HPA axis changes markedly during pregnancy. CRH is also produced by the placenta during pregnancy, and not solely the hypothalamus, as it is in a non-pregnant state. Cortisol stimulates CRH in the placenta rather than downregulating it, like it does when it originates in the hypothalamus. One recent study found that elevated CRH in pregnancy is a strong predictor of postpartum depression (Yim et al., 2009). In this study, serum samples from 100 pregnant women were assessed at 15, 19, 25, 31, and 37 weeks gestation. Serum samples were assayed for CRH, ACTH, and cortisol. Depression was assessed at four points antenatally, and one time postpartum. Elevated CRH at 25 weeks gestation predicted postpartum depression.

A study of 284 mothers from Sweden also found evidence of HPA involvement in depression (Illiadis et al., 2015). The researchers examined evening cortisol levels and assessed mothers at 18 and 36 weeks gestation, and 6 weeks postpartum. Depression was assessed with EPDS ≥10. They found that women with elevated cortisol levels were four times more likely to become depressed postpartum, even after controlling for history of depression, smoking, partner support, breastfeeding, stressful life events, and sleep problems. Women with postpartum depression had higher cortisol levels than women who were depressed during pregnancy, and non-depressed women. The authors concluded that their study indicates an altered HPA axis in postpartum depression reflected in mothers' evening cortisol levels.

Inflammatory response

The final component of the stress response is the immune system, which responds to threat by releasing proinflammatory cytokines (Corwin & Pajer, 2008; Kendall-Tackett, 2007). Researchers generally assess inflammation by measuring serum levels of proinflammatory cytokines. The proinflammatory cytokines identified most often in depression research are interleukin-1β (IL-1β), interleukin-6 (IL-6), and tumor necrosis factor-α (TNF-α). Researchers sometimes include other measures of inflammation in their studies. These include interferon-γ (IFN-γ), intercellular adhesion molecule (ICAM), fibrinogen, or C-reactive protein (CRP). Maes (2001b) described the stress–depression–inflammation connection as follows.

> The discovery that psychological stress can induce the production of proinflammatory cytokines has important implications for human psychopathology and, in particular, for the aetiology of major depression. Psychological stressors, such as negative life events, are emphasized in the aetiology of depression. Thus psychosocial and environmental stressors play a role as direct precipitants of major depression or they function as vulnerability factors which predispose humans to develop major depression. Major depression is accompanied by activation of the inflammatory response system (IRS) with, among other things, an increased production of proinflammatory cytokines, such as IL-1β, IL-6, TNF-α, and an acute-phase response.
>
> (Maes, 2001b, p. 193)

One of the original studies that established the link between chronic stress, inflammation, and premature mortality was not in a postpartum sample, but a sample of elderly men and women (average age = 70 years), approximately half of whom were caring for a spouse with Alzheimer's (Kiecolt-Glaser et al., 2003). The researchers primarily focused on IL-6, which has been linked to cardiovascular disease, type-2 diabetes, cancer, and overall functional decline. Caregivers had IL-6 levels that were four times higher than their age-matched controls. These levels remained elevated even after the spouse had died. At the end of the six-year follow-up, 78 of the 119 caregivers had died. These researchers concluded that chronic stress accelerated the risk of disease by prematurely aging the immune response.

The three systems illustrated on Figure 6.1 are interrelated, with a series of checks and balances—when the system is working normally. Inflammation influences levels of serotonin and catecholamines, and impacts the HPA axis, which secretes cortisol. However, if the system is overwhelmed, it fails (Kim & Ahn, 2015).

Depression is one state where the normal checks and balances fail. In a normally functioning system, once inflammation starts, it triggers the HPA axis to release cortisol to keep it under control. Specifically, cortisol downregulates IL-1, IL2, TNF-α, and IFN-γ

(Corwin & Pajer, 2008; McEwen, 2003). However, depressed people have either abnormally low levels of cortisol, or they become cortisol-resistant, as described in Chapter 4 (Kim & Ahn, 2015).

In a recent study, Corwin and colleagues (2015) tested whether the bidirectional interaction between the inflammatory response system and HPA axis increased women's risk of postpartum depression. Their sample included 152 women recruited during their third trimester of pregnancy. The researchers measured plasma pro- and anti-inflammatory cytokines during the third trimester, and at days 7 and 14, and months 1, 2, 3, and 6 postpartum. They also collected saliva 5 times a day before each blood draw. Depression was assessed via the EPDS ≥10. Their results indicated that family history of depression, day 14 cortisol AUC (area under the curve), and day 14 IL-8/IL-10 ratio predicted depressive symptoms. Every unit increase in IL-8/IL-10 ratio increased risk 1.8 times, and each unit increase in cortisol AUC increased risk 2 times. They concluded by noting that cytokines and the HPA axis integrate to influence postpartum mood.

Corwin and colleagues (2010) also hypothesized about a genetic component of postpartum depression that may make some mothers more vulnerable via genetic polymorphisms. These polymorphisms may make mothers more vulnerable when they are exposed to a normal postpartum stressor. According to this review, there are some genes related to central nervous system monoamine availability (particularly serotonin and norepinephrine), proinflammatory cytokines, and brain neuropeptides.

Other factors that appear related in inflammation levels include psychosocial stressors, poor diet (especially decreased omega-3 fatty acids and increased, proinflammatory omega-6s), physical inactivity, smoking, altered gut permeability, dental caries, abdominal obesity, allergic disorders, sleep, and vitamin D deficiency (Berk et al., 2013). Along these same lines, Dietert (2013) noted that changes in our environment, such as cesarean births, sanitized living, and vaccines, may be changing the gut microbiome, and increasing our tendency towards inflammatory chronic diseases. He cites natural childbirth and breastfeeding as two preventive measures. Berk et al. (2013) also noted that remission of depression is accompanied by a normalization of inflammatory markers, and that people who do not respond to treatments for depression often have persistent levels of inflammation.

In a recent review, Kiecolt-Glaser and colleagues (2015) noted that when there are predisposing factors, such as childhood adversity, stressors, and pathogens can lead to prolonged or exaggerated inflammatory responses. This can result in sickness behaviors, such as pain or disturbed sleep, depression, and negative health behaviors that lead to even more unrestrained inflammation and depression. The combination of depression, childhood adversity, stress, and poor diet can influence the gut microbiome, furthering inflammation.

Why inflammation is particularly relevant to depression in new mothers

Pregnant and postpartum women are particularly vulnerable to this effect because their inflammation levels normally rise during the last trimester of pregnancy—a time when they are also at highest risk for depression (Kendall-Tackett, 2007). Indeed, elevated cytokines in the last trimester matches the pattern of perinatal depression more accurately than the pattern of other biological markers, such as the rise and fall of reproductive hormones (Corwin et al., 2015). The findings on women's increased risk of depression during pregnancy are summarized in Chapter 1.

Immune markers remain elevated in postpartum women

Proinflammatory cytokine levels are generally elevated in women after giving birth (Corwin et al., 2015). One study found that postpartum women are generally higher in the cytokines IL-6, IL-6R, and IL-IRA than before delivery (Maes et al., 2000b).

Corwin and Johnston's (2008) sample included 38 women in the first 24 hours after delivery, and 26 provided urine for analysis of IL-1β and IL-6 at days 7, 14, and 28. Depression was assessed via CES-D (≥11). On day 14, elevations of IL-1β were associated with depression on day 28. They recommended anti-inflammatory interventions, including the use of NSAIDS, early diagnosis and treatment of subclinical infections, and careful wound care, so that these interventions might reduce the development of postpartum depression.

A study from Greece recruited 56 pregnant women, and recorded a detailed medical and obstetric history (Boufidou et al., 2009). The researchers measured postpartum blues at 1 and 4 days postpartum, and used the EPDS at 1 and 6 weeks postpartum. They obtained blood samples from 23 women, and cerebral spinal fluid (CSF) from 33 women that was collected while administering epidurals. They found that women with depressive symptoms at day 4 and 6 weeks had elevated TNF-α and IL-6 in their blood and CSF. The measure of CSF is a more sensitive measure of central nervous system activity than blood.

Physical and psychological stressors that increase inflammation and risk of depression

As described in the previous section, human bodies are designed to respond a certain way when they are threatened. These threats can be physical or psychological; the body's response is the same. Moreover, some types of stressors have both physical and psychological elements. Three stressors—fatigue, pain, and trauma—are particularly relevant to new mothers. Studies that examine fatigue and pain with regard to inflammation are described below. Trauma will be described in Chapters 6 through 8.

Fatigue and sleep deprivation

Fatigue's role in postpartum depression is often overlooked because almost *all* new mothers are tired (Bozoky & Corwin, 2002). However, fatigue can be debilitating and can decrease women's abilities to care for their babies and their enjoyment of motherhood, and dramatically increase their risk for depression (Corwin & Arbour, 2007). For example, one large Australian study found that 60 percent of new mothers reported exhaustion or extreme tiredness, and 30 percent reported lack of sleep or a baby crying in the first 8 weeks (Thompson, Roberts, Currie, & Ellwood, 2002). These problems eventually resolved, but 49 percent still reported exhaustion, and 15 percent reported lack of sleep at 24 weeks. Mothers who had cesarean sections were more likely to report exhaustion than mothers with assisted or unassisted vaginal deliveries.

Sleep disturbances and depression

Fatigue can be both a symptom of depression and a cause. Fatigue may also be the way that depression presents and can be a clue that something is amiss, particularly when women cannot sleep even when their babies are sleeping. Depression and sleep problems are mutually maintaining: poor sleep quality is a risk factor for major depression, and depression is a risk factor for the onset of poor sleep quality. Severe fatigue also predicts future depression (Posmontier, 2008b). More detailed information about sleep and maternal mental health is described in Chapter 7.

Pain

Pain is another risk factor for postpartum mental disorders that can stem from both biological and psychosocial causes. Depression and inflammation alerts the central nervous system to induce "sickness behavior," which includes increasing fatigue and pain sensitivity (Kiecolt-Glaser et al., 2015).

After childbirth, women may experience pain from a variety of sources: abdominal incisions, uterine contractions, swollen or engorged breasts, cracked nipples, episiotomies and/or perineal lacerations, back pains and headaches from spinal or epidural anesthesia, and muscle aches and pains. This pain, although transitory, can be severe and frightening. In this large sample of mothers at 8 weeks postpartum, 53 percent reported backache, 37 percent reported bowel problems, 30 percent reported hemorrhoids, 22 percent reported perineal pain, and 15 percent reported mastitis (Thompson et al., 2002). Unfortunately, postpartum pain is often undermedicated, as a study on analgesia for women who had had forceps deliveries found (Peter, Janssen, Grange, & Douglas, 2001).

Acute pain, if followed by an adaptive response, is usually followed by a rapid return to baseline. However, the response to pain can also be dysfunctional, leading to exaggerated and prolonged HPA axis activation, cortisol dysfunction, inflammation, pain, and depression (Hannibal & Bishop, 2014). What people think about their pain, and cognitive processes such as catastrophizing, rumination, and helplessness, can lead to acute pain becoming chronic pain.

A prospective study of 1,288 women found that it was the severity of the post-birth pain, rather than the mode of delivery, that predicted postpartum depression (Eisenach et al., 2008). Acute pain increased the risk of postpartum depression by 3 times. It also increased the risk of acute pain becoming chronic by 2.5 times.

Unfortunately, nipple pain appears to be common. The first sample was from Minneapolis, Minnesota. In this sample, an astonishing 50 percent of women had nipple pain at 5 weeks postpartum (McGovern et al., 2006). Another study from Toronto, Canada had similar results. In this study, 52 percent of mothers reported cracked or sore nipples at 2 months postpartum (Ansara et al., 2005).

In the study of 109 women hospitalized in a private mother–baby unit (Fisher et al., 2002), pain was also an issue. In this sample, 41 percent reported that their postpartum pain was inadequately controlled, and 41 percent described nipple pain that persisted for longer than one week. Twenty-nine percent of these mothers had experienced at least one episode of mastitis. A high-degree of postpartum pain was also associated with depression at 8 months postpartum in another study of primiparous women (Rowe-Murray & Fisher, 2001).

In a study of 465 women, Chaudron and colleagues (2001) found that women who reported ten or more somatic complaints were nearly three times more likely to develop depression than were women who reported nine or fewer symptoms. They also found a linear relationship between postpartum depression and physical or somatic complaints. The more physical complaints, the higher the depressive symptoms.

Another possible link between pain and depression is pain's impact on sleep. Sayar, Arikan and Yontem (2002) compared 40 patients with chronic pain to 40 healthy control subjects on sleep quality, depression, and anxiety. As predicted, patients with chronic pain had significantly poorer sleep quality, and more depression and anxiety. Pain intensity, anxiety, and depression were related to poorer sleep quality. However, in a multivariate analysis, depression was the only factor that was significantly correlated to sleep, explaining 34 percent of the variance.

Pain and inflammation

Depression and pain are also related to inflammation, and the relationship between pain and inflammation appears to be bidirectional. Pain increases inflammation, and inflammation increases pain. Proinflammatory cytokines (especially IL-1) are stimulated by Substance P, the neuropeptide present in patients with pain. High levels of Substance P increase proinflammatory cytokines, which increase prostaglandin synthesis, which increases pain.

In one study of 101 adults, patients with major depression or posttraumatic stress disorder had significantly higher levels of Substance P in their CSF compared to healthy controls (Geracioti et al., 2006). Moreover, the levels of Substance P rose significantly when the patients were stressed in the laboratory, showing that it responded to acute stress.

In a study of non-postpartum postoperative pain, researchers compared three methods of pain relief: pain relief with opiates on demand, patient-controlled analgesia, and patient-controlled epidural analgesia (opiates with local anesthesia, which was anti-inflammatory) (Beilin et al., 2003). Patients in the epidural group had the lowest levels of pain, with higher levels of inflammation (IL-1β and IL-6) in the other two groups.

In summary, postpartum pain is a common experience among women who have recently given birth (Ansara et al., 2005). Addressing pain promptly, and providing mothers the means to cope with their pain, can halt the cascade of stress hormones and proinflammatory cytokines, decreasing their risk of depression.

Hormonal influences

The hormonal theory of postpartum depression is the oldest, and most well-known, of the physiological theories of postpartum depression. At present, we know that women undergo substantial changes in hormone levels in the immediate postpartum period. The main controversy is whether these changes are related to depression. As I indicated in Chapter 1, research has produced mixed results, with little support for the reproductive hormonal etiology of depression. However, other hormone levels may be involved.

Hypothyroidism

Thyroid is a hormone that regulates metabolism. Low thyroid levels can cause a wide range of depression-like symptoms including an inability to concentrate, tiredness, and forgetfulness. Low thyroid can also cause intolerance to cold, persistently low body temperature, low blood pressure, weight gain, puffy face and eyes, constipation, and dry hair and skin. In mothers who are very tired, evaluating them for postpartum hypothyroidism is often prudent (Stagnaro-Green, 2012).

A study of 31 women examined the relationship between thyroid levels in late pregnancy/early postpartum, and the development of postpartum depression (Pedersen et al., 2007). Thyroid was measured at 32–35, 36, and 37 weeks gestation. All of the women had normal thyroid levels. The women also rated their mood every other week between 2 and 24 weeks postpartum. Women with lower total and free thyroxine concentrations had significantly higher depression scores, via EPDS and BDI, at all three postpartum assessment points. The researchers concluded that women with thyroxine levels in the euthyroid range may be at greater risk for developing postpartum depressive symptoms.

Another study, however, has failed to find a link between postpartum depression and postpartum thyroid dysfunction (Lucas, Pizarro, Granada, Salinas, & Santmarti, 2001). This study recruited 641 women during their 36th week of pregnancy, and followed them through the first year postpartum ($N = 444$ at the 12-month assessment). The authors found that 56 women (11 percent) developed postpartum thyroid disorder. None of these women were diagnosed with postpartum depression, using the BDI. Their sample's rate of postpartum depression was abnormally low (1.7 percent). Women with a history of postpartum depression, however, were significantly more likely to become depressed again.

The rate of postpartum thyroid dysfunction is approximately 3 percent, and postpartum thyroiditis (including both hypo and hyperthyroidism) is about 5 percent (Corwin & Arbour, 2007; Stagnaro-Green, 2012). Although screening all mothers may not be necessary, it is a low-risk test that can be helpful when working with mothers with severe fatigue. Risk factors for postpartum hypothyroidism include diabetes mellitus, and a personal or family history of hypothyroidism. Women with type 1 diabetes are at triple of the risk of postpartum thyroiditis (Stagnaro-Green, 2012).

Childhood trauma can also increase risk of postpartum thyroid disorders. In a study of 103 postpartum women from Spain with major depression, 63 percent had experienced childhood trauma, 54 percent general trauma, and 27 percent had experienced childhood sexual abuse (Plaza et al., 2010). Among women with major depression, a history of childhood sexual abuse increased the risk of thyroid dysfunction by 5 times, and increased the presence of thyroid autoantibodies by 2.5 times. In addition, women who were more than 34 years old, and who had previous postpartum depression, were at increased risk of postpartum thyroid disorder.

Screening tests for hypothyroidism include TSH levels, and free or total T4. These tests can be administered to mothers with risk factors for postpartum hypothyroidism, or to mothers with severe fatigue.

Reproductive hormones

Estrogen, progesterone, and their metabolites are the most well-studied hormones in relation to postpartum depression. Depression is hypothesized as being most likely to occur if estrogen and progesterone levels drop after partuition (Brummelte & Galea, 2016). Although this theory of postpartum depression remains popular, little evidence supports it, and it fails to explain things like the high rate of depression in pregnancy, depression in fathers and adoptive mothers, and lower rates of depression in cultures where mothers are well cared for in the postpartum period.

Hormone levels in depressed and non-depressed women

Bloch and colleagues (2000) were able to induce a postpartum-depression-like syndrome in the laboratory. They recruited two groups of eight women: women with previous postpartum depression and women with no history of postpartum depression. They simulated the high hormone levels of pregnancy with gonadotropin-releasing hormone agonist leuprolike acetate, and added back supraphysiologic dose of estradiol and progesterone for eight weeks. They then withdrew the steroids under double-blind conditions. During withdrawal, 62.5 percent of the women with a history of postpartum depression developed significant mood symptoms when the steroids were withdrawn. None of the comparison women were affected. The authors concluded that their findings constituted direct support for the involvement of reproductive hormones in the development of postpartum depression *in a subgroup of women.* They noted that women with a history of postpartum depression may be differentially sensitive to changes in these hormone levels, and develop depression as a result.

Another study measured estradiol levels in two groups of women: women with a history of postpartum depression ($n = 7$) and without a history ($n = 12$) (Schiller, O'Hara, Rubinow, & Johnson, 2013). The researchers were assessing the effects of estradiol withdrawal after birth, and identified the women with the history of depression as "high risk." They found that low levels of estradiol are related to negative mood in women who developed postpartum depression by 1 month postpartum ($n = 4$). Estradiol withdrawal was not associated with negative affect in either the high-risk or control group. Interestingly, negative mood began increasing *before* delivery, "which suggests that estradiol withdrawl did not necessarily precipitate the onset of negative mood symptoms" (p. e9). They also found, contrary to their hypothesis, that lower levels of estradiol were related to higher positive affect. Positive affect did not increase in the high-risk group after birth. These authors also argued that a certain subgroup of women may be differentially sensitive to these hormonal shifts, although their sample size was too small to draw any conclusions.

Another US study compared estradiol, progesterone, and testosterone levels in 62 women with postpartum depression, and 41 non-depressed women (Aswathi et al., 2015, in press). The researchers found no differences between the depressed and non-depressed women in estradiol and progesterone at 24–48 hours postpartum. Depressed women, however, had significantly higher levels of testosterone than the non-depressed women.

A cross-sectional study of 308 women from China measured depression and anxiety during all three trimesters of pregnancy and the first month postpartum (Fan et al., 2009). Seventy-one percent of the women were depressed, and 58 percent had clinically relevant anxiety. Women had the highest rates of anxiety and depression in the first trimester pregnancy, and in the first month postpartum. There was a sharp increase of serum estradiol in the first trimester, and a sharp decrease of estradiol in the postpartum period. The authors hypothesized that depression and anxiety increased when there were sharp changes in hormone levels, not simply when these levels decreased.

A community sample of 478 women in the first year postpartum examined the link between postpartum depression and premenstrual syndrome (Buttner et al., 2013). The researchers found that there was a significant relationship between moderate to severe premenstrual syndrome and postpartum depression, and this relationship persisted even after controlling for sociodemographic factors, suggesting an independent effect. Mothers' history of depression was also significantly related to postpartum depression, as was "not breastfeeding," which would have changed the hormonal milieu for mothers. Single marital status and non-White ethnicity also increased the risk.

A study of 166 mothers from Korea also found a link between premenstrual syndrome and postpartum depression (Lee, Yi, Lee, Sohn, & Kim, 2015). Depression was assessed via the EPDS (≥10), and BDI (>10). Fourteen percent of participants were depressed. The depressed women were significantly more likely to smoke, have a history of past psychiatric disorders, and have low marital satisfaction. Nine percent of the women had a history of premenstrual syndrome, but very different prevalence rates for the depressed women (35 percent) vs. the non-depressed women (5 percent). The researchers concluded certain women may be more vulnerable to reproductive events.

Treatment for postpartum conditions using hormones

The final strategy for studying postpartum hormonal influences involves treating women at risk for postpartum depression with hormones. Traditionally, this research is plagued by methodological issues, such as lack of double-blind trials. At first glance, these findings seem compelling, but without blinding, researchers were not able to account for the placebo effect.

For example, Ahokas and colleagues (2000; 2001) have used 17β-estradiol to treat severe postpartum depression and postpartum psychosis. In the study of depression (Ahokas et al., 2001), 23 women with postpartum major depression were recruited from a psychiatric emergency unit. They were all severely depressed and had low serum estradiol concentrations. Within a week of treatment with estradiol, the depressive symptoms had substantially diminished, and by the end of the second week, when estradiol levels were comparable to the follicular phase, the scores on the depression measure were comparable to clinical recovery.

The study of psychosis was similar (Ahokas et al., 2000). There were ten women with postpartum psychosis who all had very low levels of serum estradiol. Within a week of sublingual 17β-estradiol, symptoms were significantly improved. By the second week, when levels were almost normal, the women were almost completely free of psychiatric symptoms.

These studies are interesting, but there are serious limitations. First, the trials were open-label, which means everyone was aware of being treated. Was it estradiol that created the change, or was it the placebo effect? These studies raise some other questions, such as what are the normal levels of estradiol for postpartum women? Presumably, almost every woman is low in estradiol postpartum. How is it that only some become depressed or psychotic? Is there a certain level where we start to see psychiatric symptoms? Why are some women more vulnerable to these changes (a question several researchers have raised)?

Despite the limited evidence, proponents of this view still recommend treating postpartum depression with hormones. A recent article was astonishing because it recommends using estradiol to treat *breastfeeding* mothers, saying mothers may prefer it because it is more "natural" (Moses-Kolko, Berga, Kalro, Sit, & Wisner, 2009). Moreover, the authors recommended that future studies examine the transfer of this hormone into breast milk. The reason that this statement is so astonishing is because estrogen, and any of its metabolites, are absolutely contraindicated for breastfeeding (Hale & Rowe, 2014). This treatment option will effectively kill a mother's milk supply (breastfeeding requires that estrogen is suppressed). If this treatment is given in early postpartum, it will not matter how much estradiol transfers into breast milk *because there won't be any breast milk*. When the authors listed possible contraindications for this treatment choice, the impact on breastfeeding was not on the list. They did recommend that clinicians wait to use this treatment until "lactation is established." Only they do not indicate when this will be, nor do they mention that estrogen metabolites are generally troublesome during the entire time of lactation. The authors of this article showed a serious lack of knowledge about breastfeeding, and this treatment option would be directly harmful to breastfeeding mothers, with little evidence that it would actually treat depression.

Conclusions

Researchers to date have not established that puerperal hormonal changes are related to postpartum depression. The good news is that our models of the biological influences in depression have grown much more sophisticated, due in part to greatly increased research efforts in neuroscience and psychoneuroimmunology. I suspect we are only in the early stages of understanding the complex interplay between the immune system, sleep, neurotransmitters, and hormones. Future research promises to bring us to an even better understanding of how physiological factors can shape mood. The next chapter describes two other biological mechanisms: breastfeeding and mother–infant sleep.

Chapter 7

Physiology of postpartum depression II

Breastfeeding and
mother–infant sleep

Unfortunately, some postpartum depression advocates consider breastfeeding a risk factor for depression. Based on this belief, mothers are often urged to quit in order to recover. Some of these same providers argue that even if mothers say they want to continue, what we really need to do is give them "permission" to quit. When actress Brooke Shields experienced postpartum depression, her family strongly urged her to stop breastfeeding. She adamantly refused because she felt that breastfeeding was the one thing that was helping her to hang on to her sanity.

> Both my mother-in-law and my mother suggested that I stop breastfeeding to give myself a break. In fact, the consensus seemed to be that I give up the baby on the breast and move past that added pressure. But what nobody understood was that the breastfeeding was my only real connection to the baby. If I were to eliminate that, I might have no hope of coming through this nightmare. I was hanging on to breastfeeding as my lifeline. It was the only thing that made me unique in terms of caring for her … Without it, she might be lost to me forever.
>
> (Brooke Shields, 2005, pp. 80–81)

While advice about weaning is usually well-intended, the evidence does not support it. So the question we need to ask is whether women need to wean in order to recover from depression. When providers urge mothers who want to continue to quit, breastfeeding can become a barrier to treatment. Mothers may delay or avoid seeking treatment because they believe that they will be told to wean. In my experience, this fear is realistic: practitioners often do tell mothers to wean.

What these practitioners often fail to realize is that breastfeeding actually protects maternal mental health. If women want to continue, and it is always their choice, we should support them because it will aid in their recovery.

Breastfeeding confers survival advantage by protecting mothers' mental health

Previous studies have found that breastfeeding mothers actually have lower rates of depression than their non-breastfeeding counterparts (Dennis & McQueen, 2009; Groer,

Davis, & Hemphill, 2002). Breastfeeding protects maternal mental health because it downregulates the stress response. This downregulation confers a survival advantage by protecting the breastfeeding mother and directing her toward milk production, conservation of energy, and nurturing behaviors (Groer et al., 2002). Hormones related to lactation, such as oxytocin and prolactin, have both antidepressant and anxiolytic effects (Mezzacappa & Endicott, 2007).

A more recent review from Brazil noted that we now better understand the processes by which breastfeeding protects mothers' mental health. They described possible mechanisms by which breastfeeding might protect maternal health in more detail:

(1) by promoting hormonal processes that attenuate the cortisol response to stress (particularly the effects of prolactin and oxytocin),
(2) by regulating sleep for mother and child,
(3) by increasing mother's self-efficacy and emotional connection with her baby,
(4) by reducing difficulties related to child temperament, and
(5) by promoting better mother–infant interaction

(Figueiredo, Dias, Brandao, Canario, & Nunes-Costa, 2013)

In addition, depressed, breastfeeding mothers are less likely to have babies with highly reactive temperaments, compared with depressed, bottle-feeding mothers. Further, breastfeeding mothers have more physical contact and positive play with their infants, and vocalize more than their bottle-feeding counterparts (Figueiredo et al., 2013).

A study of 137 women from the United Arab Emirates found that formula-feeding mothers had more depressive symptoms at 2 and 4 months postpartum than their breast-feeding counterparts (Hamdan & Tamim, 2011). The researchers found that women had lower scores on the EPDS if they were "breastfeeding at all," and breastfeeding at the time of the assessment. Further, the more frequently that a woman breastfed, the lower her scores on the EPDS.

Similarly, a study of 2,072 women from Malaysia also examined the relationship between exclusive breastfeeding and postpartum depression at 1 and 3 months post-partum (Yusuff, Tang, Binns, & Lee, 2016). In this study, mothers were assessed with the EPDS. Approximately 46 percent of the mothers were exclusively breastfeeding at 3 months. The exclusively breastfeeding mothers had significantly lower EPDS scores at both time points than mothers who never breastfed, or who were not exclusively breast-feeding. This relationship remained significant even after controlling for covariates.

In a sample of 209 women from Oklahoma, researchers examined risk factors associated with a score >13 on the EPDS (McCoy, Beal, Shipman, Payton, & Watson, 2006). Formula-feeding doubled the risk of depression. Other significant risk factors included a history of depression, and cigarette smoking. Breastfeeding is associated with a significantly lower occurrence of postpartum depression. Approximately 39 percent of this sample had an EPDS score in the depressive range, possibly due to the high percentage of women living in poverty in this sample.

A prospective study of 205 pregnant women found that women who breastfed more frequently at 3 months postpartum had significantly lower depressive symptoms by 24 months (Hahn-Holbrook, Haselton, Schetter, & Glynn, 2013). Depression was measured at 5 points during pregnancy with the CES-D, and at 3, 6, 12, and 24 months with the EPDS, with a cutoff of >10. They also found that women who were depressed during pregnancy were significantly less likely to breastfeed than their non-depressed counterparts. They asked about "any" breastfeeding, number of feeds per day, the percentage of breast milk that made up the baby's diet, and the percentage of breast milk that was pumped. Mothers who breastfed at least nine times a day had significantly lower rates of depression than mothers who breastfed less than four times a day. This relationship was still true, even after controlling for possible confounding variables, such as age, income, education, social support, and employment status. Mothers who were depressed weaned their babies an average of 2.3 months earlier than mothers who were not depressed.

Breastfeeding and the stress response

A study of 43 breastfeeding women found that both breastfeeding, and holding their babies without breastfeeding, significantly decreased ACTH, plasma cortisol, and salivary-free cortisol (Heinrichs et al., 2001). Breastfeeding and holding the infant led to significantly decreased anxiety, whereas mood and calmness improved only after the baby was at the breast. In response to an induced stressor, breastfeeding suppressed the HPA axis, and provided a short-term suppression of the stress response. The researchers argued that this short-term suppression provided several evolutionary and biological advantages: it isolated the mother from distracting stimuli, facilitated her immune response, protected the baby from high cortisol in the milk, and prevented stress-related inhibition of lactation.

Groër and Morgan (2007) found, in a study of 200 women at 4–6 weeks postpartum, that depressed women were significantly less likely to breastfeed, had significantly lower serum prolactin levels, and had more life stress and anxiety. A more recent study of 63 primiparous mothers at 2 days postpartum had similar findings (Handlin et al., 2009). In this study, both ACTH and cortisol were measured. They found that breastfeeding lowered ACTH and cortisol, and that skin-to-skin contact contributed to these effects. ACTH was negatively correlated with duration sucking, but cortisol decreased in relation to skin-to-skin contact that proceeds breastfeeding. The longer the skin-to-skin contact went on, the lower the cortisol levels. Oxytocin also plays an important role in reducing ACTH and cortisol during breastfeeding.

One-hundred nineteen women were recruited during pregnancy, and followed through 6 months postpartum (Ahn & Corwin, 2015). They were assessed during the third trimester of pregnancy, on days 7 and 14 postpartum, and at 1, 2, 3, and 6 months. Pro- and anti-inflammatory cytokines were measured, as were depression and self-reported breastfeeding. The rates of breastfeeding "most of the time" were 92 percent at day 7, and 71 percent at 6 months—well over the national averages in the US. The researchers found that depression, or perceived stress, did not significantly differ for breastfeeding vs. bottle-feeding mothers at 6 months, possibly because the rates of breastfeeding were so high. However, salivary cortisol levels at 8 a.m. and 8:30 a.m. were higher (indicating that the HPA axis was functioning well), and IL-6 was lower, for the mothers predominantly breastfeeding at 6 months. One factor that may have made a difference in this study was their measure of breastfeeding. "Predominant breastfeeding" is not the same as exclusive breastfeeding from a physiological standpoint. Previous studies have found that supplementing exclusive breastfeeding lessens breastfeeding's stress-reduction effects (Kendall-Tackett, Cong, & Hale, 2011).

Breastfeeding's downregulation of the stress response appears to have long-term effects, and it likely explains another set of recent findings regarding cardiovascular disease (Schwartz et al., 2009). This study included 139,681 postmenopausal women (mean age = 63 years). The researchers found that women with a lifetime history of breastfeeding for more than 12 months were less likely to have hypertension, diabetes, hyperlipidemia, or cardiovascular disease than women who never breastfed. This was a dose–response relationship: the longer women lactated, the lower their cardiovascular risk. The authors noted that lactation improves glucose tolerance, lipid metabolism, and CRP.

Similarly, Stuebe and colleagues (2011) found that women who breastfed their first child ≥12 months were less likely to develop hypertension, and women who never breastfed were more likely to develop hypertension than women who breastfed 6 months or longer. Their sample was 55,636 women from the US Nurses' Health Study II. They concluded that 6 months of exclusive breastfeeding, or >12 months of total breastfeeding per child, reduced the risk of hypertension.

Because stress is related to the onset of depression, Mezzacappa and Endicott (2007) examined the impact of parity and whether it mediated the effect of feeding method on maternal stress. This study compared primaparae who were breast- or bottle-feeding, and multiparae who were breast- or bottle-feeding. Breastfeeding had greater stress-reducing effects, and oxytocin levels were higher, on multiparous women than primiparous women. For primparas women, 35 percent of bottle-feeding and 16 percent of breastfeeding mothers were depressed. Among multiparas women, 37 percent of the bottle-feeding and 12 percent of breastfeeding women were depressed. The authors indicated that parity was a critical factor mediating the effect of lactation on depression.

Breastfeeding appears to also influence infants' emotional development, and less exclusive breastfeeding (EBF) may bias them toward more negative information processing, which could make the infants more vulnerable to stress and depression. In a recent study of 28 8-month-olds, exclusive breastfeeding had an impact on infant brain development (Krol, Rajhans, Missana, & Grossman, 2015). Half of the infants were classed as low exclusive breastfeeding (12–152 days), and half were high exclusive breastfeeding (167–252 days). The results indicated that amount of exclusive breastfeeding was related to infants' neural processing of images of happiness or fear. Babies who exclusively breastfed longer paid more attention to happy stimuli than those with shorter duration of EBF. In contrast, infants with shorter EBF showed a negativity bias, responding more to the fear stimuli and less to the happy stimuli. The authors speculated that EBF affects central oxytocin levels in infants, and thereby impacts emotional processing. Breastfeeding plays a role in infants' socioemotional development and biases them towards either positive or negative information.

Another recent study highlights why it is important to address depression and anxiety promptly. This study examined the relationship between depression and anxiety in 81 breastfeeding mothers, and how those conditions affected the immune qualities of breast milk (Kawano & Emori, 2015). Negative mood states, such as depression and anxiety, lowered secretory IgA (SIgA) levels in breast milk, but positive mental state did not influence it. They recommended that mothers with depression or anxiety receive support, and did not suggest that they wean.

Depression and breastfeeding cessation

Women who encounter breastfeeding problems are at increased risk for depression. Conversely, depression increases the risk for breastfeeding cessation. A review by

Field (2010) found that depression impaired a wide range of caregiving practices, including breastfeeding, sleep routines, well-child visits and vaccinations, and safety practices.

Breastfeeding cessation in depressed mothers may also have a physiological basis. A study from Japan conducted an *in vitro* study on the effects of the three proinflammatory cytokines most commonly seen in depression—IL-1β, IL-6, and TNF-α—on mice mammary epithelial cells (MECs) (Kobayashi, Kuki, Oyama, & Kumara, 2016). They found that TNF-α downregulates lactose synthesis, IL-1β caused degradation of glucose transporter 1 from the membranes of the MECs, and IL-6 both upregulated and downregulated expression of lactose synthesis-related genes of the MECs. Each of these cytokines influences the lactose synthesis pathways, but in different ways. In other words, depression may have a negative impact on milk supply.

A study of 168 women in southeastern Brazil found that depressed women were more likely to stop exclusively breastfeeding at 2 months postpartum (Machado et al., 2014). The sample was assessed at 1, 2, and 4 months postpartum, and the EPDS was used at 1 and 2 months, with a cutoff ≥ 12. Depressive symptoms and traumatic deliveries both predicted lack of exclusive breastfeeding at 2 months.

A study of 226 women from Barbados also showed a relationship between depression and breastfeeding cessation (Galler, Harrison, Ramsey, Chawla, & Taylor, 2006). This study assessed women's feeding practices and attitudes in the first 6 months postpartum. If women believed that breastfeeding was better than bottle-feeding, they had lower rates of depression at 7 weeks and 6 months postpartum. Mothers with depressive symptoms were less likely to believe that breastfeeding was better for infants, and more likely to believe that breastfeeding was private and restrictive. Even after controlling for maternal feeding attitude, maternal mood at 7 weeks was still significantly associated with infant feeding practices at 6 months.

A Turkish study showed similar results (Akman et al., 2008b). In this study, 60 mothers of newborns were enrolled prospectively. Mothers and babies were assessed at 1 and 4 months postpartum. The percentage of mothers exclusively breastfeeding was high: 91 percent at 1 month and 68 percent at 4 months. Mothers with higher EPDS scores at Time 1 were less likely to be breastfeeding at Time 2.

A study from Pakistan produced results that were consistent with the other studies (Taj & Sikander, 2003). This sample included 100 women with breastfeeding-age children ranging from 2 months to 2 years. Thirty-eight percent of these women had stopped breastfeeding, and their average scores on the Urdu version of the Hospital Anxiety and Depression Scale (HADS) were 19.66, compared with 3.27 for the breastfeeding women. Of the women who had stopped breastfeeding, 37 percent reported that their depression had preceded breastfeeding cessation. The authors concluded that maternal depression caused mothers to stop breastfeeding.

Women were assessed for depression with the EPDS at 6 and 12 weeks postpartum ($N = 185$) in another study (Hatton et al., 2005). At 6 weeks, depressive symptoms were related to lower rates of breastfeeding. This relationship persisted even after controlling for prior history of depression, life stress, and current antidepressant use. There was no relationship between breastfeeding and depressive symptoms at 12 weeks postpartum. The authors concluded that depressive symptoms in early postpartum may lead to early breastfeeding cessation. They offered several possible explanations for their findings, including that depressed women may not have initiated breastfeeding, or that early depression impacted milk production or let down. They also noted that stressful life events can have a negative impact on breastfeeding, and are also predisposing factors for postpartum depression.

In a qualitative study of 12 women from Ghana, and three focus groups with new mothers, fathers, and grandmothers, the impact of depression on breastfeeding was universally acknowledged (Scorza et al., 2015). The study participants often described depression as "thinking too much" to reflect the ruminations that are common in depression. One woman described the impact on breastfeeding: "she thinks too much, the child doesn't get breast milk to suck because breast milk is not available." Grandmothers reported that women without happiness cannot, or will not, breastfeed their babies. Babies may also refuse to feed if "a woman has not happiness, her baby can see that her mother is sad by looking at the mother's face, in which case the baby would not breastfeed." Fathers also described this link by noting that depressed women become withdrawn and do not eat. If they do not eat well, they cannot produce enough milk for breastfeeding.

A US nationally representative sample of 1,271 mothers, who were part of the Infant Feeding Practices Study II, found that 31 percent met criteria for mild depressive symptoms (Bascom & Napolitano, 2016). The researchers found that women with depressive symptoms had significantly shorter overall breastfeeding, and shorter EBF. Depression was measured using the EPDS >9. Sixty-nine percent stopped breastfeeding before 6 months, with "too many household duties" cited as the most common reason. Sore nipples were also more common in the depressed mothers.

A study from Canada had similar results (Dennis & McQueen, 2007). This sample included 594 community women who were surveyed at 1, 4, and 8 weeks postpartum. The women were surveyed about their feeding method and depressive symptoms on the EPDS. The researchers found no relationship between maternal mental health and feeding method at 1 week postpartum. However, mothers with an EPDS score of >12 at 1 week postpartum were significantly less likely to be breastfeeding at 4 and 8 weeks. They were also more likely to be unsatisfied with their infant feeding method, experience serious breastfeeding problems, and report lower levels of breastfeeding self-efficacy. Mothers who thought breastfeeding was "progressing terribly" at week 1 were more likely to develop depressive symptoms. However, when depression was removed from this analysis, the effects disappeared. The authors felt these findings reflected depressed mothers' moods and cognitions, rather than objective problems. They concluded that early identification of mothers with depressive symptoms can both halt morbidity associated with depression, and increase breastfeeding duration.

One factor that might contribute to the link between breastfeeding cessation and depression is epidural anesthesia. In our study of 6,410 new mothers, women who had had an epidural had higher rates of depressive symptoms, even after controlling for other risk factors for depression (such as other birth interventions, and history of depression or sexual assault) (Kendall-Tackett, Cong, & Hale, 2015). (Our study is described in more detail in Chapter 8.) We also found that women who had had epidurals were significantly less likely to be exclusively breastfeeding.

A prospective study of 1,280 women from Australia had similar results (Torvaldsen, Roberts, Simpson, Thompson, & Ellwood, 2006). They found that women who had an epidural were more likely to be partially breastfeeding, and have breastfeeding difficulties in the first week, than women who did not have an epidural. The results of these two studies indicate a possible link between epidurals and lower rates of breastfeeding, which increases the risk of depression. Further studies will need to examine possible causal links.

Mothers' intention to breastfeed

Intention to breastfeed has also been the focus of recent studies. Mothers in the Avon Longitudinal Study of Parents and Children in the UK indicated that intention to breastfeed was an important risk factor in postpartum depression (Borra, Iacovou, & Sevilla, 2015). Depression was measured during pregnancy with the EPDS ≥14, and postpartum EPDS ≥12. In this longitudinal study of 14,000 mother–infant pairs, mothers who were not depressed during pregnancy had the lowest risk of depression if they planned to breastfeed their babies, and actually were able to do it. The mothers at highest risk were those who planned to breastfeeding and could not. They also found that mothers who had not intended to breastfeed, but actually did, were at increased risk of depression. The authors noted that depression is mediated both by breastfeeding intentions and mothers' mental health during pregnancy. They recommended that mothers be given access to skilled breastfeeding support, and mothers who intended to breastfeed, but could not, be given compassionate care.

A recent study from the US also found that mothers' expectations about breastfeeding made a difference with regard to depression. In this study, 1,501 mothers from the Infant Feeding Practices Study II were included if they intended to exclusively breastfeed (Gregory, Butz, Ghazarian, Gross, & Johnson, 2015). Only 39 percent were able to exclusively breastfeed, and 23 percent had depressive symptoms (EPDS ≥10). The researchers found that mothers who met their prenatal expectations had fewer PPD symptoms than mothers who did not. Interestingly, this was only true for the middle- and upper-income mothers, but not for the lower-income mothers. Breastfeeding pain in the first 2 weeks was also related to depression.

Nipple pain, depression, and breastfeeding cessation

A study from Melbourne, Australia found that nipple pain was relatively common in the first 8 weeks postpartum (Buck, Amir, Cullinane, Donath, & the CASTLE Study Team, 2014). This study included 340 primiparous women that were part of the prospective cohort study. After hospital discharge, 79 percent reported nipple pain. During the 8-week study, 58 percent reported nipple damage, and 20 percent reported vasospasm. By 8 weeks, the situation had improved for most of the mothers, with only 8 percent reporting nipple damage and 20 percent reporting pain. Surprisingly, despite this high rate of nipple pain, 94 percent were continuing to breastfeed.

In a study of 2,586 women who reported "ever breastfeeding," 9 percent had an EPDS score ≥13 at 2 months postpartum (Watkins, Meltzer-Brody, Zolnoun, & Stuebe, 2011). Women who disliked breastfeeding at 1 week were more likely to be depressed at 2 months. In addition, women who experienced breastfeeding pain on day 1, week 1, or week 2 were more likely to be depressed at 2 months. Severe pain doubled the odds of postpartum depression. Women who were depressed at 2 months were significantly less likely to still be breastfeeding. However, breastfeeding help appeared to protect women's mental health when the women had moderate to severe pain. The authors concluded that women who had negative early breastfeeding experiences were more likely to have depressive symptoms at 2 months postpartum, but that breastfeeding helps attenuate those effects.

Anxiety and breastfeeding cessation

Postpartum anxiety can also impact breastfeeding initiation and duration (Britton, 2007). In a study of mothers at discharge and 1-month postpartum, predischarge anxiety was inversely related to breastfeeding confidence. Mothers who were high in post-discharge anxiety were less likely to be fully or exclusively breastfeeding, and were more likely to have stopped breastfeeding at 1 month.

A study of 852 pregnant women in Brazil (Rondo & Souza, 2007) found that distress and worry about breastfeeding, concern about body changes, and work outside the home were negatively related to intention to breastfeed. However, depression and anxiety scores were not related to intention to breastfeed.

A study from India found significant levels of anxiety and depression in their sample of 85 new mothers measured by the HADS (Arinfunhera et al., 2015). The researchers found the HADS depression score, low birthweight, and lower income were all independent predictors of poorer attitudes towards breastfeeding. Anxiety did not emerge as an independent predictor of breastfeeding attitudes.

One hundred twenty-two depressed women described their breastfeeding experiences (McCarter-Spaulding & Horowitz, 2007). The researchers collected data during three home visits. They noted that in this sample, severity of depression was not related to breastfeeding, but older maternal age, living with a partner, and higher income were. Maternal education was the most important predictor of exclusive breastfeeding, and combination feeding. Depression was most severe at the 4- to 6-week assessment, dropping off after that. By 14–18 weeks postpartum, 78 percent had EPDS scores below the cutoff. All of the women were encouraged to seek outside care for their depression, but only 11–12 percent had gone to psychotherapy, and 3–6 percent had used medications.

In terms of breastfeeding patterns, by 14–18 weeks, EBF had dropped from 34 percent to 22 percent. At 14–18 weeks, 33 percent were using a combination of feeding methods, and 45 percent were exclusively formula-feeding. They noted that their findings of high breastfeeding rates, despite severity of their postpartum depressive symptoms, are consistent with previous research that suggests a link between depression and early weaning. What depression seemed to affect was EBF, which was lower than in the larger sample from which they were drawn (McCarter-Spaulding & Horowitz, 2007).

In a qualitative review of 49 articles that specifically examined the link between depression and breastfeeding, Dennis and McQueen (2009) found that in early postpartum, depressive symptoms decreased breastfeeding duration, increased breastfeeding difficulties, and decreased breastfeeding self-efficacy. Further, depressed women may be less likely to initiate breastfeeding, and to breastfeed exclusively. Mothers with depressive symptoms were more likely to discontinue breastfeeding earlier than non-depressed mothers. Depressive symptomatology was related to lower breastfeeding self-efficacy, demonstrating that depressed mothers were less confident in their ability to breastfeed.

Stuebe and colleagues hypothesized that perinatal depression and lactation failure may share common neuroendocrine mechanisms (Stuebe, Grewen, Pedersen, Propper, & Meltzer-Brody, 2012). Possible physiological mechanisms include estrogen and progesterone; oxytocin and prolactin; hormones related to stress reactivity, such as CRH, ACTH, and cortisol; pain perception; thyroid; and infant development, such as temperament and oromotor development, which can affect ability to latch. They recommended that future studies address the overlap between maternal depression and breastfeeding difficulties, understanding that they may come from the same underlying etiology.

Sleep, feeding method, and maternal mental health

As described in the previous chapter, sleep has a major impact on maternal well-being. For example, in a study of 245 pregnant women, sleep problems were the strongest predictor of poorer health-related quality of life (Da Costa et al., 2010). Depressed mood was associated with more bodily pain, and poorer general health, vitality, social functioning, and emotional health. Sleep problems also predict new-onset depression and anxiety disorders. In a non-postpartum sample of 9,683 young women from Australia, researchers found that sleep problems at Time 1 predicted that depression was two to four times more likely 3–9 years later. Anxiety risk also doubled 6–9 years later (Jackson, Sztendur, Diamond, Byles, & Bruck, 2014).

Amount of sleep also makes a difference. In a prospective study of 112 couples recruited during the third trimester of pregnancy, sleeping <4 hours between midnight and 6 a.m., spending more than 2 hours awake during that time, and napping <60 minutes during the day increased the risk of depression at 3 months postpartum (D. Goyal, Gay, & Lee, 2009). Depression was assessed with the CES-D ≥16. Twenty-eight percent had depressive symptoms. Infant temperament did affect mothers' sleep, but was not associated with depression. In addition, variables such as maternal age, income, education, sex of the infant, feeding method, delivery type, and satisfaction with their relationship with their partners accounted for 15 percent of the variance in depression.

Another longitudinal cohort study of 1,840 women from Norway followed the mothers from week 32 of pregnancy to year 2 postpartum (Sivertsen, Hysing, Dorheim, & Eberhard-Gran, 2015). The rate of insomnia was 60 percent at 32 weeks gestation and at 8 weeks postpartum, and dropped to 41 percent at year 2. Sleep duration ranged from 6 h 30 min to 7 h 16 min. Maternal depression did not explain the stability of sleep problems in these new mothers. The researchers noted that sleep problems in this sample appeared to be largely independent of comorbid postpartum depression, despite the close interrelationship of these conditions.

Sleep characteristics of depressed mothers

Ross et al. noted that several factors suggest a relationship between sleep problems and depression in postpartum women (Ross, Murray, & Steiner, 2005). These are as follows:

(1) Insomnia is a significant risk for new-onset depression.
(2) Sleep disturbances are common in most psychiatric disorders.
(3) Treatments that manipulate sleep and circadian rhythms can be used to treat mood disorders.

In a review of polysomnographic studies of postpartum women, Ross et al. (2005) noted that sleep differed in some distinct ways for women at risk for postpartum depression, or who have current postpartum depression—reduced REM latency, increased total sleep time during pregnancy, and decreased total sleep time postpartum for the women who are depressed. REM latency refers to the time during the night when REM sleep becomes the predominant pattern. A pattern of reduced REM latency means that REM occurs earlier in the nightly sleep cycle, and is a symptom of depression. As a result of these sleep disturbances, women are more fatigued during the day, and they also have more bodily pain. The authors noted that these changes may represent an underlying vulnerability to depression as they do with non-postpartum populations. They also noted that women with a history of affective disorders may be more sensitive to the normal physiologic changes of pregnancy.

A study with 425 mothers from Canada found that mothers with postpartum major depression reported substantially poorer sleep than their non-depressed counterparts at 4–8 weeks postpartum (Dennis & Ross, 2005). The mothers were assessed for depression at 1 week postpartum, and women who were depressed at that time point were excluded from the study to eliminate pre-existing depression as a cause of sleep problems. Mothers with an EPDS >13 at 1 week were more likely to report that their babies cried often, that they were woken 3 or more times a night, and that they received less than 6 hours sleep in a 24-hour period. Further, they were more likely to report that their babies did not sleep well, and that their babies' sleep pattern did not allow them to get a reasonable amount of sleep. Infant temperament mediated the relationship between infant sleep and maternal fatigue, with fussy babies sleeping less.

A Taiwanese study of 163 first-time mothers found that 50 percent were depressed at 13–20 weeks postpartum (Huang, Carter, & Guo, 2004). Depressed mothers had poorer sleep than non-depressed mothers. Half reported that their sleep quality was either "fairly bad" or "bad." The average time it took for mothers to fall asleep was 26 minutes vs. 20 minutes for non-depressed mothers. Depressed mothers had overall poorer sleep quality, took more time to fall asleep, had a shorter sleep duration, and reported more daytime dysfunctions.

In a study of 46 mothers at 6–26 weeks postpartum, data were collected via questionnaire and wrist actigraphy for 7 days (Posmontier, 2008b). Half of the mothers were depressed. Postpartum depression was measured via the Postpartum Depression Screening Scale. The author found that women with postpartum depression had substantially poorer sleep quality than non-depressed women, and that as depressive symptoms increased, so did the sleep problems. Women with postpartum depression took longer to go to sleep (longer sleep latency), were more likely to wake after sleep onset, and had poorer sleep efficiency. She concluded that for women with postpartum depression, nighttime breastfeeding demands, high-needs infants, and little nighttime support may negatively impact sleep quality, and further exacerbate depressive symptoms. This was true, even though the non-depressed group was breastfeeding and had fewer nighttime wakings than the non-depressed group.

A longitudinal study of 124 primiparous women collected data during the last trimester, and at 1, 2, and 3 months postpartum (Goyal, Gay, & Lee, 2007). At Time 1, 26 percent had clinically high depressive symptoms. Depressed women had more sleep disturbance, trouble falling asleep, daytime sleepiness, and early awakening than women who were not depressed. The mothers who had the highest depression scores reported the most difficulty falling asleep. The author concluded that delayed sleep onset may be the most relevant clinical screening question to assess risk of postpartum depression.

Sleep, depression, and feeding method

Feeding method is yet another variable that we must consider in order to understand the complex relationship between depression and sleep problems. If mothers are breastfeeding, and they have any symptoms of depression, they are frequently told to supplement at night and eliminate nighttime breastfeeding so they can get more sleep. This advice is more and more common in postpartum depression treatment programs and books written for

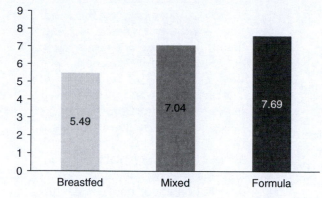

FIGURE 7.1 Hours baby sleeps at longest stretch. From Survey of Mothers' Sleep and Fatigue (N = 6,410)

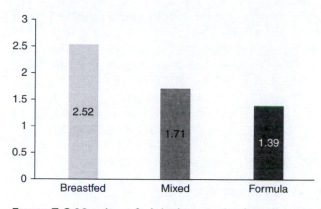

FIGURE 7.2 Number of nighttime awakenings for each feeding type. Survey of Mothers' Sleep and Fatigue (N = 6,410)

new mothers, but is this good advice? At first glance, it may seem to be. Because breast milk is lower in fat and protein than formula, we might assume that breastfeeding mothers sleep less than their formula-feeding counterparts, especially when you look at data like these from the Survey of Mothers' Sleep and Fatigue (Kendall-Tackett et al., 2011).

You see something similar when examining the number of nighttime awakenings. Babies wake more often when they are breastfed.

Looking at data like these, one could surmise that breastfeeding mothers get less sleep. However, recent research has revealed the opposite: that breastfeeding mothers actually get more sleep—particularly when the baby was in proximity to the mother.

Breastfeeding and maternal fatigue

The sleep patterns of 72 couples were compared from pregnancy to the first month postpartum via sleep diaries and wrist actigraphy (Gay, Lee, & Lee, 2004). Most of the mothers were at least partially breastfeeding (94 percent), and 80 percent were exclusively breastfeeding. Most of the babies slept in their parents' room, and 51 percent regularly slept in their parents' beds. Sleep and fatigue outcomes were not associated with

type of birth, parent–infant bedsharing, or baby's age. Mothers who were
exclusively breastfeeding had a greater
number of nighttime wakings compared
with mothers who were not breastfeeding exclusively, but slept approximately
20 minutes longer than mothers not
exclusively breastfeeding.

In a study of mothers and fathers at
3 months postpartum, data were collected via wrist actigraphy and sleep diaries (Doan, Gardiner, Gay, & Lee, 2007).
The study compared the sleep of exclusively breastfed infants vs. those supplemented with formula. In this sample,
67 percent were fed exclusively with breast

> A key question you can ask to find
> how a mother is doing is "How
> many minutes does it take for you to
> get to sleep?" If it takes her longer
> than 25 minutes, it could indicate
> that she is depressed. Asking about
> minutes to get to sleep (known as
> "sleep latency" in the sleep litera-
> ture) is a non-intrusive way to ask
> about a mother's mental well-being,
> and will give you a good deal of
> information about how she is actu-
> ally feeling.

milk, 23 percent were fed a combination of breast milk and formula, and 10 percent
were exclusively formula-fed. Mothers who exclusively breastfed slept an average of 40
minutes longer than mothers who supplemented. Parents of infants who were breastfed
during the night slept an average of 40–45 minutes more than parents of infants given
formula. Parents of formula-fed infants had more sleep disturbances. The researchers
concluded that parents who are supplementing with formula under the assumption that
they are going to get more sleep should be encouraged to breastfeed so they will get an
extra 30 minutes of sleep per night.

Dorheim and colleagues (2009) prospectively studied a group of 2,830 mothers at
7 weeks postpartum. They confirmed that poor sleep was a risk factor for depression.
When examining the risk factors for poor sleep, they identified "not exclusively breastfeeding" as one of the risk factors. In other words, if mothers supplement, they get less
sleep. The other factors associated with poor sleep included depression, previous sleep
problems, primiparity, and having a younger or male infant.

The key to understanding why breastfeeding makes a difference is understanding the
two variables that make a difference in terms of mothers' risk for depression: minutes to
get to sleep and total hours mothers report that they sleep. Three recent studies found
that new mothers' perception of their sleep was a better predictor of fatigue and depression than objective sleep measures. For example, women were significantly more likely
to report fatigue if they perceived that their sleep quality was poor, and their sleep time
was short, compared with women who were less fatigued in a sample of 109 postpartum
mothers (Rychnovsky & Hunter, 2009).

Another study included 45 new mothers from Melbourne, Australia who were at low
risk for postpartum depression (Bei, Milgrom, Ericksen, & Trinder, 2010). The researchers found that perceived sleep quality was more strongly related to postpartum depression
than actual sleep time. Similarly, Caldwell and Redeker ((2009) found that self-reported
sleep was a better predictor of psychological distress than sleep measured objectively in
115 inner-city women from New Haven, Connecticut. A recent study of 25 new mothers in North Carolina had similar results (Park, Meltzer-Brody, & Stickgold, 2013). In
this study, mothers completed self-report measures on sleep, and also measured sleep
via actigraph (a more objective measure). They found that self-report measures highly
predicted EPDS scores. Actigraph measures also predicted depression, but not as well

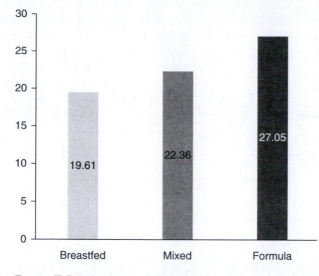

FIGURE 7.3 Minutes to fall asleep from the Survey of Mothers' Sleep and Fatigue ($N =$ 6,410)

as the mothers' self-report. The authors concluded that the subjective measures were by far the most accurate predictors of EPDS score. They also noted that disturbed sleep did contribute to postpartum depression.

In our study, the Survey of Mothers' Sleep and Fatigue, 6,410 mothers in 59 countries completed an online survey about sleep location and behaviors, and maternal well-being. Minutes to get to sleep and total sleep hours are the two best predictors of maternal mental health. Exclusively breastfeeding women do significantly better on both indicators. For example, in minutes to get to sleep, exclusively breastfeeding mothers are under 20 minutes, the time associated with better mental health. In contrast, 25 minutes or longer is associated with depression (Goyal et al., 2007; Huang et al., 2004).

On the second key variable—mothers' report of the number of hours they sleep— breastfeeding mothers also do well. They sleep significantly longer than their mixed- or formula-feeding counterparts (Kendall-Tackett et al., 2011). These findings run counter to the advice mothers are often given, which is to supplement so they can sleep more. Our findings, as well as those of Doan et al. and Dorheim et al., suggest that once a mother supplements, she actually gets less sleep, not more (Doan et al., 2007; Dorheim et al., 2009; Kendall-Tackett et al., 2011).

Doan and colleagues (2007) noted the following with regard to sleep and breastfeeding.

> Using supplementation as a coping strategy for minimizing sleep loss can actually be detrimental because of its impact on prolactin hormone production and secretion … Maintenance of breastfeeding as well as deep restorative sleep stages may be greatly compromised for new mothers who cope with infant feedings by supplementing in an effort to get more sleep time.
>
> (p. 201)

Sleep quality may also be better for mothers who exclusively breastfeed. Blyton et al.'s sleep study compared 12 exclusively breastfeeding women, 12 age-matched control

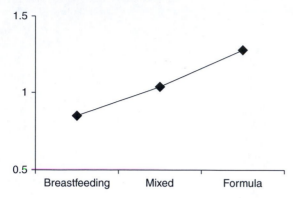

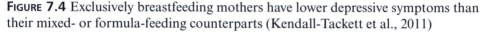

FIGURE 7.4 Exclusively breastfeeding mothers have lower depressive symptoms than their mixed- or formula-feeding counterparts (Kendall-Tackett et al., 2011)

women, and 7 women who were exclusively bottle-feeding (Blyton, Sullivan, & Edwards, 2002). They found that total sleep time and REM sleep time were similar in the three groups of women. The marked difference between the groups was in the amount of slow-wave sleep (SWS). The breastfeeding mothers got an average of 182 minutes of SWS. Women in the control group had an average of 86 minutes, and the exclusively bottle-feeding women had an average of 63 minutes. Among the breastfeeding women, there was a compensatory reduction in light, non-REM sleep.

Inflammation and sleep

Sleep disturbances and fatigue are also related to cytokine levels. Both chronic and acute sleep deprivation alter cellular and immune function (Berk et al., 2013; Kiecolt-Glaser et al., 2015). Interleukin-1β (IL-1β) was related to fatigue in postpartum women (Corwin, Bozoky, Pugh, & Johnston, 2003). Corwin et al. collected measures of fatigue, and urinary excretion of IL-1β over 4 weeks postpartum. The authors found that IL-1β is elevated during the postpartum period, and that this elevation has a significant, though delayed, relationship to postpartum fatigue.

In a study of women 4–6 weeks postpartum, Groër and colleagues (2005) found that mothers' fatigue levels correlated with their levels of stress and depression. They also found that fatigue, stress, and depression increased the risk of infection for both mother and baby. Interestingly, this same study also found that mothers who were stressed, depressed, and fatigued had lower levels of prolactin in both their serum and milk. These same mothers also had higher levels of melatonin in their milk, the hormone that regulates circadian rhythms (Groer, 2005).

In another study of 200 women at 4–6 weeks postpartum, Groër and Morgan (2007) found that depressed mothers reported more fatigue and daytime sleepiness than non-depressed mothers. The depressed mothers had abnormally low levels of cortisol, which may also cause their fatigue. The authors describe how chronic fatigue syndrome, various chronic pain syndromes, and PTSD are also associated with low cortisol levels. The depressed mothers also had more health problems since the baby was born, and had more health-related events, such as sprains, dental pain, and allergies. They had higher levels of perceived stress, anxiety, and more negative life events. The serum IL-6 levels were three times higher in the depressed mothers, but this was not a significant difference because of measurement variability.

A study of 479 women at 6 months and 1 year postpartum found that mothers averaged 6.7 hours of sleep a night (Taveras, Rifas-Shiman, Rich-Edwards, & Mantzoros, 2011b). They found that sleep duration ≤5 hours per night in the first year postpartum predicted elevated IL-6 at 3 years postpartum.

In a study of 634 pregnant women from Peru, a history of childhood abuse increased the risk of stress-related sleep quality, and doubled the odds of poor sleep quality in early pregnancy, compared to non-abused women (Gelaye et al., 2015). Women who experienced both physical and sexual abuse during childhood had 2.43 times more risk of poor sleep quality and stress-related sleep disturbance in early pregnancy. These effects were only partially explained by antenatal depression. The more abuse experiences a woman had, the worse her sleep.

Summary

Sleep disturbances and fatigue are physical stressors that increase the risk of depression. The relationship between sleep problems and proinflammatory cytokines appears to be bidirectional: sleep disturbances increase cytokines and cytokines increase sleep disturbance by delaying sleep onset, increasing daytime fatigue, and perpetuating the cycle of disturbed sleep and inflammation.

Possible interventions for fatigued new mothers

Breastfeeding mothers get more sleep and are less fatigued than mothers who supplement or wean. However, breastfeeding mothers can still be quite fatigued and may need some additional intervention to help prevent or treat depression.

Some approaches you might suggest

- Brainstorm with the mother on some strategies to help her cope with fatigue (e.g., encourage her to accept offers of help or access new sources of support).
- Treat depression.
- Use cognitive-behavioral sleep interventions.
- Use medications.
- If taking sleep medications, mothers should not bedshare with their infants.
- If mother has a trauma history, *The Post-Traumatic Insomnia Workbook* will likely be a helpful resource.

Rule out physical conditions

Severe fatigue may also be caused by an underlying physical condition. To rule out physical conditions, the following tests may be helpful.

- Blood work to rule out hypothyroidism, anemia, autoimmune disease, low-grade infection, or vitamin D deficiency.
- TSH, T3, T4, CBC, ESR (Sed rate), vitamin D.
- Possible sleep study to rule out sleep-breathing and sleep-movement disorders if other tests are negative and the mother's fatigue level has not improved.

If limiting feedings does become necessary, a stretch of 4–5 hours will meet mental health goals and be less disruptive of breastfeeding.

Reprinted with permission from Kendall-Tackett et al. (2011).

Breastfeeding, sleep location, and maternal well-being

From previous studies, we know that feeding method makes a difference in terms of how much a mother sleeps and her overall well-being. However, looking into this topic further, we recognize that where a baby sleeps is also important and could interact with feeding method. We also know that a high percentage of mothers around the world sleep with their babies at least part of the night. In the US sample from the Survey of Mothers' Sleep and Fatigue ($n = 4,789$), we found that nearly 60 percent of mothers sleep with their babies at least part of the night (Kendall-Tackett, Cong, & Hale, 2010). When these mothers were asked "Where does your baby usually sleep?" only about 40 percent indicated that their babies slept with them. However, when asked "Where does your baby end the night?" 60 percent revealed that their babies slept with them. So sleep location has the potential to play a large role in the relation between feeding method and mothers' sleep and well-being.

In a study of 33 mothers at 4 weeks postpartum, Quillin and Glenn (2004) found that mothers who were breastfeeding slept more than mothers who were bottle-feeding. Data were collected via questionnaire that recorded 5 days of mother and newborn sleep. When comparing whether bedsharing made a difference in total sleep, they found that bedsharing, breastfeeding mothers got the most sleep and breastfeeding mothers who were not bedsharing got the least amount of sleep. Mothers who were bottle-feeding got the same amount of sleep whether their babies were with them or in another room.

A recent study examined the impact of both feeding method and infant sleep location with data from the Survey of Mothers' Sleep and Fatigue ($N = 6,410$) (Kendall-Tackett, Cong, & Hale, 2016, in press-b). Mixed- and formula-feeding were combined after previous analyses revealed no significant difference between the two (Kendall-Tackett et al., 2011). The findings reveal the complex relationship between breastfeeding, sleep location, and maternal well-being. As found in previous studies, bedsharing helped sustain breastfeeding (Kendall-Tackett, Cong, & Hale, 2016, in press-a). The data revealed a main effect of feeding method (exclusive breastfeeding vs. not exclusively breastfeeding). In most cases, the exclusively breastfeeding mother has lower scores on the PHQ-2 than the non-EBF mother on most variables, especially if she is bedsharing. For example, the EBF-bedsharing mothers get more total sleep, and take less time to get to sleep than their non-EBF/non-bedsharing counterparts (Kendall-Tackett et al., 2016, in press-b).

The sleep variables are also reflected in the mothers' depressive symptoms. Overall, the EBF mothers have lower depressive symptoms regardless of sleep location, but the bedsharing-EBF mothers have the lowest rates of all.

Does taking the baby away help?

To help mothers who are very tired and/or depressed, a common suggestion is to have the baby sleep apart from the mother so she can get uninterrupted sleep. This is a suggestion that sounds reasonable, at least at first glance, but the research does not support it. To consider whether it would be helpful, we can examine studies where the babies are not with their mothers to see if it helps.

Sleep disturbances can occur in depressed mothers even when the baby is absent, or even before the baby is born. For example, we can examine the sleep of depressed mothers during pregnancy. The baby is not "there," yet the depression itself is what disturbs the sleep. In a study of 253 pregnant women, depressed women had more sleep disturbances

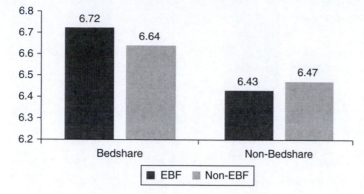

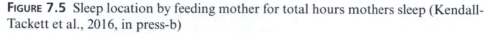

FIGURE 7.5 Sleep location by feeding mother for total hours mothers sleep (Kendall-Tackett et al., 2016, in press-b)

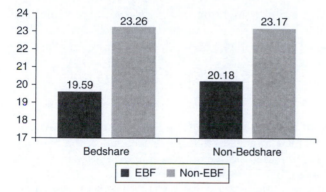

FIGURE 7.6 Sleep location by feeding method for minutes to fall asleep (Kendall-Tackett et al., 2016, in press-b)

and higher depression, anxiety, and anger scores during the second and third trimester than their pregnant, non-depressed counterparts (Field et al., 2007). The newborns of depressed mothers also had more sleep disturbance. They spent less time in deep sleep, and more time in disorganized sleep. The babies of depressed mothers also spent significantly time more fussing and crying.

In a review of the literature on PTSD and sleep, Spoormaker and Montgomery (2008) noted some specific abnormalities in the sleep of patients with PTSD. They have more stage 1 sleep, less SWS, and higher REM density. Sleep disturbances are a core feature of PTSD, and insomnia is common in people with PTSD, ranging from 40 percent to 50 percent. Conversely, disturbed sleep is a risk factor for developing PTSD. They also reported that sleep disturbances often do not respond to treatments for PTSD, and may persist even after the other symptoms have been alleviated. However, addressing sleep problems lessens PTSD symptoms. Their findings suggest that sleep disturbances may need to be addressed separately in women who have experienced PTSD in pregnancy and the postpartum period.

A study of mothers and fathers of infants in the NICU found that sleep was disturbed for both (Lee, Lee, Rankin, Weiss, & Alkon, 2007). Sleep disturbance was high for both

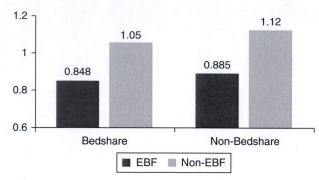

FIGURE 7.7 Sleep location by feeding method for maternal mental health (Kendall-Tackett et al., 2016, in press-b)

mothers and fathers: 93 percent of mothers and 60 percent of fathers reported disturbed sleep. Mothers had longer sleep latency, more nighttime wakings, and more subjective fatigue than fathers. Data were collected via wrist actigraphy and sleep diary. The total minutes of sleep were significantly lower for mothers than fathers, and mothers reported more morning and daytime fatigue.

Breastfeeding, sleep, and trauma

Mothers with a history of childhood abuse often feel as though they do not have the tools they need to successfully parent their own children. They may wonder whether they will perpetuate the cycle of violence. Impaired sleep can be an important trigger to the intergenerational transmission of abuse. Babies of mothers with depression or PTSD are more likely to have sleep difficulties, possibly because of mothers' elevated stress hormone levels that the babies were exposed to *in utero* (Field et al., 2007).

Intergenerational transmission of trauma is an ongoing concern. In one recent study, researchers included a group of 184 first-time mothers: 83 had a history of childhood abuse and PTSD (PTSD+); 38 had a history of childhood abuse and no PTSD (PTSD–); and 63 had no history of abuse nor any maternal pathology (control) (Hairston et al., 2011). The mothers who were PTSD+ had higher rates of both depression and infant sleep disturbance symptoms. There were two variables that predicted impaired mother–infant bonding: infant sleep difficulties and maternal depression, which predicted infant behavior problems at 18 months. The PTSD+ mothers also had more sleep impairment than the other two groups. The researchers noted that it was the maternal depression, not the mother's PTSD, that predicted the degree of mother–infant bonding impairment in the PTSD+ mothers. All of these lead to the intergenerational transmission of trauma.

Breastfeeding can have a positive effect on both maternal depression, and infant and mother sleep problems, thereby lowering the potential risk of a new mother maltreating her own children. In Strathearn, Mamun, Najman, & O'Callaghan's (2009) 15-year longitudinal study of 7,223 Australian mother–infant pairs, breastfeeding substantially lowered the risk of maternal-perpetrated child maltreatment. There were over 500 substantiated cases of maternal-perpetrated child maltreatment (abuse and neglect). Non-breastfeeding mothers were 2.6 times more likely to be physically abusive and 3.8 times more likely to neglect their children compared to mothers who breastfed for at least 4 months.

The results of our recent study may help explain why this is so. In our sample of 6,410 new mothers, 994 women reported previous sexual assault (Kendall-Tackett, Cong, & Hale, 2013). As predicted, sexual assault had a pervasive, negative effect on mothers' sleep, physical well-being, and mental health. The sexually assaulted mothers' sleep was poor overall, the mothers were more tired, they were more anxious and angry, and they had more depression. However, when we added feeding method to our analyses (feeding method × sexual assault status), we found that breastfeeding attenuated the effects of sexual assault and downregulated the stress response. There was no significant difference between mixed- and exclusively formula-feeding mothers on any of the variables in a previous study, so these two groups were combined (Kendall-Tackett et al., 2011). The rate of exclusive breastfeeding in our study was the same for sexually assaulted and non-assaulted women (78 percent for both groups). This is in line with an earlier US nationally representative sample of 1,220 mothers with children under the age of 3 (Prentice, Lu, Lange, & Halfon, 2002). In our study, exclusively breastfeeding mothers got more total sleep, took fewer minutes to get to sleep, and had more daily energy than sexually assaulted women who mixed- or formula-fed. They had less anxiety, depression, and anger. There was still an effect of the past sexual assault on the variables, but it was significantly lessened (Kendall-Tackett et al., 2013). See Figures 7.8–7.10. The effect on anger, in particular, was striking, and this might explain Strathearn and colleagues' (2009) findings about maternal-perpetrated child maltreatment cited earlier.

Although breastfeeding can be helpful in terms of lessening trauma symptoms, and lowering the risk of depression, depressed abuse survivors may be less likely to breastfeed than their non-abused counterparts, especially if they have violent partners. One large study found that women with a history of current or past abuse may breastfeed at lower rates (Sorbo, Lukasse, Brantsaeter, & Grimstad, 2015). This study included 53,934 mothers who had given birth between 1999 and 2006 in Norway. Women who experienced physical, sexual, and emotional abuse as adults were 40 percent more likely to stop breastfeeding than were non-abused women. These women also had much higher rates of postpartum depression (33 percent) than their non-abused counterparts (11 percent). Women who had experienced childhood abuse were also at high risk. The authors noted that women with a history for abuse were a high risk for early breastfeeding cessation. They only included this as a confounding variable, but found that it exerted an independent effect on breastfeeding cessation at 4 months. Childhood sexual abuse had the strongest effect.

A study from Hong Kong indicated that intimate partner violence (IPV) during pregnancy and early postpartum depression may influence breastfeeding initiation rates (Lau & Chan, 2007). This study included 1,200 Chinese mothers. Women who had no experience of IPV during pregnancy were significantly more likely to initiate breastfeeding than women who had experienced IPV, even after adjusting for demographic, SES, and obstetric variables. Early postpartum depression was not associated with breastfeeding initiation in a logistic regression model.

Mothers' experiences of breastfeeding after sexual abuse

The subjective experiences of abuse survivors who breastfeed vary quite a bit. For some, it can be quite healing. For others, it can be extremely difficult. Below are two accounts of women's experiences. In the first account, abuse survivor Beth Dubois (2003) describes how she was nervous about giving birth and breastfeeding her son. The theme of low

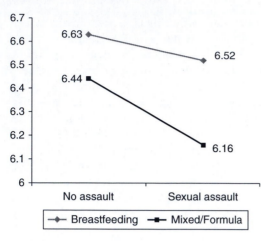

FIGURE 7.8 EBF attenuates the effects of sexual assault on hours mothers sleep (Kendall-Tackett et al., 2013)

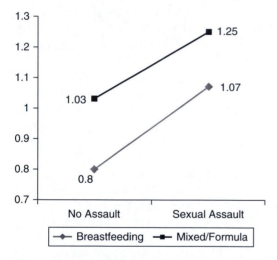

FIGURE 7.9 Sexually assaulted women had increased risk of depression, but EBF attenuated that effect

self-efficacy is evident, but she also describes how breastfeeding was healing and empowering for her.

> As the time of my son's birth approached, my worries about breastfeeding came into sharp focus. I knew the benefits of breastfeeding, and had plenty of book knowledge on the subject. I knew I wanted to breastfeed. I had been sexually abused when I was a child, however, and I was concerned. I worried that I would not be able to maintain the constant physical closeness breastfeeding would require and that breastfeeding might trigger memories of the abuse. I was especially distraught because I believed that I would be failing my child and myself if I were not able to breastfeed...

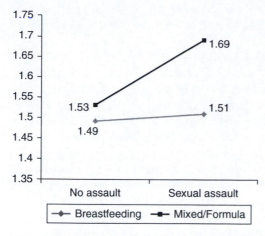

FIGURE 7.10 EBF had a dramatic effect on sexually assaulted women's anger and irritability

After describing her experiences of pregnancy, labor and delivery, she describes the positive impact breastfeeding has had on her.

> ... I now see that not only has breastfeeding been possible for me, a survivor of childhood sexual abuse, it has been immensely healing. My desire to have a fulfilling breastfeeding relationship forced me to face emotional territory I would probably have otherwise avoided. One wound left by the abuse is an underlying sense of "I can't do it. It's not even worth trying." Birthing and breastfeeding Theodore has helped to replace this with a very real sense of capability and confidence. Also, the heightened sensitivity to both myself and my son, which I gained through our breastfeeding relationship, serves us in other ways, especially now that Theodore is in the "terrific twos."
>
> (pp. 50–51)

Unfortunately, it would be negligent to only report positive findings regarding breastfeeding after abuse. Some abuse survivors struggle immensely to breastfeed, and may get to the point where they cannot continue. In a detailed case study, Beck (2009) presents the story of a woman with a history of childhood sexual abuse and rape as an adult. During Marilyn's birth, she dissociated and had a flashback to her abuse experience.

> A haze of hospital labor room, nakedness, vulnerability, pain. Silence, stretching, breathing, pain terror, and then I found myself 7 years old again, and sitting outside my parents' house in the car of a family acquaintance, being digitally raped ... my birth experience did not look traumatic at all—because the trauma physically took place 23 years before and only in my mind not the labor room.
>
> (Beck, 2009, pp. e4–e5)

After birth, her milk never came in, possibly due to the trauma of her birth or her pre-eclampsia. She felt that inability to breastfeed only compounded her sense of shame and inadequacy. What she remembered most about her postpartum experience was an incredible feeling of numbness. She felt that she could not connect with her baby, husband, life, or anything. She describes her breastfeeding experience as follows:

> Of course, I couldn't tell anyone what was really going on in my head when I tried to breastfeed. When I placed my baby to the breast, I experienced panic attacks, spaced out and dissociated. It triggered flashbacks of the abuse and a sick feeling in my stomach. I hated the physical feeling of breastfeeding. I hated having to offer my body to my child, who felt like a stranger. Whenever I put her to breast, I wanted to scream and vomit at the same time. My body recoiled at the thought of placing my baby to my breast. The thought of breastfeeding made my skin crawl. The very act of breastfeeding, which was sustaining my baby, was forcing me to relive the abuse. I resented her for needing to breastfeed … I did actually experience some relief when I expressed, rather than breastfeeding directly; however, my supply was so poor that for an hour's effort expressing, I'd only have about 10 mm of milk to give my daughter … At the moment I gave myself permission to give up on breastfeeding, things started to look up. I slowly started to feel a sense of connection with my baby, and with my life, and I even began to feel a bit like my old self again.
>
> (Beck, 2009, p. e6)

Breastfeeding can be strongly positive or strongly negative for individual abuse survivors. Even the mother in the above case illustration got to the point where she "kind of liked" breastfeeding with a second baby. Some mothers have shared with me that they never got to the point where they liked breastfeeding, but they got to the point where they could tolerate it, and that was an important goal for them. As care providers, it is important that we be open to the whole range of reactions that mothers may have and support them in their decisions to breastfeed, to pump and bottle-feed, or to simply bottle-feed.

Conclusions

Fatigue and sleep deprivation can be important signs, or even triggers for postpartum depression and psychosis. While most new mothers are tired, those who seem exceptionally tired and unable to cope may be depressed, or are at risk for depression. Sleeplessness not related to baby care can be a particularly ominous sign that requires close monitoring.

Clinical Implications

(1) Because depression is a major risk factor for breastfeeding cessation, lactation specialists should screen for it.
(2) Maternal stress and fatigue reduce prolactin levels, and may lead to breastfeeding cessation. High levels of cortisol can delay lactogenesis II.
(3) Breastfeeding difficulties, especially nipple pain, can lead to depression and need to be addressed promptly (see Chapter 6).

(4) Breastfeeding mothers actually get more sleep than their formula-feeding counter-parts. When mothers try supplementing with formula at night to get more sleep, they may encounter the opposite effect.

(5) Depressed mothers should be encouraged to continue breastfeeding because it protects infants from the harmful effects of maternal depression (see Chapter 7).

Regarding the role of healthcare providers caring for women who are breastfeeding and depressed, McCarter-Spaulding and Horowitz noted the following.

> Nurses caring for women who are at-risk, or struggling with PPD, also may feel that breastfeeding is perhaps an unnecessary burden that should be discontinued.
>
> Although nurses might expect that mothers with depression may not want to continue, or may not be able to maintain breastfeeding, such assumptions may not be accurate.
>
> (McCarter-Spaulding & Horowitz, 2007, p. 10)

Chapter 8   **Traumatic birth experiences**

The birth of a child, especially a first child, represents a landmark event in the lives of all involved. For the mother particularly, childbirth exerts a profound physical, mental, emotional, and social effect. No other event involves pain, emotional stress, vulnerability, possible physical injury or death, permanent role change, and includes responsibility for a dependent, helpless human being. Moreover, it generally all takes place within a single day. It is not surprising that women tend to remember their first birth experiences vividly and with deep emotion.

(Simkin, 1992, p. 64)

In Penny Simkin's landmark study (1991, 1992), she documented that women accurately remember details of their births 15–20 years later. Not surprisingly, birth experiences had a lasting impact on how women felt about themselves as women, and as mothers.

Incidence and prevalence of traumatic birth experiences

Many women around the world have difficult or negative birth experiences. The Childbirth Connections' Listening to Mothers' Survey II included a nationally representative sample of 1,573 mothers in the US. A stunning 9 percent met full criteria for birth-related posttraumatic stress disorder, and an additional 18 percent had posttraumatic symptoms (PTS) (Beck, Gable, Sakala, & Declercq, 2011). Nine percent might not sound too high, so it is helpful to have a comparison group: 7.5 percent of people in lower Manhattan met the full criteria for PTSD following September 11th (Galea et al., 2003). In other words, the percentage of women meeting full criteria for PTSD after birth in the US is now *higher* than it was following a major terrorist attack. Beck and colleagues (2011) noted the following:

In these two national surveys mothers did speak out loudly and clearly about posttraumatic stress symptoms they were suffering. The high percentage of mothers with elevated posttraumatic stress symptoms is a sobering statistic.

(p. 226)

Alcorn and colleagues, in their prospective study of 933 mothers in Brisbane, Australia, found a somewhat lower rate: 3.6 percent of women met full criteria for PTSD at 4–6 weeks, 6.3 percent at 12 weeks, and 5.8 percent at 24 weeks. While not everyone met criteria for PTSD, 45 percent of the mothers in this study described their births as traumatic (Alcorn, O'Donovan, Patrick, Creedy, & Devilly, 2010). That is reflected in their high rates of postpartum mood and anxiety disorders: the rates for depression ranged from 47 percent to 66 percent at 4–6 weeks; the rates for anxiety ranged from 58 percent to 74 percent.

Ayers, Harris, Sawyer, Parfitt, and Ford (2009) collected data from a community sample in the UK ($n = 502$) and online ($n = 921$). They found that 3 percent of the community sample met full criteria for PTSD and 21 percent of the online sample did. They found an interaction between sexual trauma and delivery type. Women with a history of sexual trauma were more susceptible to the negative effects of assisted delivery or cesareans.

In a study of 64 couples 9 weeks after giving birth, Ayers and colleagues (2007) found that 5 percent of men and women had severe symptoms of PTSD (avoidance and intrusion). The couples who experienced PTSD symptoms had complications, but both groups had normal vaginal deliveries. The symptoms were strongly associated within couples, and the PTSD symptoms affected neither the parent-infant bond nor the couple's relationship. The authors concluded that men and women have comparable levels of PTSD after birth, and short-term that PTSD symptoms had little impact on the couple's relationship and parent–infant bonding. The long-term effects are unknown.

A study of 229 mothers from Flanders, Belgium found that prevalence of PTSD symptoms ranged from 22 percent to 24 percent in the first week, and 13 percent to 20 percent at 6 weeks postpartum (De Schepper et al., 2016). Risk factors included Islamic belief, a traumatic birth, low income, psychiatric history, and birth complications. PTS symptoms dropped off quickly after 6 weeks. Women's sense of being in control during their labors protected them from birth-related PTSD.

When considering birth, we might argue that some negative effects are unavoidable. Birth is hard. It can be life-threatening. So there will always be some women who develop PTSD. One way to counter this argument is to examine the rates of birth trauma in countries where birth is treated as a normal event, where there are fewer interventions, and where women have continuous labor support. Sweden is one such country, and it has a much lower rate of PTSD. In a prospective study of 1,224 Swedish mothers, 1.3 percent had PTSD, and 9 percent described their births as traumatic (Soderquist, Wijma, Thorbert, & Wijma, 2009).

Rates are similarly low in the Netherlands. In a study of 907 women, 1.2 percent had PTSD and 9 percent identified their births as traumatic (Stramrood et al., 2011). The rates in both Sweden and the Netherlands are considerable lower than they are in the US. These rates may be lower because rates of birth interventions are lower. For example, in the Netherlands: 15–17 percent of women have cesareans, and 9–10 percent have instrumental deliveries.

Conversely, countries where the status of women is generally poor may have higher percentages of women reporting traumatic birth. Indeed, researchers have found precisely that. In a study of 400 women in Iran, 218 reported traumatic births at 6–8 weeks postpartum, and 20 percent met full criteria for PTSD (Modarres, Afrasiabi, Rahnama, & Montazeri, 2012).

Zaers et al.'s (2008) study of 47 women in Switzerland found that PTSD rates can increase over the first year. In this study, the rates of depression were stable from 6 weeks (22 percent) to 6 months (21.3 percent) postpartum. Rates of clinically significant PTSD increased during this same time from 6 percent at 6 weeks postpartum to 15 percent at 6 months.

Diagnostic criteria for PTSD

Posttraumatic stress disorder (PTSD) is diagnosed when someone meets the criteria established by the *Diagnostic and Statistical Manual-5* (American Psychiatric Association, 2013). Most people exposed to traumatic events are not diagnosed with PTSD. Some have no symptoms and are considered "resilient." Others develop depression or anxiety disorders, which can still cause difficulties, but they do not develop PTSD. Finally, others go on to develop PTSD. It is helpful to recognize symptoms of trauma and its possible sequelae so you can provide information and resources to mothers. The following is a brief description of the diagnostic criteria for PTSD and a listing of possible symptoms.

Exposure to traumatic events

The first criterion that someone must meet before they are diagnosed with PTSD is exposure to a traumatic event. A traumatic event is defined by death or threatened death, actual or threatened injury, or actual or threatened sexual violation (Friedman et al., 2011). Unfortunately, birth can include all three. During labor, women might believe that they, or their babies, might die. This can happen whether or not it is "medically true." If women believe they are in peril, there are likely to be sequelae. People can be exposed to traumatic events by directly experiencing them, by witnessing them (and this would include the experiences of partners, labor and delivery nurses, doulas, and others in attendance), or by hearing about the traumatic experiences of a close friend or relative (Friedman et al., 2011).

Lauren, a breastfeeding peer supporter in London, describes how she believed her baby had died and how that belief impacted her. Her father had passed away only two weeks before her baby was born. Lauren's mother was also present at the birth and thought she had witnessed the death of her first grandchild only two weeks after losing her husband.

> I was 28 when I had William. My father was very ill throughout my pregnancy, and died two weeks before my baby was born. William was named after him and was his first grandchild. The funeral was on my due date. Fortunately, William was born two weeks late.
>
> My labor with William was very slow, and after 48 sleepless hours of slow back labor, the hospital reluctantly admitted me even though I was only 3 cm. My husband and mother were both with me. I was told that my waters would be broken to speed things up. William's heart rate was slowing with contractions, so he was monitored and I was asked to lie a particular way as pressure was causing him distress. I was given an epidural, managed to get a few hours sleep, and then woke to the news I was nearing the magic 10 cm. I don't know how long I pushed for, but it must have been a long time as there was eventually discussion of taking me for a forceps delivery. But William started to make his way just before that. He delivered back to back in front of a room full of people as the alarm bell had been set off for a third time. William took in a deep breath of meconium as his head turned, and my first view of him was of a blue, motionless baby descending onto my chest from a great height, being vigorously ruffled on me and taken

away again. I thought, "that baby is dead." That image is still what I think of when I recall his birth.

Attempts were made to get him breathing again as I was stitched up, as I'd torn quite badly. The room was silent. Jonathan held my hand and my poor mother sat in the corner of the room, watching. Then the man stitching me up said, "he's pinking up. I can see him pinking up." Then they took William away for an hour or two, and apparently he started breathing on his own on the way to the SCBU. When he came back to me, they had put a purple hat on him. He was wide eyed, but hardly interested in breastfeeding. I thought he was brain damaged, and I still expected him to die.

We stayed in the hospital for 4 days. He did not latch on for the first 48 hours, and he was cup-fed. I remember ringing for help in the middle of the night and saying, "he won't go on." The night attendant told me, "well, you have to feed him, or we have to give him formula." She took him, poured the expressed colostrum into his mouth, and handed him back. "There you go," she said, as if this was a problem solved. On the morning after my third sleepless night on the shared ward, I broke down. They moved me to a private room, where I was finally given help latching him on. Both William and I were traumatized.

I don't know when I stopped expecting him to die. He was such a miserable newborn, and I remember thinking that he didn't seem to want to be alive, just as my father felt in the last weeks of his illness. He was uncomfortable to be around. At no point during my pregnancy, birth, or postnatal period was I offered any sort of psychological support.

When William was 6 months old, I regained enough self-awareness to know that I needed help, and took bereavement counseling at my local surgery. Having someone say, "what you went through was AWFUL" gave me permission to grieve, and allowed me to feel sorry for myself retrospectively. I look back on that time and can't believe we, William and I, got through it. But you do, don't you? I breastfed for almost a year.

This may not be the type of story you're looking for, but in any case, it rather helps me to retell it now and again. William is now a wonderfully kind and sensitive 6-year-old boy, and a great big brother to his 4-year-old sister and 1-year-old baby brother. (All back-to-back vaginal deliveries, but numbers 2 and 3 were a walk in the park!!)

Amanda, a hospital-based lactation consultant, was sexually assaulted during her second birth. She experienced symptoms for several years after it occurred, as she describes.

To my great disappointment, the birth of my first-born ended in a cesarean section. The long separation afterward took a long time to heal from. When I became pregnant with my second child, I did a lot of research and decided to plan a homebirth. Unfortunately, due to some complications with the baby's heart tones, we transferred to the hospital. When I arrived, the obstetrician on call came into the room while I was having a contraction during transition. He began yelling at me that he knew that I was only there to sue him. He told me that he was going to insert the internal monitor, or he would call the attorney and make me. I was trying to tell him "Wait, No!", but he refused. He pulled my legs open and inserted the monitor. I felt extremely violated. I began having a panic attack during labor. He didn't care what I wanted; he would do what he wanted to do because he had the power.

The theme of sexual assault is remarkably common in mothers' accounts of their labors. In Beck's (2011) meta-ethnography of six qualitative studies on birth trauma, she noted that the three most common themes were being "stripped of protective layers, invisible wounds, and insidious repercussions." Being stripped of their protective layers made them feel exposed and vulnerable. Many reported feeling like rape victims.

Symptoms of PTSD

In addition to being exposed to a traumatic event, people need to also have symptoms in four clusters to meet full criteria. Even if someone does not meet full criteria, she may still experience some of these symptoms, which can negatively affect her transition to motherhood.

Intrusion symptoms

Intrusion symptoms include recurrent involuntary and intrusive memories of her birth. These can also be experienced as flashbacks or nightmares, or just a running loop of thoughts about their births that they cannot stop (Friedman et al., 2011; National Center for PTSD, 2014a). A common statement could be something like, "every time I close my eyes, I am re-experiencing my birth." There could also be intense or prolonged psychological distress and/or marked physiological reactions when something reminds them of their births. Amanda experienced intrusion symptoms for several years after the sexual assault (described above) that she experienced during her birth.

> For years after the assault, I had trouble being intimate with my husband. When we tried, I would feel trapped and panicked. I couldn't go to a doctor for a long time. I hyperventilated and nearly passed out at my first postpartum check-up. Every time I thought about the birth, my hands would shake, my breathing would get ragged and I would end up in a panic state. Yet, I was in denial. I told myself that I was overreacting. Yes, he was unkind, but I couldn't bring myself to call it anything more sinister. Finally, when referring to my birth experience, a friend called it a sexual assault. Then things began to click for me. I finally began to see a therapist, who diagnosed me with PTSD. She taught me some coping mechanisms to enable me to begin to heal. I will never be fully healed from the sexual assault, but now I call myself a survivor. I still have to face the gut-wrenching panic attacks, especially near the anniversary of the assault. The worst part is, my child's birthday isn't the day of complete joy that it should be. It is also the day I was sexually assaulted.

Avoidance symptoms

After a traumatic birth, mothers may avoid things that remind them of it, such as activities, places, or people associated with their births. This can even include disengaging from their babies.

Avoidance symptoms are also common following a traumatic birth. Women may avoid everything that reminds them of their traumatic births, including not returning for medical appointments, or avoiding their doctors, medical offices, and the hospital where their births occurred. These effects can become chronic. Beck (2015) synthesized the results of 14 studies and described the middle-range theory of the long-term consequences of birth trauma. Mothers in these studies described numbing symptoms as just going through the motions of caregiving, and being a shadow of their former selves. Because their infants were constant reminders of what they went through, some found themselves distancing themselves from their babies. Symptoms can also flair again during the anniversary of the trauma.

Negative changes in cognitions and mood

Trauma may also bring about negative changes in mood and cognitions. Women must have three or more of the following symptoms to meet full criteria.

- An inability to remember an important aspect of the traumatic event.
- A persistent or exaggerated negative expectations about themselves, others, or the world.
- A persistent distorted blame of self or others about the cause or consequences of the traumatic event. These negative beliefs can include a pervasive negative emotional state, such as fear, horror, anger, guilt, or shame.
- A markedly diminished interest and participation in significant activities.
- A feeling of detachment or estrangement from others.
- A persistent inability to experience positive emotions
                        (Friedman et al., 2011; National Center for PTSD, 2014a).

After Amanda's birth (described above), she reported not remembering the doctor's name or face after her birth.

> To this day, 6-plus years later, I do not remember the name of this doctor. I don't remember his face. Every once in a while, I will look him up online to remind myself (and then can't sleep for a couple of days after), but I quickly forget again. I have been told that this is a mild form of dissociative amnesia. I am guessing that his image and name disturbs me so greatly, that my mind blocks it for protection. However, I am terrified that I will run into him unawares, now that I work in that hospital system as an IBCLC. This is why I keep looking him up.

Negative changes in mood and cognition overlap considerably with depression, and can directly impact how a woman feels about her baby and partner. Jessica describes her self-blame for having a cesarean.

> I feel like it was probably my own fault that that happened—that, basically, I didn't do the things I needed to do in order to give birth—and that because it is my own fault, it's wrong for me to feel bad about it and I should just suck it up, and not feel sad that I failed, or that there is a very real possibility that I will never get to give birth in the future either, and will just end up with another C-section.

Ayers et al. (2006) found that women who had traumatic births described rejecting behavior towards their babies immediately after birth. Many reported eventually bonding with their babies *in one to five years*, with avoidant or over-anxious attachment styles being the most common. This is a particularly concerning symptom and one that professionals can gently help mothers address.

Changes in arousal and reactivity

This symptom cluster is perhaps one of the most characteristic of PTSD, and these symptoms must have begun or worsened after their births. Women must have three or more of the following symptoms.

- An increase in anger, irritability, or aggressive behavior.
- Reckless or destructive behavior.
- Hypervigilance.
- Exaggerated startle response.
- Problems with concentration.
- Sleep problems, specifically difficulty falling or staying asleep, or restless sleep.

Jessica experienced a highly traumatic birth, where she almost died. She describes how it impacted her physical and mental well-being. She felt abandoned by her husband, even though she recognized that he had no choice about returning to work. She also received no help from her family of origin. Her hyperarousal symptoms compounded the normal challenges of new motherhood, and her significant health problems were also exacerbated.

Even before we left the hospital, I was having severe anxiety and depression. I was beyond what the word "exhausted" implies … Add to that no sleep, baby's needs, and breastfeeding, and I was barely hanging on. I either didn't know or didn't understand that my husband had to go back to work two days after we got home from the hospital. It was not a case of him not wanting to be with us. He had to go back to work or they would have fired him. They couldn't have cared less that his wife just had a baby, and that he watched his wife and baby almost die. We needed the money and he had to go. Not only did he have to work, he had to work extremely long, stressful hours.

I was terrified to be away from him. I was already experiencing posttraumatic stress episodes. The anxiety was worse than it had ever been in my life. I don't know what I was afraid of, but I was scared and lonely all the time. I would panic several times an hour. My body became more depleted by the day. The headaches I had every day only got worse after delivery, and the fibromyalgia I had dealt with all my life was in a full flare. I was a wreck. I was diagnosed with hypothyroidism and rheumatoid arthritis.

My family was nowhere to be found. They didn't want to think about how scary things were. They wanted to pretend that everything was fine. I was on my own all day with a newborn. I would beg my husband not to go. He had to go. He felt guilty, and was scared, and confessed much later that he had been terrified I was going to die from the day I told him I was pregnant. He has always been a realist. That fear explained why he had been a checked-out jerk for most of my pregnancy. I realize now that it was ripping his heart out to see me so depressed and sick, and to have to leave anyway, but he left to keep a roof over our heads. He went to a job where he was treated like crap, and came home to a wife who hated him. We were both miserable.

I got around the house on my hands and knees, dragging my baby behind me on a blanket, because I didn't have the strength, and was in too much pain, to walk. I was depressed, hurting, and afraid. When my husband got home, I would hand him the baby without saying anything, and I would go lay down and cry. My husband was completely confused. I wanted a baby. I had a baby. Why was I mad at him? And why was I so sad? We weren't talking at all. He was hurt because I didn't understand that he was trying to take care of us financially, and I was hurt because he wasn't at home to take care of me physically.

Risk factors

Which factors increase women's risk of having a traumatic birth experience? Slade (2006) proposed a model that included predisposing (pre-pregnancy/pregnancy), precipitating (perinatal), and maintaining (postpartum) factors. These can be internal (within the individual mother), external (from the environment), and an interaction between both internal and external. Below are some of the factors that have been studied most often.

Predisposing factors
Prenatal depression, anxiety, or PTSD

A study from Finland (Saisto, Salmela-Aro, Nurmi, & Halmesmaki, 2001) found that women who had been depressed during their pregnancies were significantly more likely to be disappointed with their deliveries and develop postpartum depression. Similarly, a study from Switzerland (Zaers et al., 2008) found that anxiety and psychiatric symptoms in late pregnancy were predisposing factors to both depression and PTSD postpartum. Trait anxiety also predicted childbirth-related PTSD in a study of 372 couples from the UK at 6 weeks and 3 months postpartum (Iles, Slade, & Spiby, 2011). Pain in labor and emergency cesareans were the strongest predictors of disappointment with delivery.

A prospective study of 298 women attempting vaginal births found that prenatal stress was associated with cesarean delivery (Saunders, Lobel, Veloso, & Meyer, 2006). Highly stressed women were more likely to receive analgesia, which increased the risk of surgical delivery. Women who received both meperidine and an epidural had the highest rates of cesarean delivery. One possible explanation has to do with the role of stress in prolonging pain, lowering pain tolerance, and exacerbating physical reactions to acute pain. Data analysis controlled for previous cesarean, diabetes, primiparity, advanced maternal age, BMI >40, medical induction, preeclampsia, and meconium staining—all potential confounds.

In contrast, a Dutch study of 354 healthy nulliparous pregnant women found no psychosocial risk factors predicted instrumental deliveries or cesarean births (van de Pol et al., 2006). Specifically, they found that social support during pregnancy, lack of depressive symptoms and specific pregnancy traits did not protect against instrumental and cesarean delivery. In contrast, characteristics of the labor itself were: higher fetal weight, non-occiput anterior presentation, advanced gestational age, and fetal distress. They found no independent contributions of personality characteristics or depression on mode of delivery. Oddly, they found that having a better relationship with their partners was predictive of higher rates of instrumental and cesarean deliveries, but had no explanation for this finding.

Sexual abuse/prior trauma

A study from Montreal of 308 women found that birth PTSD was more likely if women had anxiety in pregnancy and a history of sexual trauma (Verreault et al., 2012). The women were assessed at 25–40 weeks gestation, 4–6 weeks, and 3 and 6 months postpartum. Of these women, 6 percent met full criteria for PTSD, and 12 percent met partial criteria. PTSD was three times more common in women with a history of sexual assault.

A study of 933 women in Australia examined a number of factors that could predict birth-related PTSD (O'Donovan et al., 2014). Forty-six percent reported that their births were traumatic, and 8 percent of these women developed PTSD between 4 and 6 weeks postpartum. The researchers found 16 pre-birth and birth-related predictor variables significantly distinguished women who thought birth was traumatic compared with those who did not, and 11 distinguished between those who developed PTSD and those who did not. They found that prior trauma was the "single most important predictive factor of PTSD" (p. 935).

Trauma history was also an important factor in high-risk pregnancy in a study of 1,071 Jewish women from Israel (Lev-Wiesel, Chen, Daphna-Tekoah, & Hod, 2009). The researchers found that a higher percentage of women with high-risk pregnancies had a history of trauma. Further, a history of trauma, prenatal PTS, and subjective pain during delivery were related to PTS postpartum. Consistent with previous studies, prenatal depression was related to birth complications.

A prospective study of 138 women in the UK found that support and control during labor did not decrease posttraumatic symptoms for the sample as a whole (Ford & Ayers, 2012). Overall, they found that control beliefs, level of intervention during birth, and depression in pregnancy were risk factors for acute PTS, and that depression in pregnancy predicts chronic PTS. Support and control during labor did lower risk for PTS for the subset of women who had a history of prior trauma at both 3 weeks and 3 months after birth, accounting for 16 percent of the variance. Low support from practitioners predicted postpartum posttraumatic stress in women with a history of trauma who had more intervention during birth. The authors concluded that one-on-one care during labor and birth maximized positive outcomes for postpartum women.

History of childhood abuse was also one of the predisposing factors identified for dissociation during birth in a sample of 564 primiparous women (Choi & Seng, 2016). Dissociation allows someone to escape from a situation when normal fight or flight is not possible. Dissociation can happen to anyone during an overwhelming stressful event when usual coping mechanisms do not work. Dissociation in labor is when women feel detached from their bodies or minds in response to a birth-related traumatic stressor. The other predisposing factor was a history of pre-existing psychopathology. The precipitating factors included perception of care and negative appraisal of labor. The prevalence of dissociation in labor was 7 percent.

Perinatal factors
Objective factors

Cesarean vs. vaginal

A study from Israel of 1,844 low-risk women found that 21 percent reported high levels of depressive symptoms on day 2 postpartum (Weisman et al., 2010). The researchers found that type of delivery influenced symptoms. The rate of depressive symptoms was

23 percent for cesareans, 21 percent for assisted vaginal, and 19 percent for unassisted vaginal. In addition, 13 percent reported high levels of trait anxiety.

Researchers from Iran compared 50 women who had unassisted vaginal deliveries and 50 who had cesareans (Torkan, Parsay, Lamyian, Kazemnejad, & Montazeri, 2009). The researchers found that quality of life for both groups improved between Time 1 (6–8 weeks postpartum) and Time 2 (12–14 weeks postpartum). Women who had vaginal deliveries had a better mental-health functioning at the first assessment, and physical functioning at Time 2. There was no significant difference on most of the other measures. They excluded women with histories of depression, who had instrumental deliveries, a low birthweight baby, major life stressors, or medical conditions (including chronic constipation, low back pain, or urination problems).

A study of 5,332 women from the UK found that women who had forceps-assisted births or unplanned cesareans, had a number of significant sequelae at 3 months postpartum (Rowlands & Redshaw, 2012). These women had the poorest health and well-being, and were more likely to report PTS later in the postpartum period. The women who had forceps deliveries were more likely to report ongoing physical problems than were women who had cesareans. In contrast, the women who had unassisted vaginal deliveries, or planned cesareans, had fewer negative sequelae following the birth.

Mauri describes her experience with both forceps and a cesarean, and how her traumatic birth influenced her emotional state and her ability to bond with her baby. She was post-dates and threatened with an induction. She went into labor on her own.

> I went into labor naturally on Sunday. I had horrific back labor and begged for the epidural I swore I wouldn't get. The night midwife broke my water in a misunderstanding about a fetal heart rate monitor that I did not want screwed into my child's head, and a series of pelvic checks took place overnight and into the morning. The morning midwife ended up being the one who had called us back at 11 p.m. the Thursday before, so she wasn't especially compassionate to my situation. After more pelvic exams than I had wanted, an OB in training came in and told me she would be doing another. I told her I didn't want another, and she basically told me she was doing one anyway. After Pitocin, and an internal contraction monitor, and oxygen, and a failure of antiquated external monitors, which the staff all swore indicated my baby's heart rate fluctuating (though moving the monitors always showed her to have moved), and another more passionate attempt to use an internal fetal heart rate monitor, I got to 10 cm and was able to push. I pushed for an hour and half and the baby was stuck. They brought in forceps, one of my truly dreaded interventions. It felt like they were going to split my pelvis in half, and I had an effective epidural. They failed, and I spiked a fever, no doubt influenced by the number of hands inside of me over the course of this ordeal. As I was sobbing on the way to the OR and begging for horizontal cuts, the OB told me not to worry, she would give me a cute bikini cut. I was wanting horizontal incisions for a chance at ever having a VBAC. I woke up high as a kite on morphine, itchy, and desperate for orange juice. I didn't care at all about the baby my husband held, and I struggled to bond with her for months. She just didn't feel like she could be mine after all of that.
>
> At her 48-hour visit, I filled out the postpartum depression survey honestly. I felt like I was drowning. The pediatrician looked at my file, noted the C-section, and told my husband, not me, that she thought I was fine, just shaken up by the

experience. I was invalidated and undermined by every person who was sup-posed to help me because, "the baby is healthy." I haven't been diagnosed with post-traumatic stress, but now that I'm pregnant for the second time, I'm scared to death of dealing with labor and delivery professionals.

One study compared 40 women with four types of births: spontaneous vaginal, induced vaginal, instrumental vaginal, and emergency cesarean (Maclean, McDermott, & May, 2000). Women who had had an instrumental delivery with episiotomy rated their birth as more distressing, and were less satisfied with the efficacy of pain relief during labor, than were women in the other three groups. In contrast, women with emergency cesareans reported little distress, lower perceived risk of injury, and significantly greater satisfac-tion with pain relief. There was no significant difference between the groups on depressive symptoms.

Cesarean delivery impacted women's responsiveness to their babies in another study (Swain et al., 2008). This study used functional magnetic resonance imaging to view mothers' responses to the crying of their own babies. Mothers needed to differentiate between the cries of their babies' and the cries of others. They compared six moth-ers who had cesareans to six mothers who had had vaginal deliveries. They found that women who had vaginal deliveries were more responsive in the relevant areas of their brains (e.g., hypothalamus, frontal cortex, and basal ganglia) at 2–4 weeks postpartum than mothers who had cesareans. They also found that independent of mode of delivery, parental worries and mood were related to specific brain activations in response to their own babies' cries.

Another study randomized mothers who were expecting twins into planned vaginal vs. planned cesarean conditions (Hutton et al., 2016). The study included 2,804 women from 25 different countries. Using the EPDS ≥12, they found a rate of depression of 14 percent for both groups. Breastfeeding rates were high in both groups, and the women had similar scores on all other measures of well-being and quality of life. There was no increase in depression for mothers who had planned cesareans.

Kuo and colleagues (2014) studied specific trajectories of 139 women who had elective cesareans in Taiwan. The overall rate of depression and anxiety among these mothers was quite high: 27 percent with an EPDS ≥12, and 36 percent with high STAI scores. However, that is not the whole picture. The researchers demonstrated that there were four distinct subgroups of women, ranging from low to high, and that these groupings were stable over the first year postpartum. Further, depression and anxiety were highly correlated, with anxiety being more common than depression. Surprisingly, women with higher BMIs before pregnancy, and poor sleep in the third trimester, were more likely to have symptoms of both depression and anxiety throughout the postpartum year.

Birth practitioner

A study of 281 women at 1 month postpartum in Japan compared women's perceptions of their births when attended by midwives vs. obstetricians (Iido, Horiuchi, & Nagamori, 2014). Overall, the women in the study rated both types of care highly, but women who had midwives rated them significantly higher, and were more satisfied with their care, than women who had OBs. Women in the OB group had higher rates of induction, aug-mentation, amniotomy, and episiotomy than women in the midwife group. Women in the midwifery group also appreciated longer prenatal appointments and more individualized care. Significantly more women were breastfeeding in the midwifery group. There was no significant difference on EPDS scores, but women in the midwifery group had lower rates of maternity blues. There were no adverse outcomes for women in the midwives' group.

Epidural anesthesia

In our cross-sectional study of 6,410 mothers from 59 countries, women who had epidurals had higher levels of depressive symptoms on the PHQ-2 (Kendall-Tackett et al., 2015). In bivariate analyses, women who had the most common birth interventions, such as epidurals, other pain medication, or induction, had significantly higher depressive symptoms. In multivariate analysis, controlling for income, education, parity, all the birth interventions, history of sexual assault, and history of depression, only three interventions were still significantly related to PHQ-2 scores: postpartum hemorrhage, postpartum surgery, and epidurals.

In contrast, a study from China found that epidurals were actually related to *lower* levels of depression (Ding, Wang, Chen, & Zhu, 2014). Ding et al.'s study included 214 pregnant women who were planning vaginal births. Fifteen percent of mothers in the epidural group had depressive symptoms compared with 37 mothers (35 percent) in the non-epidural group. Depression was measured via EPDS >9. They also found that attending childbirth classes and breastfeeding were also associated with decreased depression.

A study of 351 women from Taiwan found that delivery type significantly impacted maternal mental health (Chang et al., 2015). Women who had cesareans had higher depressive symptoms at 3 months postpartum, and higher levels of pain at all time points up to 6 months, compared with women who had vaginal deliveries. At 4–6 weeks, the prevalence of depression was 49 percent for the whole sample, and 56 percent for the women who had cesareans. By 12 months, the percentage of women who were depressed dropped to 33 percent.

A study of 319 women from New Zealand who identified themselves as having experienced birth trauma found that 62 percent indicated that they had unexpected outcomes, such as emergency cesareans, and that these outcomes were related to their birth trauma (Sargent, 2015). They also identified other risk factors, including fearing for their own or their babies' lives (53 percent), poor care from the midwife or doctor (47 percent), poor pain management or other physical trauma (42 percent), and baby in the NICU (27 percent). Interestingly, only 4 percent of women identified past abuse as related to their birth trauma. Of the women who experienced poor maternity care, 45 percent developed a mistrust of midwives, doctors, and/or the maternity care system.

A study of 876 women in Nigeria at 6 weeks postpartum found that the rate of PTSD was 6 percent (Adewuya, Ologun, & Ibigbami, 2006). Birth type strongly increased women's risk of PTSD. Women at the highest risk were those who had been admitted to the hospital due to pregnancy complications. Women who had either instrumental deliveries or emergency cesareans were almost 8 times more likely to develop PTSD. Manual removal of the placenta increased risk almost five-fold. The authors noted that maternity care is poor in Africa, as reflected by the high rates of maternal mortality and morbidity. Yet, their rate of PTSD is comparable (or lower) than is typical in US studies. Interestingly, only 15 percent of mothers in this sample delivered in the hospital. Others delivered at home, primary health centers, or with traditional birth attendants. Twenty-three percent had no antenatal care.

In a study of 60 women who had cesarean births, 37 percent described their experiences as entirely positive (Karlstrom, Engstrom-Olofsson, Norbergh, Sjoling, & Hidlingsson,

2007). In contrast, 63 percent reported having a mixed or entirely negative experience. Women who had emergency cesareans were twice as likely to describe their experiences as negative than women who had planned cesareans.

A study examined the objective characteristics of births to determine whether they were related to postpartum depression, maternal functional status, and infant care at 2 weeks postpartum (Hunker, Patrick, Albrecht, & Wisner, 2009). Data were collected from OB charts and collected via the Peripartum Events Scale (PES). The categories included precipitous labor, traumatic or life-threatening events, cesarean section due to a medical emergency, midforceps or vaginal breech delivery, significant lacerations, abnormal fetal heart rate, and several other variables related to length of labor or abnormal fetal-monitoring results. In this study, 46 percent were identified as having an adverse unplanned event at their births. Depression rates were also high: 26 percent were depressed during pregnancy and 21 percent were depressed at 2 weeks postpartum. The findings of this study indicated that women with adverse, unplanned events during labor or delivery had varying outcomes regarding depression, functional status, and infant care at 2 weeks postpartum. The authors concluded that adverse birth events were not related to postpartum depression, even after controlling for depression during pregnancy, antidepressant use at delivery, education, age, and parity.

Subjective factors

Sense of control

In a sample of 876 women from Nigeria, mothers' lack of control during labor increased their risk of PTSD by almost five times (Adewuya et al., 2006). Ford and Ayers (2009) found that staff providing supportive care influenced mothers' anxiety, mood, and perceived control during labor. Supportive care had a greater effect than stressful events during birth, and increased mothers' sense of control.

Beck's (2015) synthesis of 14 studies found that women's "terrifying loss of control" was a key issue for women who experienced traumatic births. Women reported feeling powerless and helpless, that their bodies had been seized and controlled by the labor and delivery staff, and no longer belonged to them. Staff often did not communicate with them, which increased their sense of vulnerability and powerlessness. They felt that they could survive only through obedience.

Women in Elmir et al.'s (2010) meta-ethnography of ten qualitative studies also felt out of control, powerless, vulnerable, and unable to make informed decisions about the care they received. They felt betrayed by their providers. Some agreed to procedures, such as epidurals and vacuum extractions, to make the trauma stop.

In a sample of 319 women who experienced birth trauma in New Zealand, mothers reported being bullied and coerced (Sargent, 2015). One mother reported that she was "physically forced to do things against my wishes." Another mother said, "I was bullied into an elective C-section" (p. 7), and that her partner was extremely unsupportive as well. Other mothers described that their voices "fell on deaf ears," that their needs and wants were not listened to, and that much of the conversation with healthcare providers was downright disrespectful. One mother described how her midwife came and forced her to get out of bed after the birth. She screamed and told the midwife that she was in too much pain. The midwife looked disgusted and left. It turns out that the mother had fractured her pelvis during the birth. It took over a year to heal.

Perception of caregiving

> Respectful care is an essential component of safe care.
>
> (Prochaska, 2015, p. 1015)

The actions of care providers during labor speak volumes, and have a tremendous impact on whether women will feel positively about their births, or be traumatized by them. In a statement on the human rights of birth, Prochaska (2015) cited the White Ribbon Alliance, Charter for Respectful Maternity Care, which makes the same point.

> A woman's relationship with her maternity providers is vitally important. Not only are these encounters the vehicle for essential lifesaving health services, but women's experiences with caregivers can empower and comfort, or inflict lasting damage and emotional trauma.
>
> (p. 1015)

Women in the 14 studies Beck (2015) synthesized had much to say about the care they received. They felt stripped of their dignity. Some of the women did not feel that they or their babies were in danger, but they felt degraded and disrespected, and that they had been raped on the delivery table. They also felt abandoned and alone, unsupported and offered no reassurance at a time when they were very vulnerable. They described the process of birth as cold and unfeeling, like a "piece of meat on an assembly line" (p. 4). The mothers often reported that their care was unsafe and they were powerless to rectify or get out of the situation. They were treated like they were nothing, and they were terrified (Beck, 2015).

Similarly, women in Elmir et al.'s (2010) meta-ethnography of ten qualitative studies described the care they received as dehumanizing, disrespectful, and uncaring. They tended to be more negative if they felt "invisible and out of control." They used phrases such as "barbaric," "intrusive," "horrific," "inhumane," and "degrading." They were distressed when large numbers of people were invited to watch their birth without their consent.

A qualitative study of 42 mothers from Sweden, which generally has low rates of traumatic birth, showed that quality of caregiving also made a difference (Tham, Ryding, & Christensson, 2010). Women who had higher symptoms of posttraumatic stress also reported that their midwives were nervous or not interested. These mothers felt intense fear and shame during delivery, and that there was not enough postpartum follow-up. Finally, they indicated that their partners did not provide adequate support. Similarly, a study of 372 couples at 6 weeks and 3 months postpartum (Iles et al., 2011) found that dissatisfaction with partner support increased risk of both postpartum depression and posttraumatic stress.

A study from Italy including 160 women who had had normal vaginal births were assessed at 48 hours, and 3 to 6 months postpartum (Cigoli, Gilli, & Saita, 2006). They found that 1.3 percent had clinically relevant PTSD following birth, and 29 percent had symptoms in at least one PTSD subscale. Women were more likely to have traumatic stress symptoms if it was their first delivery, they had low levels of support from family members and medical personnel, or they had a history of anxiety or depression. Women perceived their deliveries as violent events, in which they feared destroying the baby and being destroyed by him.

Physical injury

Priddis and colleagues (2014) conducted in-depth, qualitative interviews with 12 women who experienced severe perineal trauma (i.e., third and fourth degree lacerations) during their births. They identified three themes: (1) *the abandoned mother*, where they felt exposed, vulnerable, and disempowered. The women reported feeling disconnected from their bodies. Their broken bodies were messy, leaking, and "dirty"; (2) *the fractured fairytale*, which describes the disconnect between their expectations of birth and life with a new baby, how it really is, how this impacts their ability to mother, and their sexual identities. Despite the trauma, they were proud that they gave birth vaginally; and (3) *a completely different normal*, which is their pathway to rediscover and redefine their sense of self following their injury.

Delivery preference

A study from Norway of 1,700 mothers examined PTSD based on birth type (Garthus-Niegel et al., 2014). Surprisingly, they found higher rates of PTSD in women who preferred a cesarean, but delivered vaginally. Prenatal fear of childbirth likely contributed to this reaction. Depression and anxiety in pregnancy also increased the risk. Interestingly, they did not find a similar effect for women who preferred a vaginal delivery, but had a cesarean. However, another recent study of 160 women found that women who strongly preferred a vaginal birth, and had a cesarean, were at higher risk for depression at 8–10 weeks postpartum (Houston et al., 2015). Depressive symptoms were measured via PHQ-9. The stronger the preference, the more depressive symptoms they had. There was no difference based on preference in depressive score by 6 months postpartum.

Postpartum factors
Pain

Women's pain postpartum can also influence their perceptions of their births. A study from Australia compared the experiences of 203 primiparous women who had either vaginal, assisted vaginal, or cesarean births (Rowe-Murray & Fisher, 2001). The authors found three variables related to postpartum depression at 8 months: a high degree of postpartum pain, a perceived lack of support during labor and birth, and a less-than-optimal first contact with their babies. These factors accounted for 35 percent of the variance in depression.

Sixty women undergoing cesarean births reported on their postpartum pain levels (Karlstrom et al., 2007). Seventy-eight percent of the women reported that their pain was a 4 or higher on the Visual Analog Scale (VAS), which indicated that their pain was inadequately controlled. There was no difference in pain level between women who had planned vs. elective cesareans. However, the risk of a negative birth experience was 80 percent higher for women who had emergency cesareans, and postoperative pain had a negative effect on both breastfeeding and infant care. The authors described how adequate pain relief was essential to facilitate a swift recovery from surgery and emotional bonding with the baby. Women who expected high levels of pain before birth scored higher on the VAS after birth. Sixty-two percent reported that their pain interfered with baby care in the first 24 hours, and one-third indicated that it influenced breastfeeding. In a logistic regression, the two predictors of a negative birth experience were emergency cesarean and experiencing a higher level of pain than they expected.

In another study of post-birth pain, Eisenach and colleagues (2008) found that severity of post-birth pain, but not mode of delivery, predicted postpartum depression. This study was a prospective, longitudinal study of 1,288 women who were hospitalized for either a vaginal or cesarean delivery. Acute pain increased the risk of persistent pain by 2.5 times, and caused a three-fold increase in postpartum depression. Persistent pain at 8 weeks was also related to postpartum depression. The authors indicated that pain is often undermedicated because of limited nursing staff and a hesitancy to use adequate pain medication in breastfeeding women. They noted that opioids and NSAIDs, long the mainstays of acute pain treatment, have warnings about their use during breastfeeding. However, these warnings are likely unnecessary. Mothers who had had surgical or instrumental vaginal births with perineal lacerations had higher pain scores. Ten percent of women who had cesarean births had persistent pain at 8 weeks.

Another study examined the relationship between maternal fear prior to delivery, partner's level of fear, and level of postoperative pain for 65 women having planned cesareans (Keogh, Hughes, Ellery, Daniel, & Holdcroft, 2006). Within this sample, mothers who had negative expectations before birth, and who were fearful before delivery, had higher levels of postoperative pain. Partners' fear and anxiety also influenced maternal postoperative pain. In regression analyses, mother's fear was related to partner's fear, and when mother's and partner's fear were both entered into the equation, partner's fear exacerbated mother's pain. Interestingly, the mother's level of fear was not related to her pain.

Pain catastrophizing also increased pain intensity during labor, and at 2 days postpartum in a sample of 82 Israeli women (Ferber, Granot, & Zimmer, 2005). In this study, pain catastrophizing had three elements: *rumination* (focusing on increasing pain), *magnification* (a tendency to exaggerate the consequences of the pain), and *helplessness*. At 6 weeks postpartum, pain catastrophizing was related with both postpartum depression, measured by the EPDS, and social functioning. A high pain score was not related to either variable.

Breastfeeding

Not surprisingly, traumatic birth experiences can make breastfeeding much more difficult, and possibly undermine it completely. For example, a national survey of 5,332 mothers in England at 3 months postpartum found that women who had forceps-assisted births and unplanned cesareans had the highest rates of PTS, and the most breastfeeding difficulties (Rowlands & Redshaw, 2012).

Some of the mothers in Beck's study describe how breastfeeding triggered flashbacks to their traumatic births.

> The flashbacks to the birth were terrible. I wanted to forget about it and the pain, so stopping breastfeeding would get me a bit closer to my "normal" self again.

> I had flashbacks to the birth every time I would feed him. When he was put on me in the hospital, he wasn't breathing and he was blue. I kept picturing this; and could still feel what it was like. Breastfeeding him was a similar position as to the way he was put on me.

> (Beck, 2011, p. 306)

Traumatic or difficult births can also delay lactogenesis II. A study from Guatemala found that highly stressful births were related to increased cortisol levels, which delayed lactogenesis II by as much as several days (Grajeda & Perez-Escamilla, 2002). If professionals are aware that this delay is possible, they can anticipate it and work with mother to lessen its impact.

In contrast to the stories cited above, breastfeeding can also be enormously healing. With gentle assistance, breastfeeding can work even after the most difficult births. For some mothers in Elmir et al.'s (2010) study, women reported that breastfeeding provided women an opportunity to overcome the trauma of their birth experiences and "prove" their success as mothers, as these mothers describe.

> Breastfeeding was a timeout from the pain in my head. It was a "current reality"—a way to cling onto some "real life," whereas all the trauma that continued to live on in my head belonged to the past, even though I couldn't seem to keep it there.
>
> (Beck, 2011, p. 306)

> Breastfeeding became my focus for overcoming the birth and proving to everyone else, and mostly myself, that there was something that I could do right. It was part of my crusade, so to speak, to prove myself as a mother.
>
> (Beck & Watson, 2008, p. 233)

> My body's ability to produce milk, and so the sustenance to keep my baby alive, also helped to restore my faith in my body, which at some core level, I felt had really let me down, due to a terrible pregnancy, labor, and birth. It helped build my confidence in my body and as a mother. It helped me heal and feel connected to my baby.
>
> (Beck & Watson, 2008, p. 233)

Characteristics of traumatic birth experiences

Elizabeth describes how the social environment of their hospitals contributed to her psychic distress and physical pain. In a chart, this birth probably appears "fine." However, the mother's subjective experience of it was quite different.

> I had 25 hours of labor. It was long and hard. I was in a city hospital. It was a dirty, unfriendly, and hostile environment. There was urine on the floor of the bathroom in the labor room. There were 100 babies born that day. I had to wait 8 hours to get into a hospital room post-delivery ... There were 10 to 15 women in the post-delivery room waiting for a hospital room, all moaning, with our beds being bumped into each other by the nursing staff. I was taking Demerol for the pain. I had a major episiotomy. I was overwhelmed by it all and in a lot of pain. I couldn't urinate. They kept catheterizing me. My fifth catheterization was really painful. I had lots of swelling and anxiety because I couldn't urinate. My wedding ring was stuck on my finger from my swelling. The night nurse said she'd had patients that had body swelling due to not urinating and their organs had "exploded." Therefore, she catheterized me again. They left the catheter in for an hour and a half. There was lots of pain. My bladder was empty, but they wouldn't believe me. I went to sleep and woke up in a panic attack. I couldn't breathe and I couldn't understand what had happened.

In Elizabeth's story, we see themes of helplessness, pain, and dissociation. This birth was still vivid when she described it to me, even though several years had elapsed since it occurred, and she had had a subsequent positive birth experience. This birth also occurred in a well-known hospital, where the medical care is purported to be top-notch.

Human rights in childbirth

In 2014, the World Health Organization issued a statement on disrespect and abuse during childbirth, which called for reform of many birthing practices (World Health Organization, 2014). They noted that there is a growing body of literature that reflects the negative experiences women encounter during pregnancy and postpartum. Women are particularly at risk while they are giving birth. WHO cited numerous problems that women have reported during their births, including physical and verbal abuse, humiliation, coercive, and unconsented procedures, withholding pain medication, gross violation of privacy, and ignoring and neglecting women when they have life-threatening complications. They described these practices as a violation of women's fundamental human rights.

The WHO (2014) calls for professionals to design maternal health programs with a strong focus on respectful care as an essential component of quality care. Quality care includes support during labor with the companion of her choice, mobility, access to food and liquids, informed choice, and providing women with information about their rights. It provides a mechanism for redress if a mother's rights have been violated. There also needs to be evaluation of these health systems to ensure that providers are accountable for the treatment they provide during childbirth.

> The surge of interest in human rights in childbirth reflects a new international consensus that respectful maternity services are critical to ensuring the health of women and babies. It also reveals the enduring universal power of human rights principles that apply to all women in all countries. A human rights approach to maternity care offers the chance to enrich relationships between women and caregivers by focusing on individual, not institutional care.
>
> (Prochaska, 2015, p. 1016)

Possible interventions for traumatic birth experiences

If you are concerned that a mother has had a traumatic birth, you may want to ask her some questions about it. Alder et al. (2006) recommended screening women for PTSD and PTSD symptoms in the first 3 weeks after birth. Some possible questions that can be asked about the birth, and the presence of PTS, are listed below (Alder et al., 2006). Regarding the birth:

- What was your experience of pain during labor and was your pain adequately addressed?
- Did you feel involved in the decisions that were made regarding your care? Did you have support from your partner or healthcare team?
- Did you feel that you or your baby might die during the birth?

Regarding trauma symptoms, questions could include:

- Do you avoid thinking about your birth?
- Have you had negative dreams about your birth?

- Do you find yourself thinking about your birth without meaning to?
- Are you having any problems falling or staying asleep?
- Have you been more tense, nervous, irritable, or anxious?
- Are you avoiding people and places that remind you of your birth?

For women who have had emotionally difficult births, follow-up has been helpful. In one study, parents were interviewed regarding their distress following childbirth (Alder et al., 2006). If they were distressed, they were randomized into intervention and normal-care groups. The intervention was a 40–60-minute counseling session at 3 days, and a follow-up telephone call at 4–6 weeks postpartum. At 3 months, women in the intervention group had lower PTSD total symptoms than women in the standard-care group. The intervention group also had lower depression and self-blame, and higher confidence scores about having another baby. The authors recommended that interventions include counseling about subsequent pregnancies and birth options, and strategies that help lower patient anxiety. A final component is relaxation training, including muscle relaxation and guided imagery.

Debriefing

A similar type of intervention is debriefing. Debriefing is when a midwife or other health-care provider talks to women about their births, and allows them to ask questions and discuss any of their feelings of sadness, guilt, anger, or confusion. In theory, this intervention should help women process their experiences. In reality, the results have been mixed. An Australian study of 917 women who had had either cesarean sections, or vaginal births using forceps or vacuum extraction, found that a slightly *higher* percentage of debriefed women were depressed and in poorer health at 6 months postpartum than women assigned to standard care. These differences between the groups were not significant, however. Indeed, the overall percentages of depressed women were small (17 percent vs. 14 percent for debriefed vs. standard care, respectively) (Small, Lumley, Donohue, Potter, & Waldenstrom, 2000). Interestingly, these results occurred even though mothers reported that the intervention had been helpful to them. A higher percentage also reported that depression had been a problem for them since the birth (28 percent vs. 22 percent). The authors concluded that debriefing was ineffective, and expressed some caution about its use.

In discussing this study, Boyce and Condon (2001) noted some methodological points that temper these findings. First, they noted that debriefing is for the prevention of PTSD, not depression. Given that, it is not surprising that this intervention did not have an impact on depression. They also noted that women who had had elective vs. emergency procedures were grouped together, and that may have obscured the findings. Finally, they questioned the usefulness of having a midwife debrief who had not been present at the birth. They wondered how she could answer women's questions when they had not been there. They also pointed out that even though this particular intervention was not effective, women need to have the opportunity to discuss their experiences.

A review of the literature on midwife-led debriefing found there was insufficient evidence as to the effectiveness of debriefing (Gamble, Creedy, Webster, & Moyle, 2002). The methodological issues Gamble et al. raised included the lack of a standardized debriefing intervention, comprehensive outcome variables, including the non-inclusion of trauma symptoms, and lack of inclusion of the woman's partner in the debriefing. The authors concluded that a single-session intervention would probably be insufficient to deal with the problem. Meades and colleagues (2011) raised similar concerns about the inconsistency in the use of the term debriefing, its purpose, timing of the intervention, and what it entailed.

Gamble and colleagues (2002) acknowledged that women may benefit when they can talk with a person about their births. On the other hand, women who had been most deeply traumatized by their births may have been so numb from the experience, or may have desired so strongly to "just get back to normal," that any intervention immediately after the experience would have been pointless.

Rowan and colleagues (2007), in their review of eight randomized controlled trials of debriefing for women with difficult births, noted that hospitals in the UK were already offering debriefing as part of routine maternity care. In their review, Rowan et al. found that in six of the eight studies, there was no significant difference in outcomes in women who were debriefed vs. ones who were not. They did note a number of methodological issues, including inconsistent definition of debriefing. They found that women valued the opportunity to talk about their births, but how this differed from formal debriefing was unclear. The authors indicated that it was appropriate to offer all women a chance to discuss their births, but that formal debriefing was not supported by the evidence.

Meades and colleagues (2011) worried that in getting rid of debriefing, we may have thrown out "the baby with the bathwater." They conducted a trial comparing 46 women who met criterion A for PTSD and requested debriefing to 34 women who had given birth at the same hospital, met criterion A for PTSD, and had not requested debriefing. PTSD symptoms lessened for women in both groups over time, but there were greater decreases in the women who requested debriefing. Debriefing did not affect depressive symptoms. This study did not account for some important pre-existing differences between the group that requested debriefing and the group that did not. Debriefing might have led to the reduction in symptoms. Or the group that requested help might have been higher in characteristics like self-efficacy, that could have increased their ability to recover from trauma. They did account for women's appraisals of their births and perceived social support. Both were worse in the debriefing group. They also found that women waited, on average, 16.5 weeks before requesting debriefing, suggesting that previous studies may have been attempting to debrief too soon after birth for mothers to find it helpful. This study does at least raise the possibility, however, that debriefing might be very helpful *for some women*, suggesting that it might not be time to completely "throw out" the practice.

Conclusion

Women who have had traumatic or difficult birth experiences must acknowledge their trauma if they are ever to move past it. Trying to "just forget it" is not an effective strategy, and trauma that is not acknowledged and dealt with can manifest itself in a variety of destructive and negative behaviors. Women who have not processed their birth experience may manifest symptoms, such as depression, blunted affect, and inability to empathize with others (including their infants), helplessness, self-destructive behaviors, somatic complaints, sexual dysfunctions, marital difficulties, anger, and hostility. They may also become pregnant again before they are physically and emotionally ready to do so, in order to do things differently "this time." Working through trauma is difficult, but it is the only route to healing.

As a result of working through trauma, a woman has acknowledged it and given herself permission to feel pain and anger following her experience. She may need a period of time to grieve over her experience. As trauma and grief are reclaimed, she can give meaning to the events and move forward. She may even come to value her experience and try to do something to help other people.

In summary, the research literature on recovery from traumatic events contains a message of hope: people can and do recover from traumatic events. The most important components of any intervention focus on helping women acknowledge and accept their experiences, and helping them regain a sense of self-efficacy. More specifics on trauma-related treatment are found in Chapter 17.

Chapter 9　　**Infant temperament**

Developmental psychologists once believed that mothers influenced their babies, but that the reverse was not true. Eventually, researchers discovered what now seems glaringly obvious; that babies bring quite a lot to the interaction, and could indeed be a major influence on their mothers' emotional state. Infant temperament, in particular, has a substantial influence on mothers' mental health. Temperament includes how much babies cry, how shy they are, how distractible, irritable, soothable, and active. Broadly defined, temperament is a behavioral style and characteristic way of responding to people and the environment.

Temperament is a stable characteristic of newborns that is later shaped and modified by children's experiences, including how well their personalities match those of their mothers. If the mother and baby's temperament are in synchrony, there is said to be "goodness of fit." If mothers and babies don't seem to fit together, there is said to be asynchrony between mother and baby (McGrath, Records, & Rice, 2008).

The baby with a "difficult," or high-needs, temperament is central to the topic of the infant's impact on postpartum depression. Infants with high-needs temperaments have strong emotional reactions; cry for long periods of time; are hard to comfort; slow to accept new people, foods, or routines; and less easy to predict or regulate in their eating, sleeping, or elimination schedules. Mothers might describe these babies as "colicky." Babies with difficult temperaments can be challenging to care for. When babies have difficult temperaments, mothers may conclude that they are not effective or competent, and begin to resent their babies. In addition, they are often afraid to share their feelings with others, as this mother describes.

> My first baby screamed from the day he was born. He screamed all the time, even in the hospital. He reacted oddly to all kinds of different things. The pediatrician said he was a "difficult" child. Even now, he has to have things always the same … When I went back for a check-up at 2 weeks, a nurse asked me how the baby was. She said "aren't they wonderful?" I didn't know what to say. I thought he was the pits.

Mothers feel ambivalent toward their high-needs babies, or start to resent them, which makes them feel guilty. When mothers feel this way, they often withdraw from others. Temperamentally difficult infants may disrupt many aspects of a woman's life, as Barbara describes.

> When the baby started throwing up, I felt terrible. I wouldn't go any place with her because I didn't want people to see her screaming. I wanted to be the perfect

mother ... My mother-in-law said "you've got to relax. She's picking up on your cues" ... The baby had a difficult temperament. Even now, she's very stubborn and strong-willed. The control issue is big for me. I'm a perfectionist and always have been. I don't want the baby to experiment with food, even though I know it's normal. I don't want her to do it ... I wanted this baby so bad. When she came, I hated her. I thought of throwing her out the window. I just wanted her to die. I spanked her when she was 3 or 4 weeks old, and I'm still dealing with the guilt of it ... I'd yell at her, right in her face "I hate you. I wish you would die."

A study of 74 first-time mothers, and 58 first-time fathers in Switzerland, examined the relationship between stress, depression, psychopathology, and child difficulty during pregnancy, and at 1, 3, 12, and 18 months postpartum (Perren, von Wyl, Burgin, Simoni, & von Klitzing, 2005). The researchers assessed psychopathology on the German version of the Revised Symptom Checklist. Infant difficulty did increase stress, but only for some parents. Surprisingly, fathers were more stressed by infant temperament than mothers. Contrary to prediction, child difficulty did not increase depression. Overall, depressive symptoms decreased over the 18 months, but stress did not decrease.

Infant crying and colic

Infant crying is the most salient behavior in babies with high-needs temperaments, and can be very challenging for new parents to cope with. It is one of the most common reasons for pediatric visits in the first 3 months. Colic is usually diagnosed using the "Wessel" criteria: crying or fussing that lasts more than 3 hours a day, occurring on more than 3 days in any week, for 3 weeks or longer (Pauli-Pott, Becker, Mertesacker, & Beckmann, 2000). Colicky crying can even persist past the first 3 months (Wolke, Rizzo, & Woods, 2002).

Bond and colleagues (2001) found that 116 mothers of colicky babies were highly stressed and anxious. Moreover, the mothers reported low self-efficacy, less attachment to the baby, and less satisfaction with lives since having their babies. Social support did not ameliorate the effects.

A mother who is depressed in pregnancy is already more vulnerable to depression in the postpartum period. One possible mechanism for this relationship could be the mother's response to infant cries. A study from the UK of 72 pregnant women examined mothers' autonomic response to the sound of an infant crying (Pearson, Lightman, & Evans, 2012). They found that depressed pregnant women ($n = 22$) had a larger increase in systolic blood pressure in response to infant crying than did pregnant women who were not depressed. The depressed women were actually more sensitive to the sounds of infant distress than women who were not depressed.

Crystal describes her experience with a colicky baby. Her baby's fussiness interfered with her initial ability to bond with her baby. Once she identified the cause, a dairy allergy, her baby's symptoms improved and she was able to attach to her baby.

My daughter was born in 2005, and in hindsight, I know that something was not right right away. She was my second child, and fortunately, initiating breastfeeding was easy.

Early on, I had mastitis, which I had not had with my first child. It was horrible. On top of the developing mood issues I was having, I felt like all I could do was rock in the recliner with a blanket up to my neck and shiver. Breastfeeding was toe-curlingly painful, but I kept up with it and pumping, hoping to rid my body of this infection. Fortunately, the antibiotics kicked in quickly, and I felt physically better soon.

Kira continued to be a fussy, unhappy baby. She would scratch at her face, and pull her legs up to her stomach to push out a poop every few days. She would cry, spit up ... none of this helped my bonding with her.

Around 5 weeks postpartum, I decided to cut dairy out of my diet. That, and getting her started on a medicine for reflux, started to turn things around. For her. I found myself obsessively reading food labels, researching articles online, thinking about what else I could do. I cut out soy and nuts for a while too, after reading about connections with milk and soy proteins. Friends and family encouraged me to wean, but no, this was something I could DO. Something to take my focus away from how awful I was feeling, and reassure myself that I was a good mom.

The good news was that the changes I made did help Kira. And over the following few weeks, the beautiful, happy little girl was allowed to come out, and I slowly felt myself able to start bonding with her.

I continued with my elimination until she self-weaned around 10 months. I learned a lot, and felt like I was a good mom.

Longitudinal findings

Twenty-two percent of babies had infant colic in a prospective, longitudinal study, and 13 percent of their mothers had an EPDS score >13 (Akman et al., 2008a). Mothers of colicky babies had significantly higher scores on the EPDS than did mothers whose babies were not colicky. Colic also influenced attachment: 63 percent of colicky infants had an insecure attachment, compared with 31 percent of non-colicky infants. The authors concluded that infant colic was associated with both depressive symptoms and insecure attachment style.

Similarly, Pauli-Pott et al. (2000) found that even when babies did not meet Wessell criteria, extended crying made mothers feel angry and nervous. The mothers believed that their babies were dissatisfied with them, and rejecting them. The mothers reacted with anger and disappointment.

A US study of 662 mothers found that mothers at 8 weeks postpartum were more likely to be depressed if they have a colicky baby, or a baby that refuses feeding (Dagher & Shenassa, 2012). Depressive symptoms were measured as a continuous variable on the EPDS. Mothers also had more depressive symptoms if they felt stressed out by parental responsibilities, and had a hard time balancing their responsibilities.

In a longitudinal study of 139 women, women were assessed at 8 months gestation, and at 2 and 6 months postpartum (McGrath et al., 2008). Depressed mothers reported that their infants had more difficult temperaments at both postpartum points. These differences were still apparent even after controlling for mothers' history of abuse or anxiety disorders. Depressed and non-depressed mothers reported equal levels of childcare stress and social support. The author recommended interventions that increased goodness of fit between mothers and babies.

A qualitative study of 30 Canadian couples, where the mother had an EPDS >12, identified nine factors that they believed caused the depression, one of which was child health and temperament challenges (Habel, Feeley, Hayton, Bell, & Zelkowitz, 2015). The other causes included lack of social connection, mother's physical health problems, disappointing childbirth, life stress, and past history of depression. Interestingly, only the fathers mentioned "societal pressures on women" as a possible cause.

An Australian study of 232 mothers of colicky babies at 12 months assessed women with the EPDS, MINI, and an assessment of psychosocial risk (Christl et al., 2013). Thirty percent were depressed (EPDS >12), 41 percent had high trait anxiety, 44 percent had past mental health problems, 38 percent had perfectionistic traits, and 32 percent had experienced past abuse. Mothers of colicky babies had twice the rate of anxiety disorders compared to the general population of mothers. The authors noted that some mothers were at higher risk for experiencing problems, especially if they had unresolved issues around their own parenting, or if they had a trauma history.

Canadian researchers examined the relationship between mothers' psychosocial resources, such as her security in relationships, and infant health problems, fussing, and crying at 12 months (Sawada et al., 2015). Using longitudinal data from 5,092 mothers, the researchers identified 135 mothers who reported infant fussing and crying at 12 months, or who had health problems at birth. Using confirmatory factor analysis, they identified a variable called "felt security," which includes mothers' attachment, relationship quality, self-esteem, and social support. Infant health alone did not predict fussing and crying at 12 months. Rather, felt security during pregnancy interacted with infant health problems at birth to predict fussing and crying at 12 months.

Infants who cry a lot are also at higher risk for being abused. In a study of 84 parents, 32 were at high risk for physically abusing their children (Crouch, Skowronski, Milner, & Harris, 2008). High- and low-risk parents were asked to watch a video of an infant crying. As predicted, high-risk parents rated the crying infant more negatively, and had more hostile feelings after they watched the video, than did low-risk parents.

Persistent crying in infancy may also be related to problems in school. In a prospective study of 64 infants referred for persistent crying, Wolke et al. (2002) followed up with them at 8–10 years of age, and compared them to a matched sample of 64 age mates. At follow-up, 19 percent of the children referred for persistent crying had hyperactivity problems compared with only 2 percent of the control children. Parents, and the children themselves, reported more conduct problems. Parents of the persistent criers rated their children's temperaments as more negative, difficult, and demanding. The academic achievement of persistent criers was significantly lower than that of the control children. This was especially true for those with hyperactivity. There was no difference in current depression for mothers.

Depression-related distortions

An issue that frequently arises in the study of infant temperament is whether the difficulties are real, or simply a matter of depressed mothers seeing their children in a more negative light. Mothers' depression may also color their perceptions of the babies in a negative way. They may perceive that their babies are difficult, even when they are not, and this can influence how mothers respond to them. If mothers are inconsistent in responding to their infants, or respond to them in an angry and intrusive way, mothers can even *cause* fussy and unsettled behavior in their infants. In one study (Rosenblum, McDonough, Muzik, Miller, & Sameroff, 2002), mothers' beliefs about their infants had an impact on infant affect regulation over and above the impact of maternal depression. Rosenblum et al. also found that mothers with distorted representations of their infants were more likely to also report depressive symptoms.

A study from Sweden found a subgroup of infants who were genuinely colicky by objective measure (Canivet, Jakobsson, & Hagander, 2002). Interestingly, women who indicated, during late pregnancy, that there was a risk of spoiling a baby with too much contact were more likely to have a colicky baby. Infants of these mothers were more distressed, even when given the same amount of physical contact as other babies.

Mothers' perceptions of older children

The effects of depression on mothers' perception of their children lasts well past infancy. Maternal depression led to negative biases in reporting children's symptoms of ADHD, general behavior problems, and their own negative parenting styles, compared with laboratory assessment, in a sample of 96 6- to 10-year-olds (Chi & Hinshaw, 2002).

Mothers who were depressed or anxious were also more likely to report behavior problems in their children at 14 years of age (Najman et al., 2000). There was a systematic difference in the way mothers reported on the behavior of their children. Because there was no outside verification of the children's behavior in this study (such as teacher or friend report), the authors had no way of knowing whether the children actually did have more behavior problems. The authors suggested that mothers who are depressed may have more difficulties in coping with their children's behaviors, and may perceive them as more negative across the board.

Impact of maternal depression and elevated cortisol

There is some debate in the field about whether mothers' depression and/or stress can physiologically alter babies' temperament, either prenatally or via breastfeeding. If breastfeeding mothers had higher cortisol levels, their babies had higher levels of fear behaviors in a study of 253 2-month-olds (Glynn et al., 2007). This relationship was not observed among the formula-feeding mothers. Glucocorticoids easily pass the blood–brain barrier, and can be passed to infants via breast milk. The limbic regions of the brain are highly sensitive to the effects of glucocorticoids. The mothers in the breastfeeding and formula-feeding groups had similar mean cortisol levels. Cortisol was not directly assessed in the milk, but was assessed in maternal plasma. The findings were based on maternal report of infant temperament, so this variable could be more accurately called "maternal perception of infant fear." The authors concluded that breast milk is a potential avenue by which mothers' fear can be communicated to their infants. However, the design of this study did not allow the researchers to conclude that (a) there was actually more fear in the infants (vs. the mothers believing that it was there), and (b) that the mechanism of transmission was via breast milk vs. the mothers' behaviors.

In contrast to these findings, breastfeeding has also been shown to increase babies' resilience to psychosocial stress (Montgomery, Ehlin, & Sacker, 2006). These data were part of a longitudinal birth cohort study from the UK. The researchers found that babies who were breastfed were less susceptible to stress following their parents' divorce than babies who were not breastfed. The outcome variable was anxiety at 10 years of age. This effect held even after controlling for possible confounding factors. Although this study is intriguing, the measure of breastfeeding was pretty poor, and it does not appear that amount of breastfeeding was responsible for the effect. The authors themselves felt that breastfeeding may simply be a marker for other resilience factors in women's lives. They also felt that breastfeeding may have had this effect because it downregulated the HPA axis and likely prevented maternal depression, which would have improved the mother–infant bond.

Summary

Infants with difficult temperaments can have a negative impact on their mothers' emotional state. However, a mother's depression can also influence how she sees her child's behavior. As described in Chapter 4, interventions that address depression and give mothers tools to cope with the behavior of their children are more likely to be effective than simply treating depression alone.

Chapter 10   **Prematurity, infant health problems, and disability**

My first child was premature. He was born at 35 weeks with severe Hyaline Membrane Disease ... He was in the hospital for five months; in the NICU for four months and in intermediate care for one month ... The depression started around the time he was 3 or 4 weeks old ... Up until that time, everything had been so urgent. He had had a couple of arrests. It was overwhelming. Suddenly my son was doing better. Why was I feeling so bad? I had difficulties going to sleep. I was up several times during the night. It was difficult to wake up in the morning. I didn't want to do anything during the day except sleep and call the NICU to check in. I started not to eat well. I felt an impending sense of doom. The depression lasted about a month.

... About a month after he came home, I felt physically depressed, same as in the initial postpartum period. I brought home a very sick baby. I think it was a delayed reaction, reliving the early part. [Patricia]

Infants with health problems can also influence their mothers' emotional state. Yet, postpartum depression, and other conditions, are often overlooked in women whose babies are not healthy. It is important that we don't overlook depression because feelings from the postpartum period can have a long-term impact on how a mother copes, how she sees her child, and her level of attachment. I will first describe prematurity, then illness and disability.

Prematurity

The birth of a premature infant precipitates a psychological crisis. Women who give birth prematurely must face the reality of an infant who may be sickly or fragile when they themselves are psychologically and physically depleted. Mothers may experience guilt for an early delivery, or anxiety regarding the viability and morbidity of their infants. The babies may also be born following a history of infertility, difficult pregnancy, or an emergency delivery.

Some of the aspects associated with medical care of a premature or sick newborn may contribute to the mother's grief and depression. Jan, who had a very difficult pregnancy and delivery, described her feelings after the birth of her daughter. Her daughter was delivered 6 weeks premature, via emergency cesarean section, after Jan developed eclampsia.

> They took her away right after delivery. I never got to hold her, after all that [the difficult pregnancy and delivery]. They brought her back, but my arms were tied to the delivery table. I wish they had released at least one arm. It was really hard … Leaving the hospital without the baby was really bad. I left early because I didn't want to leave at 11 a.m. with all the other moms and babies … I shouldn't complain because she only had a few preemie problems. Others in the nursery were so sick. But it was very stressful. It was awful to see them putting the feeding tube down her throat, hearing her gagging and crying. It makes me cry now just to think about it.

Depression can take place at many different times throughout an infant's illness. Mothers may be particularly at risk immediately following their deliveries, after any medical crisis with the baby, when she must leave the hospital without the baby, when the baby is about to be discharged, or after the baby is home. A mother's risk of depression is further increased if the baby is transferred to another hospital, particularly if the hospital is in another city. If mothers follow their babies to these other hospitals, they may be cut off from their normal support systems, including their partners, returning every night to an empty hotel room.

In some cases, especially with babies who are very sick, mothers may experience anticipatory grieving, and begin to mourn the loss of their infants. In this process, they may distance themselves from their babies in order to prepare themselves for their babies' eventual death. When babies recover, this process of mourning is interrupted, and mothers have to readjust.

There is often little acknowledgment of what the parents have gone through, and how it impacts their current functioning and subsequent childbirth. These negative effects can be compounded by insensitive hospital policies and lack of compassion from healthcare providers (Sargent, 2015).

Heather describes how she was told that she had miscarried during her second week, only to find out a week later that she was still pregnant. She experienced a similar type of grief, and then struggled to reconnect.

> My second pregnancy started off with tears. We went in for our first ultrasound and were told (and saw with our own eyes) that we had miscarried. The midwife showed where the gestational sac was breaking apart and there was nothing in it when we should have seen a heartbeat. We went home and cried, just waiting for the miscarriage to start. After a week of waiting, and running to the bathroom every time thought I felt any sort of discharge, we went back in for a follow-up ultrasound to see if I needed a DNC. Up on the screen popped a baby, and a heartbeat. The previous week, I had tried to emotionally separate myself from this baby. I found it hard to reconnect and be excited. The entire pregnancy I was plagued with the feeling that something was wrong.

Mothers of preterm infants often have birth experiences that are frightening. And they may struggle with the care provided in the NICU. Often, their feelings about these experiences are not acknowledged because they are dealing with a baby with serious health problems, and that takes precedence. Their reactions may surface months later, once their babies are out of danger, as Heather describes.

At 30 weeks pregnant, I started experiencing what I figured were Braxton Hicks contractions. We went to the hospital at the urging of my midwife because they were able to be timed at 5 minutes apart. The hospital confirmed I was in pre-term labor. Since I was at the hospital my midwife did not have rights at, I was mainly seen by a resident whose bedside manner and wording of sensitive situations were lacking …

After 4 days of labor we couldn't stop it any longer and my little girl was born at 31 weeks. She was born by repeat C-section as our area hospitals don't allow VBAC. Since she was so ready to come out vaginally (they waited until the last possible minute), the surgeon had to pull on her neck and shoulders with more pressure than usual. He finally ended up doing a T-incision on my uterus, making future pregnancies extremely dangerous, to be able to pull her out. Minutes later, when I first saw her, her face was extremely purple from the bruising. The nurses said she looked like a domestic violence survivor.

The following 27 days in the NICU felt like a constant battle between what I knew was best for my daughter and not wanting to make the doctors mad, inevitably lengthening our stay. We battled with the required bottle-feeding and needed supplementation, and not being allowed to nurse. My biggest concern for my husband and I was if we got sick, we suddenly wouldn't be allowed to see her for days. And what if that happened to me when we were finally allowed to nurse? They weren't going to delay feeding by mouth while I got better, and would they not allow my milk?

After 27 days, she came home. My husband and I felt like zombies and were still so concerned about illness. We both showed signs (and still a year later, we both suffer) from what seems to be depression and PTSD.

Severity of illness and prematurity

Severity of illness or degree of prematurity can also influence maternal mental health. The range of illnesses or problems of premature infants varies from minor to life-threatening complications. Some babies are hospitalized for only a few days, while others may be in intensive care for several weeks or months. Whatever the circumstances, having a preterm infant can increase the mother's risk of depression, anxiety, and PTSD.

Acute Stress Disorder (ASD) is the precursor syndrome to PTSD. ASD has been found in high rates among mothers and fathers with infants in the NICU. For example, a study from Boston Medical Center compared 59 low-income mothers with babies in the NICU to 60 similar mothers with well babies at 1 week postpartum (Vanderbilt, Bushley, Young, & Frank, 2009). The researchers measured depression, ASD, and lifetime trauma exposure. Thirty-nine percent of mothers with babies in the NICU screened positive for depression compared with 22 percent of mothers of well babies using the EPDS ≥10. They found that 24 percent of mothers with babies in the NICU met criteria for ASD compared with 3 percent of mothers of well babies. This difference was significant even after controlling for depression and lifetime trauma.

A study of 40 parents of babies in the NICU found that 44 percent of the mothers met full criteria for ASD, while none of the fathers did (Shaw et al., 2006). ASD was also associated with changes in the parental role, family cohesiveness, and emotional restraint. Parents had more ASD if they felt that they were not able to help, hold, or care for their infants, protect their infants from pain, or share their infants with other family members.

What mothers believed about the seriousness of their infants' illness was a better predictor of the mothers' reactions than the objective disease characteristics. This is similar to other findings regarding PTSD related to other medical conditions. If the mothers had a supportive family and a positive coping style, they were less likely to have trauma symptoms. If their family was not supportive, and they had a negative coping style, they were significantly more likely to have trauma symptoms. The authors recommended that care providers help parents feel more involved and less helpless, even with severely ill infants.

Another study by this same group of researchers extended their previous findings (Shaw et al., 2009). In the more recent study, 18 parents completed a measure of ASD at baseline, and a measure of PTSD at 4 months. At baseline, they found that 55 percent of mothers met criteria for acute disorder, but none of the fathers. At 4 months, 33 percent of fathers, and 9 percent of mothers, met criteria for PTSD. The researchers noted that fathers showed a more delayed trauma response, but were at even higher risk.

Very low birthweight infants

A study of 21 mothers of very low birthweight (VLBW) babies in Quebec found that 23 percent of mothers were in the clinical range for PTSD at 6 months corrected age (Feeley et al., 2011). Birthweight, and severity of infant complications, were related to the severity of symptoms in the mother. Mothers with more PTSD symptoms were less sensitive in their interactions with their infants.

A US study had similar findings with a sample of 24 mothers of VLBW infants, and a comparison group of 22 mothers of normal infants, at 2–3 years postpartum (Ahlund, Clarke, Hill, & Thalange, 2009). Using the Impact of Events Scale, the researchers found that the mothers of the VLBW infants had significantly higher trauma symptoms on all three trauma subscales (intrusion, avoidance, and hyperarousal) than did mothers of normal weight babies.

A study from Germany compared 50 mothers with VLBW infants to 30 control mothers whose babies had normal birthweights (Kersting et al., 2004). Mothers were assessed at 1–3 days, 14 days, 6 and 14 months postpartum. They completed multiple measures of PTSD, depression, and anxiety. The mothers of VLBW infants were higher on trauma symptoms, depression, and anxiety at all time points except 6 months. None of the mothers met full criteria for PTSD, however. In addition, mothers of the VLBW infants had no significant reduction in PTS, even at 14 months. The authors concluded that giving birth to a VLBW baby is not a single traumatic event. Rather, it is a complex, longer-lasting type of trauma.

Another recent study from Germany included 230 mothers, and 173 fathers, and compared depression scores for parents of VLBW infants ($n = 111$) and parents of full-term infants ($n = 119$) at 4–6 weeks postpartum (Helle et al., 2015). The researchers assessed depression with clinical interviews, the EPDS ≥13, and the Beck Depression Inventory. They found that depression scores that were 4–18 times higher in mothers of VLBW babies (depending on the measure), and 3–9 times higher in fathers. Parents of VLBW infants were also at higher risk if they had a history of psychiatric disorder, and had low social support.

A longitudinal study of 30 VLBW babies examined the relationship between medical complications and developmental outcomes at 36 months (Miceli et al., 2000). Social support data were collected at 4 months, and developmental measures were taken at 4 and 13 months corrected age, and 36 months chronological age. Medical complications heightened the risk for depression in the early months, but not at 36 months. Maternal social support was not related to infant outcomes at 4 and 13 months, but was related to child language function and internalizing behaviors at 36 months. Similarly, maternal distress was not related to outcomes at 4 and 13 months, but was related to internalizing and externalizing at 36 months.

Late preterm infants

Mothers can have difficulties even when their babies are born closer to full-term. One recent study compared 29 late preterm infants with 30 mothers whose babies are born at term (Brandon et al., 2011). Mothers of the late preterm infants experienced more distress after birth than did mothers of full-term babies, and this distress continued throughout the first postpartum month. They had more depression and posttraumatic symptoms. The babies also had more health problems and were in the hospital for a longer time, and the mothers worried about their health more. Mothers also described that lack of time to prepare for the birth. These babies often have difficulty breastfeeding, and mothers expressed concern about that as well. The authors recommended that practitioners not treat late preterm deliveries like they are term deliveries, and recognize that these mothers may be suffering from considerable stress.

Preterm birth and infant behavior problems

Preterm birth, and mothers' subsequent depression or PTSD, can influence how mothers interact with their infants. A study from Switzerland examined the impact of prematurity and mothers' PTSD on mother–infant interaction at 6 months corrected age (Forcada-Guex, Borghini, Pierrehumbert, Ansermet, & Muller-Nix, 2011). The researchers compared 47 mothers of preterm infants with a gestational age of <34 weeks and 25 mothers of full-term infants. They found that mothers of preterm infants with PTSD symptoms were more controlling in their interactions with their babies. In contrast, mothers of full-term babies were more likely to follow a cooperative interaction style. The controlling interaction style leads to less positive infant outcomes. The mothers of preterm infants with low PTS were more likely to be disengaged from their infants. This style, too, is associated with less positive outcomes. The authors cautioned that their sample size was small, but also emphasized that parents need supportive interventions after giving birth to a preterm infant.

A sample of US racial/ethnic minority mothers examined the link between preterm birth, mother's depression, and infant's negative affect at 3 and 10 months (Barroso, Hartley, Bagner, & Pettit, 2015). The participants were 102 predominantly Black and Hispanic mothers. Compared to normative samples, these mothers had high rates of preterm birth. Low birthweight and preterm birth were directly related to postpartum depression, which predicted negative infant affect, using path analysis.

Low birthweight and prematurity can also lead to other problems in children, including ongoing health problems and chronic conditions. In one study, low birthweight was related to the development of attention-deficit hyperactivity disorder (ADHD). In this study (Mick, Biederman, Prince, Fischer, & Faraone, 2002), 252 children with ADHD were compared with 231 children without ADHD. The results indicated that children with ADHD were three times more likely to have been born low birthweight than were comparison children. These findings held even after controlling for prenatal exposure to alcohol and cigarettes, parental ADHD, social class, and comorbid disruptive behavior of family members. Low birthweight appears to be an independent risk factor of ADHD, but children with low birthweight are a relatively small percentage of children with ADHD.

A study of 27 children, ages 18–60 months, who were born prematurely (<37 weeks), examined the link between cortisol reactivity, and internalizing and externalizing problems (Bagner, Sheinkopf, Vohr, & Lester, 2010). The findings indicated that children with a hyperreactive cortisol response had more attentional problems, anxiety, depression, and emotional reactivity than children in the sample without cortisol reactivity. The children with high cortisol yelled, whined, and talked negatively during a lab activity more than did children with low cortisol. Studies with children who were preterm also show that internalizing and externalizing behaviors are more common in children with cortisol reactivity.

Another study conducted a cognitive assessment at 18 months, and compared cortisol levels for three groups of infants: 25 infants at extremely low gestational age (ELGA: 24–28 weeks), 26 at very low gestation age (VLGA: 29–32 weeks), and 22 full-term (Brummelte et al., 2011). The ELGA infants had higher pretest cortisol levels, and a different cortisol response pattern, compared to the other two groups. This pattern was associated with dysfunctional mother–infant interaction and more internalizing behaviors. In addition, maternal interaction influenced cortisol levels in the ELGA children, but not in the other groups. Positive maternal care lowered cortisol levels in preterm children, but cortisol was not related to care for full-term children. The authors hypothesized that altered programming of the HPA axis occurred, especially for the ELGA infants. They also noted that the VLGA infants seemed to cope better with early-life challenges, and need to be distinguished in studies from ELGA infants.

Reproductive technologies and prior infant loss

Mothers who have premature babies may also have a history of infertility, miscarriage, or fetal loss, and this can also increase their risk for depression and anxiety with subsequent pregnancies.

Women are at risk for depression after using assisted reproductive technologies (ART) as well (Monti, Agostini, Fagandini, La Sala, & Blickstein, 2009). Italian researchers compared a sample of 48 parents who used ART (25 mothers, 23 fathers) with 39 non-ART mothers at 30–32 weeks gestation, and at 1 week and 3 months postpartum. The researchers found that the ART mothers were more depressed at all assessment points than were the non-ART women, with the highest rate during pregnancy. Interestingly, the men in ART couples were not depressed at the first two assessment points, but were at month 3. They concluded that women using ART are more vulnerable to depression that may persist until after delivery, and suggested ongoing monitoring for this possibility.

In a study of 36 mothers and fathers, prior loss increased the risk for PTSD, depression, and anxiety with a subsequent birth (Armstrong, Hutti, & Myers, 2009). While depression and anxiety decreased over time, PTSD remained in the moderately high range throughout their pregnancies, and actually increased from the third trimester of pregnancy to 6–8 months postpartum. Mothers and fathers had similar rates of posttraumatic stress symptoms.

Karin describes her experience with a traumatic stillbirth and her subsequent high-risk pregnancy and preterm birth. Her baby was in the NICU for 13 days. She eventually developed postpartum OCD at 6 months postpartum.

After a traumatic stillbirth at 19 weeks, I found myself immediately pregnant with baby number 2. I was overwhelmed. I did not know that I could even get pregnant that soon after a birth (2 weeks), and I was in my first year of marriage where we were both full-time students. I dropped out of school. It was simply too much.

But I had to soldier on.

My doctor recommended a procedure to ensure a healthy delivery at a better time for our son. I was told that most women can resume normal activities (with the exception of "pelvic rest") 2 weeks after this procedure: a cerclage. We would have it done as soon as the 1st trimester was over to allow for the highest success. When the 2 weeks had passed after the cerclage, I went back to work part-time. I ended up in preterm labor and it was stopped with drugs. I had to quit my job and begin complete bedrest.

For 17 weeks, I laid in my bed and hoped my baby would stay in for one more day. I obsessed about how far along I was, if I had felt my baby move recently, and how many contractions I was having. The thought that I would have to bury another baby was exhausting.

I couldn't read books as I didn't have the brainpower to concentrate. I couldn't do needlework, crossword puzzles, or anything like it. Just about the only activities I could do were to watch TV, and read the big stack of *Reader's Digest* back issues my thoughtful sister-in-law had brought for me. Because I was in bed all day, I also didn't sleep well.

At 33 weeks, I started experiencing back labor, so my OB/Gyn gave me a dose of betamethasone at my prenatal appointment with the instructions to come in the next day for an NST and the second dose. The next day, the contractions continued, and my blood count came back with a high white cell count. I had an infection. My husband had left me at the hospital to go take a final exam, and while he was gone, it was decided that the baby needed to be born. Except that he was transverse. A cesarean delivery was prepared. As soon as my husband walked in, they dressed him in scrubs and rolled me back to the OR.

While Zeke had a high 1 minute APGAR, he started struggling almost immediately after that. He was intubated and taken to the NICU. I first saw him as I was wheeled past his isolette after surgery.

The day after the birth, my husband's siblings came to visit. None of them had children. They stayed so long that I missed a pumping session. Then they went to the NICU without me due to the visitor limits, and the NICU staff allowed my husband to be the first to hold him. Even 16 years later, I am angry at the NICU staff for knowing that was an important time, and not waiting for me. I was so young (21). I didn't know how to be an advocate for myself or my son. For 13 days, he stayed there.

Jared would take me when he went to class, and I would stay until he was done. Then we would go home, and my parents would take me in the evening when Jared was at work. That was a shorter visit. Sometimes, while I was up in the middle of the night pumping, I would call the NICU and ask for an update on his progress.

He was called a "feeder/grower," and even though we didn't have to worry too much about future problems, the constant vigilance to the monitors and mLs of milk was exhausting. His ET tube was pulled within 24 hours, and his NG tube was pulled on day 12. We took him home on preemie formula fortification on my milk, with very little instruction. It felt like we were being tossed to the wind. We had never done his daily care for longer than an hour at a time. The experts had done it. We felt so alone and unprepared for taking this tiny human home. It took 7 weeks to get him fully breastfeeding, which was done without any direction or help from any HCP.

By the time he was 6 months, he had caught up to his same age peers in development and by the time he was 18 months, he had also caught up in size.

Mothers can also experience trauma during an ultrasound following a previous perinatal loss (O'Leary, 2005). A descriptive phenomenologic study of 12 mothers explored mothers' and fathers' experiences of ultrasound. All had lost babies in the previous year. The current ultrasound reminded the parents of when they had learned that their babies had died, or had seen their babies die on the previous ultrasound. Many aspects of the experience reminded them of that prior event: the smells, sights, feelings, and sounds of the ultrasound room. During the ultrasound, some mothers experienced flashbacks to when they lost their previous babies—even when the current baby was healthy. Both the fathers and the mothers showed equal levels of trauma following the ultrasound. Based on her research, O'Leary (2005) recommended recognizing that parents may be remembering their previous babies when undergoing testing for a current pregnancy. She also recommends preparing parents for possible flashbacks during ultrasound. Let them hear the heartbeat first before the ultrasound. Acknowledge and validate the parents' concerns while assuring them that the current baby is healthy. Finally, recognize that fathers may be as traumatized as the mothers.

A study from Germany examined mothers' grief after a pregnancy termination for fetal anomalies (Kersting et al., 2005). This study compared the reactions of 83 women who had undergone a termination 2–7 years previously, 60 mothers who had undergone a termination 14 days prior, and 65 women who had had a full-term baby. Contrary to the researchers' expectations, they found that there was no difference in traumatic symptoms between the two groups who had a termination. Both groups differed significantly from the mothers who had full-term babies, and were significantly higher on all three subscales of the Impact of Events Scale (hyperarousal, avoidance, and intrusion). The events experienced as traumatic were the invasive medical procedures, waiting for labor pains to begin, and delivery of a dead fetus. The authors noted that mothers experienced intense grief reactions, in addition to trauma symptoms. They concluded that these terminations had been emotionally traumatic events that led to severe posttraumatic stress responses that persisted for years.

In another study, these same researchers replicated their earlier findings (Kersting et al., 2009). They compared 62 women who had late-term terminations for fetal anomalies, with 43 mothers who had VLBW babies, and 65 mothers of healthy infants. At 14 days, they found that 22 percent of the mothers in the termination group had psychiatric disorders (PTSD, depression, and anxiety), compared with 19 percent of the mothers of VLBW infants, and 6 percent of the mothers with full-term infants. At 14 months, the rates were still elevated for the mothers in the termination group (17 percent), and preterm-infant group (7 percent). None of the mothers of full-term infants had psychiatric conditions at 14 months. The authors concluded that both late termination, and giving birth to a very preterm baby, can cause substantial psychological distress, even up to 14 months later.

Reproductive loss can be life-threatening for mothers as well. Van Pampus and colleagues (2004) described three case studies where mothers developed trauma symptoms after their experience with HELLP syndrome. HELLP syndrome is a serious form of preeclampsia that includes hemolysis, low platelets, and liver damage. HELLP syndrome is a potential cause of mother and infant mortality and morbidity. Even several years after the event, the women in the study were still highly fearful, and did not want to become pregnant again for fear of what might happen. They noted that women who experienced HELLP syndrome may suffer from significant emotional sequelae, and need extra support.

Mothers who received support after a stillbirth had less anxiety and depression than mothers who did not receive support (Cacciatore, Schnebly, & Froen, 2009). This study was a survey of 769 mothers in the US who had had a stillbirth in the last 18 months. If they received family support after the stillbirth, they had less anxiety and depression than did mothers who did not receive support. The authors noted that while nurses, physicians, and support groups were cited as being helpful for mothers, they did not have a significant effect on anxiety and depression. However, family support did.

Elaine describes the loss of her first son, Noah, who was born prematurely, and her difficult second pregnancy and emergency cesarean. She felt disconnected from and in a daze for the first 7 months of her baby's life before she finally got the help she needed.

In 2008, I lost my first baby, a son named Noah, when I went into labor at 24 weeks. He passed away after two hours because his lungs were not developed enough for him to survive. I struggled with a deep grief after that, the very worst feelings I have ever experienced in my life.

When I became pregnant again two years later my pregnancy was filled with anxiety, constant ultrasounds, bed rest and worry. When I went into labor at 41 weeks, I was so excited and proud to have reached that point. My labor progressed and seemed to be going well until my OB called a code red, cord prolapse, everything turned to panic as I was rushed to the ER having to leave my husband behind. I remember stopping the nurse before I passed out, asking her to tell me if my baby was OK, and her answer was "we can't tell you that."

Thankfully, my son, Darragh, was perfect, but I spent the next few months in a daze. When he was 7 months old, I finally asked my doctor for help. I felt out of control, panicked, and so isolated. She sent me to a psychologist and I was prescribed Celexa. I had never done the "drugs" thing before, and felt like a failure. But it helped so much. A cloud and weight was lifted.

I thought it was strange how different grief and depression are. Depression was unexplainable. It didn't make any sense.

I have had another two boys since, I'm still on Celexa and have not had any significant PPD.

Fathers can also become depressed following infant loss. In a review of 17 studies, Badenhorst et al. (2006) found that fathers experienced classic grief symptoms, but less guilt than mothers. Fathers also experienced anxiety and depression, but at a lower level than mothers, and may also develop PTSD. The authors concluded that fathers may also be traumatized by stillbirth or neonatal death, and need help in their own right before they can support their partners.

Kangaroo care

One technique that can be useful for mothers of premature infants is kangaroo care. Kangaroo care involves placing the baby, wearing only a diaper, between the mother's breasts, or on one breast, under her clothing. The babies are held in a sling or pouch. Fathers can also do kangaroo care. The benefits for babies appear almost immediately. The babies are calmer and their body temperature is stable. They cry less, thereby conserving precious calories. The babies do better physically, and are discharged from the hospital earlier. Mothers also benefit. They feel more confident in caring for their babies, and are more likely to form secure attachments.

Parmar and colleagues (2009) studied families of 135 babies from India, with an average birthweight of 1460 g, and a gestational age of 30 weeks. Kangaroo mother care (KMC) was started in the first week of life. Infants in KMC had improved oxygen saturation levels, their temperature and respiration stabilized, and heart rate was lowered by 3–5 beats. Ninety-six percent of the mothers, 82 percent of the fathers, and 84 percent of other family members accepted KMC as a treatment. In addition, healthcare workers found it an acceptable and conservative treatment for babies in the NICU. The mothers reported that they felt closer to their babies, and that KMC elevated their mood, although they were initially frightened about trying it. The mothers also reported increased confidence in handling their babies. Healthcare workers reported that it made mothers feel more confident, and it increased breastfeeding. Babies also cried less and slept more.

A study from Israel showed similar results with a larger sample (Feldman, Eidelman, Sirota, & Weller, 2002). This study randomly assigned preterm infants to either the kangaroo care (KC) or standard care. The mothers were matched for birthweight, gestational age, medical severity, and demographics. At 37 weeks gestation, mothers in the KC group had more positive affect, touch, and adaptation to their infants' cues. The infants showed more alertness and less gaze aversion. The mothers were less likely to be depressed and to report that their infants were abnormal. At 3 months, mothers and fathers were more sensitive and provided a better home environment (based on their score on the HOME inventory). At 6 months, the KC mothers were more sensitive to their babies' cues, and their infants scored significantly higher on the Bayley Mental Developmental Index, and the Psychomotor Developmental Index. The authors speculated that KC influenced infant development directly by having a positive impact on infants' perceptual–cognitive and motor development. There may have also been an indirect impact because KC improved maternal mood, perceptions of their infants, and their interactive behavior. In another study, KC was related to successful lactation in mothers of VLBW infants, even after controlling for maternal age, race, marital status, and education beyond high school (Furman, Minich, & Hack, 2002).

In a case study, Dombrowski and colleagues (2001) found that KC was helpful for a mother at very high risk for depression. She was 22 years old, single, and had given up a previous baby for adoption. She and her younger brother were removed from their home when she was 5 because of repeated physical and sexual abuse by her father. She and her brother were adopted at age 9, after four years in multiple foster homes. The mother had an active history of substance abuse. Immediately after her baby's premature birth, she was severely depressed. However, within 24 hours of starting KC, she was no longer depressed. She was assessed at 6 weeks, 3 months, and 7 months, and was neither depressed, nor abusing substances at any of these assessments. In describing her experience, she noted the following:

It was important to both of us for bonding. It made me feel closer than I felt holding her regular, you know, wrapped. It calmed her down a lot more and made her more secure. It made me close to her and I was scared to be a mother, but it gave me a sense of peace that I could do it (take care of the baby). It made me less stressed and able to relax—a "time out" together kind of thing. I was able to forget everything else. It worked well for both of us on stress. I felt like I needed something and being a recovering drug addict, I needed this to help. (p. 215)

KC was also helpful for full-term babies in another study from Iran (Kashaninia, Sajedi, Rahgozar, & Noghabi, 2008). In this study, 100 healthy neonates were assigned to either the KC or control groups. The infants in the KC group were held in KC 10 minutes before an injection, and during the procedure. The KC infants had significantly lower scores on the Neonatal Infant Pain Scale than did the control groups. This scale measured facial expression, cry, breathing pattern, arm and leg movements, and state of arousal. The control infants were significantly higher on all measures, including duration of crying, than were babies in the KC group.

Social support interventions

In addition to KC, providing specific social support improved outcomes for mothers of premature babies (Jotzo & Poets, 2005). In this study, mothers were randomly assigned to a crisis intervention 5 days after birth, or they received usual care. The intervention took place in the NICU two times a week, for 5–15 minutes. The crisis intervention included helping mothers reconstruct the events before and after their births, teaching them relaxation techniques, explaining stress and trauma responses, providing them with support during "emotional outbursts," discussing with them personal resources and current support, and offering them possible solutions for concrete problems. At discharge, mothers in the intervention group had significantly lower trauma symptoms than mothers who received standard care.

Prematurity is only one type of health issue that can influence mothers. Infants' long-term health problems, such as disability and chronic illness, can also affect mothers' mental health.

Infant disability or chronic illness

Disabilities, or infant illness, also vary considerably in how much they impair a child's functioning, and how that impairment impacts mothers. In a sample from India, infant hospital admission was highly significantly associated with postpartum depression (Patel et al., 2002). Similarly, serious infant health problems were a risk factor for Turkish women at 6 months postpartum (Danaci et al., 2002). Even relatively minor problems can lead to mothers being separated from their babies, increasing the risk of depression.

Chronic health problems in children can influence mothers' emotional health, as found in a study of mothers of children with epilepsy (Mu, Wong, Chang, & Kwan, 2001). The children in this study ranged in age from 1 to 19 years old. The authors found that there were three factors associated with maternal depression: boundary ambiguity, uncertainty, and mother's age. These three factors accounted for 21 percent of the variance in maternal depression. Uncertainty refers to inadequate ability to structure or categorize an event due to lack of sufficient cues. Epilepsy, by its unpredictable nature, makes it difficult to predict. Boundary ambiguity refers to an uncertain role of the child in the family. Because of the child's illness, parents are unsure what role their children can fulfill. For example, should they be assigned household chores? Caretakers may be either inadequately or excessively involved. Mothers' age also made a difference, with younger mothers having more difficulty coping with their children's illness.

Similarly, mothers' feelings that they could not manage their children's asthma increased the likelihood of hospitalization for their children's asthma (Chen et al., 2003). In this study, 115 children (ages 4–18) were followed for a year. All the children had had at least one hospitalization during the study period. If parents thought there was nothing they could do to manage their children's asthma, or they felt overwhelmed by caring for their children, their children were more likely to be hospitalized for acute attacks. This effect was found even after controlling for baseline severity of asthma, medications, and child age. Some other characteristics related to increased hospitalization included greater levels of family strain and conflict, and greater financial strain.

Social support for mothers of infants with health issues

Social support can attenuate many of the negative effects of having a baby or child with a health problem. Social support can take many forms, including information, practical assistance, and emotional support. However, sometimes "support" is stressful for mothers of babies or children with health problems.

> I found it difficult to speak with my husband and family about being depressed, and about my constant concern and worry. They kept trying to be positive, saying what they would do with him when he got well. I don't know if my medical knowledge made it worse. I knew how serious it was. It made me more depressed when my family was upbeat and tried to deny how serious it was. I had to deal with their denial and I felt they were heaping expectations on me.
> … I got lots of support from a couple we're friends with. She's a NICU nurse. They would offer to sit at the hospital for us so we could go out. They also made meals for us. They were people who understood the medical issues. They didn't say everything would be OK. They realized it could be fatal. [Patricia]

Why "social support" is sometimes stressful

When considering whether a woman is receiving adequate support, it is easy to be fooled by appearances. We might assume that a woman who knows a lot of people, or is receiving functional assistance, is experiencing social support, but this is not always the case. People in a woman's social network might not offer to help. Even if they help, the woman may not *perceive* it as support. Unwanted help can undermine a woman's confidence in her mothering abilities, threaten her self-esteem, and engender dependency on the person providing the help. Even when a woman is grateful for the assistance, she may be uncomfortable accepting it if she is an independent or private person and is used to doing things for herself. Christine describes how having her mother, and her in-laws, come to help after the baby was born made her uncomfortable.

Everyone was really helping with the baby but me. They were too supportive. I know my husband wouldn't want to think that. I felt like they were taking over everything, that I had to be able to do it all. I kept trying to be the perfect wife. I'm a very private person. I felt like everything was exposed.

Summary

Both mothers and at-risk babies bring special challenges to the mother-infant relationship. Mothers may be in the process of grieving when they are forced to deal with babies who are different from what they expected, and may be difficult to handle. In spite of these difficulties, attachment can develop between mother and baby, especially if the mother is given adequate support—and she perceives it as support. You can do much to facilitate these types of positive reactions. Helping mothers feel competent in caring for their at-risk babies is vital for reducing risk for postpartum depression, and helping mothers to become attached to their babies.

In the next two chapters, I describe psychological risk factors for postpartum depression.

Chapter 11 **Psychological risk factors I**

Attributional style, self-esteem, and psychiatric history

Many psychological factors either increase women's risk of depression or increase her resiliency. These factors include a woman's attributional style; her expectations about what it will be like to be a mother; her self-esteem; and how competent she feels as a parent. She may also have factors that make her vulnerable, such as a history of loss, previous psychiatric illness, and a dysfunctional or abusive family of origin. Each of these increase women's risk of depression, and may co-occur. The first factor described has to do with how mothers see the world.

Attributional style

People have different ways of looking at the world. They are either "optimists" or "pessimists." A pessimistic attributional style increases vulnerability to depression because people learn to interpret events in a way that makes them more stressful and negative. Specifically, pessimists are more likely to become depressed after a negative event because they maintain internal, global, and stable attributions about why negative events occurred. Internal attributions mean that the cause of the negative event is within the person's control. Negative events can also be attributed to stable ("I am stupid") or unstable ("I was tired") characteristics. Global attributions mean that a person feels that the negative event affects many areas of their lives, while persons who make specific attributions realize that the negative event only affects one or two areas. Stable attributions mean that the person feels the negative situation will never change. Barbara's story shows characteristics of the pessimistic style.

> I hadn't handled a lot of babies. The nurse was yelling at me, saying, "What's the matter, haven't you handled a baby before?" I was offended and hurt. All I could think of was "I'm a bad mother." … When [the depression] was really bad, I thought "I'm a bad person. I should have never had a baby, never gotten married. I'm a bad mother. I'm crap." I talked about it all the time until others were sick of hearing about it … At one point, my mom said to me "I don't know what you are worried about. One baby is no work." All I could think was "I'm a failure." [Barbara]

While the research cited above refers to depression in general, attributional style has also been studied in relation to depression in new mothers. An Australian study of 65 primiparous women found that dysfunctional attitudes were related to depression at 6 weeks postpartum. This was especially true for women with high amounts of postpartum stress, or whose babies had high-needs temperaments (Grazioli & Terry, 2000). Negative thinking, and thoughts of death and dying at 1 month postpartum, predicted depression at 4 months in another study of 465 postpartum women (Chaudron et al., 2001). The authors considered thoughts of dying as a prodrome of later depression. Interestingly, although breastfeeding and bottle-feeding women did not differ in their rates of depression, women who *worried* about breastfeeding were significantly more likely to become depressed than those who did not worry.

Optimism was found to influence birth outcomes in a medically high-risk sample of 129 women (Lobel et al., 2000). In this study, prenatal stress and optimism were examined in relation to birth outcomes (birthweight and gestational age), controlling for risk and ethnicity. Women who were less optimistic had babies who weighed significantly less, even when controlling for gestational age. Prenatal stress did not have an effect once optimism was added to the model. Some of this difference may have been behavioral. Optimists were more likely to exercise, and exercise lowered the risk of preterm birth.

Self-esteem, self-efficacy, and personality traits

> The truth of the matter is that I'm ashamed. Why is it so hard for me and looks so easy for other mothers? I saw other full-time mothers always doing things better. I felt I couldn't keep up. I used to be able to "run with the guys." … Now, I'm in a traditional mommy role, but I'm not relating to this role. So where does this leave me? Not fitting into either role … I'm used to being the best at what I do. But I felt I couldn't [function as a mother]. Especially when I look at other moms. I can't seem to understand why I can't do this … I was depending on other people's expectations. Maybe even my own expectations were too high. This led to feeling down, out of control. That's when the depression really started. Doubting I could do it. It got to where I was scared to death, nervous, chest tightness, crying, not wanting to eat.

Self-esteem, self-efficacy, and the mother's pre-existing personality traits can influence her adjustment to her role as a mother, what she expects of herself, and how competent she feels. In a meta-analysis of 84 qualitative studies, Beck (2002) found that self-esteem had a moderate effect on postpartum depression. Low self-esteem at 1 month postpartum predicted depression at 4 months in another study of 465 women (Chaudron et al., 2001). A prospective study of 191 low-income, inner-city women found that self-esteem was related to lower levels of depression in both the prenatal and postpartum periods (Ritter et al., 2000).

Perfectionism

In a meta-synthesis of 18 qualitative studies, Beck (2002) found that beliefs about motherhood played a large role in postpartum depression. Mothers, and professionals who care for them, often harbor the belief that motherhood brings total fulfillment to women. This expectation, without acknowledging the difficulties, sets standards that are impossible to meet. Women may try to be "perfect" mothers, and when they cannot, they feel that they have failed. Women in the studies Beck reviewed often did not confide in others because they believed that no one else ever felt the same way. She noted that first-time mothers were more prone to the myth of the perfect mother, whereas multiparous women's expectations focused on trying to cope with the new addition to their families.

In contrast, a study from Portugal of 386 pregnant women did not find a link between perfectionism and postpartum depression (Maia et al., 2012). The researchers excluded women who were depressed in pregnancy from the study, which likely influenced their findings. They measured self-oriented perfectionism, others' high standards, and conditional acceptance, and found that none of the variables they measured predicted depression at 3 months postpartum. They concluded that perfectionism was not a risk factor for postpartum depression.

Women's expectations about their babies can also lead to depression. In a sample of 68 at-risk African American women, those who worried about spoiling their babies reported more depression, and had more inappropriate developmental expectations of their babies than mothers who worried less about spoiling. These findings suggested that fear of spoiling may influence responsiveness in mothers who are at-risk, and may lead to potentially disturbed mother-infant relationships (Smyke et al., 2002).

Breastfeeding self-efficacy is a variant of the construct of self-efficacy. Breastfeeding self-efficacy refers to a mother's belief that she possesses the ability to breastfeed her baby. A recent study from Norway examined whether breastfeeding self-efficacy had an impact on postpartum depression (Haga et al., 2012). In this online, longitudinal survey of 737 mothers at 6 weeks, 3 and 6 months postpartum, the researchers examined breastfeeding self-efficacy, along with perception of social support, and three cognitive processes (rumination, self-blame, and catastrophizing), and their impact on postpartum depression across time. They found that EPDS scores dropped between 6 weeks and 3 months postpartum, and that rumination, catastrophizing, and self-blame were related to higher depression scores. In addition, women with higher breastfeeding self-efficacy scores had lower rates of depression at all three time points. Finally, women with a higher need for support had more depression, whereas women who perceived that they had a higher level of support had significantly less depression.

Personality traits

A study from Leuven, Belgium had a sample of 403 pregnant women, and assessed their depression during each trimester pregnancy, and at 8–12 weeks, and 20–25 weeks postpartum (van Bussel et al., 2009). The researchers found that two personality traits predicted depression in pregnancy and postpartum: neuroticism, and regulator orientation. Neuroticism describes high sensitivity to stress and encompasses anxiety, fear, moodiness, worry, frustration, jealousy, and loneliness. Women high in regulator orientation fear that motherhood will change their lifestyles and identities too much, so they show more detachment during pregnancy and postpartum. The facilitator orientation was only weakly correlated with depression. These women often have high expectations for themselves as mothers, and were hypothesized as being vulnerable to depression when the reality of early motherhood does not match up with the idealized version of it. Depression was highest during pregnancy, and decreased after childbirth at both postpartum points, consistent with previous studies. Depression was measured with the EPDS and HADS-D. Both were scored as continuous variables.

A study of 277 pregnant women from the Netherlands found that neuroticism was related to postpartum depression (Verkerk et al., 2005). Introversion and neuroticism were measured at 32 weeks gestation, and depression was measured at 3, 6, and 12 months postpartum. A high neuroticism score indicates feelings of tension, emotionally lability, and insecurity. A high introversion score indicates inhibition and shyness in social interactions. Only the combination of high neuroticism and high introversion predicted depression across the first year postpartum. In contrast, a personal history of depression only predicted depression at 3 months.

Psychiatric history

Women's history of previous depression, anxiety, or PTSD can increase their risk of postpartum depression. A study in Canada ($N = 622$) found that women with a previous psychiatric history were almost four times more likely to be depressed at 8 weeks postpartum (Dennis & Ross, 2006a). Family psychiatric history was not a significant risk factor. The strongest risk factors at 8 weeks were maternal antenatal depression, maternal history of postpartum depression, and an EPDS >9 at 8 weeks. This model accounted for 42 percent of the variance in depression scores. In this sample, 45 percent reported a personal psychiatric history, and 62 percent had a close family member who had a history of psychiatric illness.

Previous psychiatric history may increase risk of depression because of a heightened inflammatory response to current stressors (Maes et al., 2001). A study of 16 women with a history of depression, and 50 without depression at 1 and 3 days postpartum, measured IL-6, sIL-6R, and sIL-1R. After delivery, IL-6, sIL-6R, and sIL-1RA were elevated in all women. As hypothesized, women with a history of depression had even greater increases in serum IL-6 and sIL-1RA in the early postpartum period than did women without a history of depression. The authors concluded that the major depression sensitized the inflammatory response system, increasing risk of subsequent depressive episodes.

Depression during pregnancy

Researchers have consistently found that women depressed during pregnancy are at very high risk for depression postpartum (Beck, 2001). In a large sample ($N = 9,028$), depression rates were highest at 32 weeks gestation and lowest at 8 months postpartum (Evans et al., 2001). In a low-income minority sample ($N = 802$), 37 percent of the women had depressive symptoms, and 7–9 percent had major depression at 3–5 weeks postpartum. Fifty percent of these women were also depressed during pregnancy (Yonkers et al., 2001).

A recent study from Australia of 5,219 postpartum women found that 15 percent of mothers reported experiencing postpartum depression with at least one child (Chojenta et al., 2016). The two strongest predictors were postpartum anxiety and depression during pregnancy. Other risk factors included history of depression, emotional distress during labor, and breastfeeding for less than 6 months.

A longitudinal study from Baltimore found rates of depression increased from the first (12 percent) and second (14 percent) trimester to be highest in the last trimester (30 percent) (Setse et al., 2009). It was 9 percent postpartum. Depression was assessed using the Center for Epidemiologic Studies-Depression, with a cutoff of ≥16.

A US nationally representative sample of 3,051 pregnant women found that 8 percent reported poor antenatal mental health (Witt et al., 2010). A history of mental health problems increased the risk 8.45 times (OR = 8.45, 95 percent CI, 6.01–11.88). Women with low social support, in poor health, or with a history of mental illness were at increased risk of mental health problems during pregnancy. However, this study had some limitations, including the vague definition of mental health problems, which makes the findings difficult to interpret. Mothers were categorized as having a "mental health problem" if they indicated that they had a mental health condition, or if they indicated that they felt "sad, blue, or anxious about something," or were in "fair" or "poor" mental health. The mothers were also asked to rate their overall mental health on a five-point scale.

In a sample of 80 women, 25 percent were depressed during pregnancy, and 16 percent were depressed at 4–5 weeks postpartum (Da Costa et al., 2000). Women who were depressed postpartum reported more emotional coping, and higher state and trait anxiety during pregnancy.

Similarly, a study from Germany of 273 healthy pregnant women found that 13 percent had elevated depressive symptoms on the Edinburgh Postnatal Depression Scale, and 8 percent with the Patient Health Questionnaire (Gawlik et al., 2013). A study from Florence, Italy of 590 pregnant women found that 22 percent had an EPDS score ≥10, and 13 percent in the postpartum period (Giardinelli et al., 2012). There were also high rates of anxiety during pregnancy: 25 percent were positive for state anxiety on the STAI. The most important risk factors include foreign nationality, conflict with family or partner, and lifetime psychiatric disorders. The risk factors for postpartum depression included depression during pregnancy, and use of reproductive technologies.

In Malawi, a study of 583 pregnant women found that the percentage of women with a current major depressive episode was 11 percent, and 21 percent had minor depression (Stewart et al., 2014). Risk factors for major depression included low social support, and intimate partner violence. Other factors associated with depressive symptoms included being unmarried, the father of the baby reacting negatively about the pregnancy, previous pregnancy or labor/delivery complications, and lower levels of education. Women who were beaten by their partners were 19 times more likely to be depressed.

In a sample of 252 mothers from India, 23 percent had postpartum depression (N = 252). Seventy-eight percent of these women were also depressed during pregnancy. Only 21 percent developed depression for the first time during the postpartum period, when they were assessed at 6 weeks postpartum. Fifty-nine percent of women depressed at 6 weeks were still depressed at 6 months postpartum (Patel et al., 2002).

Although previous episodes of depression increased the risk for depression postpartum, it is by no means inevitable. Mothers with previous episodes are at higher risk, so they should alert their caregivers during pregnancy, arrange for follow-up postpartum, and get extra help and support after their babies are born. Depending on the severity of the episode, prophylactic use of antidepressants may be appropriate as well. Recognizing risk and taking steps to counter it can often prevent a recurrence.

Disaster and postpartum mental health

A number of recent articles have addressed the issue of disaster in the pre- and postpartum periods, including the impact of terrorist attacks and natural disasters on mothers' mental health and infant distress. A recent review found that experiencing disasters during pregnancy can negatively impact fetal growth, but that they do not appear to impact gestational age (Harville et al., 2010). The amount and severity of exposure predicts maternal mental health. Not surprisingly, maternal mental health is the key factor contributing to child developmental outcomes following disasters.

In a study of 317 new mothers who survived the Sichuan earthquake, 20 percent had PTSD symptoms, and 10 percent met full criteria for PTSD. Twenty-nine percent were depressed at 8 months postpartum (Qu et al., 2012). These rates were not higher than in the general population. Consistent with the results of other studies, women with high exposure to the earthquake had significantly higher rates of PTSD and depression. Other risk factors for PTSD were low income and living on a farm. Risk factors for depression were low income, unemployment, and poor sleep quality.

Brand and colleagues recruited a sample of 98 pregnant women who had had direct exposure to 9/11, and assessed their salivary cortisol levels and PTSD symptoms (Brand et al., 2006). The mothers who developed PTSD following 9/11 had cortisol levels that were lower in the morning and evening than the women who did not develop PTSD. The lower their morning cortisol levels, the higher the mothers' ratings of infant distress and negative responses to novelty at 9 months, such as loud noises, new foods, or unfamiliar people. In addition, if mothers had PTSD, they were more likely to say that their infants had a negative response to novelty. These mothers did not rate their infants as having an overall negative temperament, just a negative response to something new. The authors described this as a possible epigenetic effect provided by trauma exposure during their pregnancies.

A study that analyzed data from birth records in the State of California in the six months following September 11 found an increase in negative birth outcomes for women with Arabic last names. The researcher did not find this effect for any other group (Lauderdale, 2006). These women were compared with women who gave birth one year earlier, including those with Arabic last names. Following 9/11, women with Arabic names were twice as likely to have low birthweight babies compared with other groups. The findings are consistent with the hypothesis that ethnicity-related stress during pregnancy increases the risk of preterm and low birthweight.

A study of mothers following Hurricane Katrina had similar findings (Tees et al., 2010). This study included prospective cohort of 288 women who gave birth in New Orleans or Baton Rogue in 2006–2007 (Hurricane Katrina occurred in 2005). Mothers reported on their experiences during the hurricane, their mental health, and their infants' temperament. Infants were identified as having "difficult" temperaments if they were in the top quartile for three or more of the subscales of the Early Infant and Toddler Temperament Questionnaire. Tees et al.'s findings indicated that hurricane exposure was not related to infant temperament, but the mothers were significantly more likely to report that their infants had difficult temperaments if they had PTSD, depression, or were high in hostility. Depression increased the risk by more than three times, measured by the EPDS ≥12. The authors noted that it was maternal mental health, not exposure to a disaster, that predicted difficult infant temperament. Black women, and women with lower education, were more likely to have had severe experiences with the hurricane (Harville et al., 2009). Severe impact on property, injury to a family member, and feeling like their life was in danger all increased the risk of PTSD and depression.

Another study with this sample compared PTSD and depression rates of pregnant women with high vs. low hurricane exposure (Xiong et al., 2010). The researchers noted that almost the entire population of New Orleans experienced severe and chronic stressors, including relocation, discontinuity in medical care, disruption of social networks, and loss, or potential loss, of lives, jobs, and property. The researchers found that

14 percent of women with high hurricane exposure had PTSD compared with 1 percent of women with low exposure. In addition, 32 percent of the women with high exposure were depressed compared with 12 percent of women with low exposure.

Unfortunately, the effects of a disaster can be long-lasting. A longitudinal study of 532 low-income mothers from New Orleans measured posttraumatic stress symptoms and psychological distress one year before Hurricane Katrina, and 7–19 months, and 43–54 months after (Paxson et al., 2010). Eighty-four percent of these mothers were African American, and 32 percent reported that they had a friend or relative who died as a result of the hurricane. Some mothers' posttraumatic stress symptoms were long-lasting, and 30 percent had high enough scores to indicate "probable mental illness" at the 43–54-month assessment. Hurricane-related home damage was especially associated with more posttraumatic stress symptoms. Higher income and social support were somewhat protective.

Donna describes how the events of September 11 influenced her during her pregnancy, and made her vulnerable to depression.

> We had a joint baby shower on September 8. September 11 was three days later. My sister was injured, and they couldn't find her for several hours. I was getting bits and pieces of information. I think my depression started then. I didn't get really bad until after delivery … I've been seeing a psychologist, sometimes twice a week. We're dealing with the disappointment with my difficult pregnancy, my birth, the guilt about not being the perfect mother, September 11. My sister had severe eye lacerations, and my dad still works down there.

Loss

Previous loss can also increase the risk of depression and takes many forms. Childhood illness and childhood abuse can also represent loss of a "normal" childhood. Childbearing loss can also increase the probability of depression during subsequent pregnancies, and after a new baby is born. Recent loss of a partner through death or divorce, or loss of a parent, can also predispose a woman to postpartum depression.

A qualitative of 28 mothers from Victoria and New South Wales, Australia indicated that "loss and frustration" were the major themes in women with postpartum depression (Highet et al., 2014). The women indicated dissatisfaction with the pregnancy and motherhood experience that included difficult pregnancies, difficulties in infant care, and conflict with their partners. The symptoms they identified included disconnection, isolation, and unhappiness. They also reported sleep disruption, impaired decision-making, and feeling overwhelmed. Their anxiety symptoms included excessive worry and impaired social functioning. Some of the mothers reported:

> Having zero enjoyment for life … nothing made me smile, and mothering made me happy.
>
> (p. 182)

> I've always been very organized, in control, all of the rest and along came this baby that threw me into utter chaos. I didn't know what I was doing. I felt like I had no control.
>
> (p. 181)

> The first eight weeks in particular was a shock. Tahlia had reflux, she was a very unsettled baby ... I was exhausted and not getting enough sleep.
>
> (p. 181)

Loss was also a theme in Beck's (2002) meta-synthesis of 18 qualitative studies of postpartum depression. She noted, "loss permeated deep into the crevices of depressed mothers' lives. It insidiously seeped into the very fiber of their beings" (p. 466). There were several types of loss that women in these studies described. The first was the loss of self. This consisted of two components: loss of who you are and loss of a former self. Women didn't know who they were after they had had their babies, and described how they had lost their sexuality, power in the family, personal space, intellectual ability and memory, and occupation. Related to this is loss of identity. This was especially an issue for women who had worked outside the home before they had their babies.

Beck (2002) also described loss of relationships. Women agonized over lost relationships with their infants or other children, partners, friends, and family. They felt depression had robbed them of the positive feelings they should have for their babies. Sometimes women described how they resented and became angry with their babies. Loss of relationships also occurred with women's older children. They suddenly became resentful of their older children's needs, and felt that their older children were "suffocating" them. Women's relationships with their partners became strained. Women admitted resenting their partners, and wishing that their partners would take the initiative to help them. On the other hand, many were ashamed that they were struggling because it meant they were inadequate, or failures as mothers. These feelings of inadequacy kept them isolated from other mothers, whom they assumed were doing a much better job than them.

The final loss Beck (2002) described was loss of voice. Mothers suffering from depression made a conscious effort to silence their own voices. They feared the reaction of others if they admitted how they had been struggling. They didn't want to burden friends or family, and feared being rejected or misunderstood. One mother described her experience as "imprisoned in my own prison" (p. 468). When they did find their voice, partners or others often silenced or rejected them, contributing further to their loss of voice.

Summary

The above-cited studies demonstrate that how a woman feels about herself, her general outlook on life, and her family history can either protect her or make her vulnerable to depression in the puerperium and beyond. Psychological factors, such as prior trauma and loss, a negative attributional style, and unrealistic expectations can all contribute to a mother's risk of depression.

Depression in pregnancy also raises some issues about how we conceptualize postpartum depression. It appears, from this research, that depression during pregnancy is at least as likely as postpartum depression. If that is the case, then it is inaccurate to consider postpartum a time of unique vulnerability. On the other hand, it might be useful to conceptualize postpartum depression in lifespan perspective—to see vulnerability to depression as occurring over the life of a woman, and that both pregnancy and postpartum are vulnerable times. On a more hopeful note, even with significant risk factors, depression is not inevitable.

It is now time to turn our attention to another psychological stressor that is, unfortunately, quite common, and that is violence against women.

Chapter 12   **Psychological risk factors II**

Violence against women

Violence against women (VAW) is an unfortunate fact of life for millions of women around the world. This too can increase the risk of depression and other perinatal mood disorders. Mothers who have a history of adverse childhood experiences (ACEs), or a currently abusive partner, are at increased the risk of depression in the perinatal period.

Adverse childhood experiences

Adverse childhood experiences increase the risk of depression across the lifespan, including the perinatal period. A recent review of 43 studies found that women abused as children, or by their partners, had more lifetime depression, and more depression during pregnancy and postpartum (Alvarez-Segura et al., 2014). If women experienced both childhood abuse and partner violence, they had more severe depression and it lasted longer. In a study from New York, 884 women were followed from their first prenatal visit to 6 weeks postpartum (Silverman & Loudon, 2010). The strongest predictors of postpartum depression were a history of physical or sexual abuse that occurred during pregnancy, a history of psychiatric disorders, and a psychiatric diagnosis at the first prenatal visit.

A study of 332 postpartum women in Toronto found that 14 percent reported a history of child sexual abuse, 7 percent reported child physical abuse, 13 percent reported adult sexual abuse, 7 percent reported adult physical abuse, and 30 percent reported adult emotional abuse (Ansara et al., 2005). In a study of 79 pregnant and parenting adolescents (Gilson & Lancaster, 2008), 20 percent reported either physical or sexual abuse. In their study, there was not a higher rate of depression or anxiety during pregnancy. However, by 6 weeks postpartum, those who had been physically abused, or both physically and sexually abused, had higher rates of depression and anxiety. By 6 months, there was significantly more depression and anxiety for women who had been physically abused, or both sexually or physically abused, than for their non-abused counterparts.

A study that included two distinct samples found a relationship between abuse and prenatal depression with an EPDS score ≥ 13 (Rich-Edwards et al., 2011). One of the samples was from an affluent suburb ($n = 1,509$), and the other from an urban population ($n = 2,128$). In the urban sample, 54 percent reported physical abuse and 20 percent reported sexual abuse. In the suburban sample, 42 percent reported physical abuse and 13 percent reported sexual abuse. Seventy-five percent of the women who reported sexual abuse also reported physical abuse. Women with a history of abuse had a 63 percent increased odds of depression during pregnancy. The odds were higher if women were abused as adults. Socioeconomic status did not alter the results.

Maternal psychosocial adversity led to shorter gestation length in a study from the Danish National Birth Cohort (N = 78,017) (Tegethoff et al., 2010). The researchers found that both life and emotional stress decreased gestation length. Interestingly, psychosocial stress increased infant birthweight, abdominal circumference, and head circumference, controlling for length of gestation. The authors noted that their findings indicate that the fetoplacental–maternal unit can possibly regulate fetal growth in response to psychosocial adversities. Insulin is one possible mechanism regulating fetal growth in response to stress.

Seng et al.'s (2013) longitudinal study prospectively examined the impact of PTSD in pregnancy and its relationship to postpartum depression. Their study included 566 mothers divided into three groups: PTSD+, trauma-exposed resilient, and non-trauma-exposed. The women were interviewed at 28 weeks gestation, and 6 weeks postpartum. The results indicated that PTSD in pregnancy, alone or with comorbid depression, was associated with postpartum depression. Further, postpartum depression, alone or with PTSD, impaired bonding. If women reported higher quality of life, there were better outcomes. However, dissociation during labor was associated with worse outcomes. Child maltreatment was the largest risk factor for developing PTSD in pregnancy. They noted that there is a cycle of vulnerability, and the possibility of transmission of interpersonal violence in the childbearing year.

There is also some evidence that mothers who have been abused may pass along some of the changes to the HPA axis through their pregnancies. A study of 126 mothers, 30 percent of whom had been physically or sexually abused as children, tested cortisol levels for the women and their babies (Brand et al., 2010). The mothers and infants were stressed through a series of procedures in the lab. The abused mothers had steeper declines in cortisol, and the infants had lower baseline cortisol. Current maternal depression, PTSD, or life stressors were significantly related to cortisol changes. If a mother had a history of abuse, and currently had PTSD, there were greater changes in cortisol for her infant.

A study of 44 pregnant women explored the impact of child maltreatment on women's experiences of pregnancy, and in the first year postpartum (Lang et al., 2006). They found that mothers' history of sexual abuse and emotional neglect were related to psychopathology during pregnancy. Physical abuse and neglect predicted poorer maternal outcomes at 1 year postpartum.

In a sample of 116 pregnant teens, a history of childhood abuse, and ever having had an alcoholic drink, both predicted depression in pregnancy (Tzilos et al., 2012). Fifty-three percent of the sample reported a history of physical or sexual abuse. History of abuse remained a significant predictor of depression even after adjusting history of depression, and for drug and alcohol abuse.

A study of 559 pregnant women in Israel found that 27 percent reported childhood sexual abuse (CSA; Lev-Wiesel & Daphna-Tekoah, 2007). Women in the sexual abuse group also reported more miscarriages than women with no history of abuse. Forty percent of women in the CSA group had also experienced other types of trauma. The abused women had significantly higher levels of PTSD, but not depression. Women who experienced sexual abuse, and other types of trauma, had more symptoms of depression than women who experienced sexual abuse alone.

Another study by these same researchers of 837 women compared women with a history of CSA to those who had experienced other types of trauma (Lev-Wiesel et al., 2009). The women were assessed mid-pregnancy, and at 2 and 6 months postpartum. The initial sample was 1,586 women, 323 of whom had been sexually abused, 868 who experienced at least one traumatic event, and 152 with no trauma history. They found that child sexual abuse increased women's intrusion and arousal symptoms after birth, whereas other types of trauma had no impact on PTSD scores. CSA women had more dissociation before and after birth, and birth-related PTSD was higher for the CSA group. The authors did not feel, however, that their findings demonstrated that birth retraumatizes women. Rather, they concluded that child sexual abuse had a greater negative effect than other traumas on a population of pregnant women.

A study in the Netherlands examined the impact of CSA on birth (van der Hulst et al., 2006). This study included 625 women with low-risk pregnancies. Of these women, 11 percent had a history of sexual abuse. Compared to the non-abused women, the abuse survivors had more emotional distress, internal beliefs about their health, and pelvic pain. The abused women were more likely to smoke and to have lower incomes. The sexually abused women also reported higher levels of autonomy, and, interestingly, had significantly *lower* rates of episiotomies. Rates of pharmacologic pain relief and cesarean births were similar between the abused and non-abused groups. The authors also found no significant difference in rates of major birth-related obstetric technical interventions, but there were trends towards more assisted deliveries, and higher frequencies of augmentation among the abuse survivors.

A history of childhood abuse increased the risk for intimate partner violence in one study from Lima, Peru (Barrios et al., 2015). This study included 1,556 pregnant women. A stunning 70 percent of the women had been physically or sexually abused as children. The abuse survivors had poorer overall health than women who were not abused. Women who experienced either physical or sexual abuse had more than twice the risk of lifetime IPV. The abuse survivors had seven times the risk of lifetime IPV, and triple the risk of IPV that occurred in the past year. Childhood abuse doubled the risk of antenatal depression, except for women who experienced sexual abuse alone. That group had no increased risk of depression, contrary to previous findings.

Val describes how her past history of sexual abuse related to her postpartum depression, and how it manifested in obsessive thoughts of harming her twin babies.

> My depression started three days after birth. It came on very suddenly. My husband was coming to the hospital. We were going to give the babies a bath. As we were giving [my daughter] a bath, I was suddenly afraid that I might abuse her. I had been sexually abused as a child. I didn't tell anyone until the next day … It started with "Oh my God. I was abused. I could abuse them." Then it was more general. Everything was a danger. Everything could hurt the kids … I can't tell you how surprised I was. I haven't done anything to hurt the kids. I first visualized my son being thrown into the fire. Then it was me throwing him in. I worried about plastic. I'd have thoughts of smothering the kids with pillows. There were certain rooms in the house I couldn't even go in. I couldn't drink coffee. I'd have thoughts of pouring it on the kids. Through all of this I never neglected my children's needs, no matter how difficult … No one ever questioned that I would hurt the kids. I'm the only one. I feel it could be from the sexual abuse. I obsess

and worry about things. I've had times and traumatic events that I've worried about before, but it's always been just me.

Intimate partner violence

All around the world, women are beaten and raped by their intimate partners. The Centers for Disease Control and Prevention estimates that 4.8 million women are beaten by their partners each year in the US (Centers for Disease Control and Prevention, 2006). Women are also vulnerable to IPV in the perinatal period. Neither pregnancy nor the postpartum period offers protection from abuse, as the studies below indicate, and this too increases mothers' risk of depression. In a recent review, IPV was the strongest predictor of depression in the perinatal period (Alvarez-Segura et al., 2014).

Three recent, large, population-based studies found that many women are beaten during pregnancy and the postpartum period, but no clear pattern emerged about which was the highest-risk time. In a Chinese study that included 32 communities, 9 percent of women were beaten before pregnancy, 4 percent during pregnancy, and 7 percent after pregnancy (Guo et al., 2004). In North Carolina, 7 percent were beaten before pregnancy, 6 percent during pregnancy, and 3 percent postpartum (N = 2,648) (Martin et al., 2001). Finally, in Bristol, Avon, UK (N = 7,591), 5 percent were beaten during pregnancy, and 11 percent postpartum (Bowen et al., 2005). In this sample, the more social adversities a woman reported during pregnancy, the more likely they were to be victimized postpartum. Women who experienced one social adversity during pregnancy were 2.73 times more likely to report physical victimization. Women who reported five or more social adversities were 15 times more likely to report postpartum victimization.

A study of Latina women in the US included 118 women with no history of IPV, and 92 women who had experienced IPV (Valentine et al., 2011). The women were assessed during pregnancy, and at 3, 7, and 13 months postpartum using the BDI. Forty-four percent met criteria for depression at one or more of the assessment points. The results revealed that in multivariate analyses, the two strongest predictors of postpartum depression were depression in pregnancy and recent IPV. They found that recent IPV was a stronger predictor of postpartum depression than prenatal depression, which has traditionally been one of the strongest. Recent IPV increased the risk of postpartum depression by over five times compared to three and a half times increased risk for prenatal depression.

A study of 774 migrant women in Canada found that 8 percent experienced violence associated with their pregnancies (Stewart et al., 2012). The women who were beaten had significantly higher rates of depression, anxiety, somatization, and PTSD. They reported more pain of all types, and were more likely to soak through three or more pads in 24 hours at 1 week postpartum. In addition, they reported significantly fewer health behaviors during their pregnancy. They started prenatal care after 3 months gestation, did not have up-to-date vaccinations, and did not take folic acid before conception. The women were less likely to use contraceptives after the birth, more likely to have had a miscarriage, and less likely to have social support. There was no difference in the health of their infants, however, contrary to some earlier findings.

A recent review of 67 published research articles sought to estimate the prevalence of violence in the perinatal period, and the prevalence of perinatal mood disorders (Howard et al., 2013). The results indicated that violence during pregnancy increased the risk of postpartum depression by three times. It also increased the risk of PTSD, and prenatal and postpartum anxiety. In addition, antenatal depression also results in a woman being 3–5 times more likely to experience domestic violence. There was no link between domestic violence in pregnancy and postpartum psychosis.

A study of 1,127 women from Canada found that women who were refugees or asylum-seekers were more likely to experience violence during their pregnancies than were immigrants, or women born in Canada (Gagnon & Stewart, 2014). They found that some of these women actually had lower rates of depression on the EPDS. Therefore, the researchers conducted in-depth interviews of 10 mothers. All were migrants. All reported being beaten or raped during their pregnancies. They described three major factors that aided in their resiliency. The first was internal psychological resources, such as self-esteem, self-efficacy, hope, and optimism. The second resiliency factor was social support from family, friends, church, work, or school. Finally, systemic factors made a difference. These included daycare, healthcare (physical and mental), legal services, language lessons, and social services. Interestingly, one of the hindrances to resilience that the women mentioned was "being in love." Other hindrances included repeating their stories to various social service agencies, further violence, and trying to be strong.

A study of 570 teen mothers showed the continuity between antenatal and postpartum violence. The prevalence of IPV was highest at 3 months postpartum (21 percent), and lowest at 24 months (13 percent). Seventy-five percent of mothers beaten during pregnancy were also beaten during their first 2 years postpartum. And 78 percent of women who experienced IPV at 3 months postpartum had not reported IPV during their pregnancies (Harrykissoon et al., 2002).

Lutz (2005) also described the continuity between past and present violence in her qualitative study of 12 women who were survivors of IPV during at least one childbearing cycle. Among these women, depression, PTSD, and anxiety were common. The study participants reported many types of violence during their lives: childhood physical, emotional, and sexual abuse; neglect; parental intimate partner violence and substance abuse; current intimate partner violence; adult sexual assault; and community violence. The women experienced each exposure to violence as influencing and flowing into the next. They viewed IPV during the childbearing year as just part of the continuum of abusive experiences in their lives.

In a sample of rural women, Ellis and colleagues (2008) found that women who were experiencing partner violence sought care for their babies more often in the first 6 weeks postpartum, and had significantly higher levels of stress, than did non-abused women. There was no difference between the groups in the type of healthcare consultations they sought. Not surprisingly, the abused women were also more depressed, and had less support. An important intervention that care providers can offer is screening for partner violence at all prenatal and postpartum visits.

Abuse and the inflammatory response

Experiencing violence increases the inflammatory response, and this can also increase the risk of depression. Previous child maltreatment was related to high C-reactive protein levels when they were assessed 20 years later (Danese et al., 2007). The participants ($N = 1,037$) were part of the Dunedin Multidisciplinary Health and Development Study, a birth-cohort study of health behavior in New Zealand. Researchers assessed the participants every 2–3 years throughout childhood, and every 5–6 years through age 32. The impact of child maltreatment on inflammation was independent of other factors that could have accounted for the findings, such as co-occurring life stresses in adulthood, early life risks, or adult health or health behavior. It was a dose–response effect: the more severe the abuse, the more severe the inflammation.

A similar finding resulted from a study of women abused by intimate partners. In this study, 62 women who had had abusive partners 8–11 years previously had significantly higher interferon-gamma (IFN-γ) levels than did non-abused women (Woods et al., 2005). The women also had high rates of depression (52 percent) and PTSD (39 percent). Even several years after their abuse had ended, these women were still manifesting significant physical symptomatology. Inflammation was also found to be elevated in a study of 15 women who had been raped 24–72 hours after their assault, compared with 16 women who had not been sexually assaulted. Sexually assaulted women had higher ACTH, C-reactive protein, IL-6, IL-10, IFN-γ than had women in the non-assaulted group (Groer et al., 2006).

Abuse history and parenting difficulties

Women who have been abused as children or adults may also have difficulties parenting, and problematic relationships with their children. In one study, women with a history of CSA were more anxious about the intimate aspects of caring for their own babies, including activities such as diapering. These mothers were more worried that their normal parenting behaviors were inappropriate—or that others would see them that way. Finally, they reported more parenting stress than did their non-abused counterparts (Douglas, 2000). This lack of confidence eroded the mothers' mental health, increasing their risk for depression.

Dubowitz and colleagues (2001) found that when mothers have experienced multiple types of abuse, they were more likely to be depressed. They also used harsher discipline, and had more problems with their children ($N = 419$). Mothers abused as children and as adults, or who were both physically and sexually abused as children, had worse outcomes than mothers who experienced only one type of abuse. Mothers' depression and harsh parenting were associated with internalizing and externalizing behavior problems in their children. The authors speculated that mothers who have been victimized may be less attentive to their children, and less emotionally available. These mothers may also have less tolerance for the day-to-day stresses of parenting, and may be more inclined to view their children's behaviors as problematic. The authors concluded that a mother's history of victimization appears to be highly prevalent in high-risk samples. More than half of the mothers in their sample had been physically or sexually victimized at some time, and half of the mothers victimized during childhood or adolescence were revictimized as adults.

A study of primiparous women included 107 women with a history of CSA and 156 comparison mothers (Schuetze & Das Eiden, 2005). The mothers were re-interviewed when their babies were 2–4 years of age. CSA was associated with both maternal depression, and higher rates of partner violence. CSA women also had higher rates of parenting difficulties, but these disappeared when the researchers accounted for depression and partner violence.

A study comparing 670 non-abusing families with 166 abusive families found similar results (Gracia & Musitu, 2003). The families in this sample were Colombian and Spanish. The authors found that in both cultures, abusive parents showed lower levels of community integration, participation in social activities, and use of formal and informal organizations than parents who were providing adequate care for their children. The abusive parents tended to be more socially isolated and negative in their attitudes towards their communities and neighborhoods.

A qualitative study of 32 mothers from Canada described the difficult process that trauma survivors go through as they become mothers (Berman et al., 2014). The researchers described this process as "laboring to mother." When asked if their past traumatic experiences could affect their ability to mother, the women all agreed that it would, and they went through a process of healing so that it would not spill over into their relationship with their children. They described "forgetting and forgiving," and the importance of growing from their pain, letting go of anger, and learning from the past. Without this, they could not be the mothers they wanted to be. Other women deliberately contained their trauma so that it did not affect other areas of their lives, and so they could protect their babies. Unfortunately, some of the women described using a range of harmful coping behaviors that included substance abuse, self-harm, and eating disorders. Even with difficulties and challenges, many of the women were determined to create stability for them and their families. They wanted an idealized version of their families that was so different from their family of origin. Many expressed fierce determination to not be like their mothers. Their idealized version of what they would provide for their children was often very different from the lived reality of what they could provide. Although difficult, many of the women in the study demonstrated enormous personal strength and resourcefulness.

Summary

Abuse survivors have a higher lifetime risk for depression than the general population. Therefore, we should not be surprised when they are at increased risk during the postpartum period. As I described with previous psychiatric illness, past abuse is a risk factor for depression, but depression is not inevitable. It can be helpful for mothers to check in with their care providers periodically, as well as any mental health providers that they have seen in the past. You might also want to have a list of referral sources ready for mothers who are dealing with past abuse for the first time in the postpartum period.

Chapter 13   **Social risk factors**

Women do not become mothers in a vacuum. They live in families, extended families, cultures, and societies. At each of these levels of social connection, mothers can be protected from, or made more vulnerable to, depression. The social factors related to depression include the amount of help she has with her baby and other children; the amount of emotional support she receives from her partner and others around her; her socioeconomic and immigration status; and her exposure to stressful life events. Research on these social risk factors is described below.

Immigration

Recent studies have identified that immigrant women are a group at very high risk for pre- and postpartum depression. For example, a recent iterative review of eight studies notes that up to 42 percent of immigrant, asylum-seeking, and refugee women had postpartum depression compared with 10–15 percent of native-born women (Collins et al., 2011). Stressful life events prior to or during their pregnancies were common risk factors for depression. For refugee women, these events could also include life-threatening events, such as violent death of family members or sexual violation, and leaving behind other children in their home countries. Even under good circumstances, navigating a new country, and possibly new language, culture, and customs can be highly stressful. Migrating may also mean that they are separated from support that would have been available in their home countries. The authors recommended that healthcare providers should regard all recent immigrant women as at high risk for postpartum depression.

A more recent review of 24 studies had a more conservative estimate of postpartum depression (Falah-Hassani et al., 2015). Falah-Hassani and colleague pooled the results from 18 studies ($N = 13,749$ women). They found that the rate of postpartum depression in immigrant women was 20 percent, and that immigrant women were twice as likely to experience postpartum depressive symptoms compared with non-immigrant women. Risk factors included shorter length of residence, lower level of support, poorer marital adjustment, and insufficient income.

In a population study of 736,988 women who were classified as native Danes, or first- or second-generation immigrants, found that first- and second-generation immigrants had a higher rate of treatment for depression during pregnancy and in the postpartum period (Munk-Olsen et al., 2010). Although there was a higher rate, the rates were overall quite low: only 504 first-generation and 242 second-generation immigrants were identified as having received either in-patient or out-patient treatment for depression and other psychiatric conditions (anxiety or schizophrenia) during pregnancy or postpartum.

A study from Ontario, Canada included 519 immigrant women who were part of a prospective cohort study that examined the predictors of depression in the first post-partum year (Ganann et al., 2016). The women were assessed at 6 weeks, 6 months, and 1 year postpartum. When the cutoff on the EPDS was ≥12, the rates of postpartum depression (PPD) were 8–10 percent at all time points. Lowering the cutoff to ≥9 doubled the rate. The factors that predicted depression were living in Canada ≤2 years; perceiving their pre-pregnancy health as good, fair, or poor; pregnancy complications; perception of poor health since delivery; and previous depression. Low level of support was also a factor. In addition, living in communities with a high prevalence of immigrants and low income was also associated with PPD. Surprisingly, the researchers did not ask about previous sexual assault or loss of family members (especially violent deaths) in their home countries.

A study from Montreal considered the role of violence in depression in pregnant immigrant women (Miszkurka et al., 2012). This study included 5,162 pregnant women, 1,400 of whom were born outside Canada. They found that 15 percent reported IPV, and IPV happened more frequently among the poorest pregnant women. There were strong associations between more than one episode of depression and abuse, and IPV and depression. The authors concluded that violence against pregnant women was not rare in Canada, and when it occurred, it increased the risk of depression. The combination of being an immigrant, and being abused more than once, increased the risk of depression by seven times. In comparison, for native-born, Canadian women, being abused more than once increased the risk of depression by 4.78 times.

Acculturation

Acculturation refers to the cultural adaptation people must experience when they immigrate to a new country, often due to fleeing a war or other political situation that makes life in their home country untenable. Not surprisingly, degree of acculturation is specifically related to mental health. Some aspects of acculturation include ability to perform adequate skills in the new country (such as learning the language or how to navigate essential systems, such as housing); preservation of the original culture; social integration into the new society; the moral attitudes of the new country; and loss feelings concerning the country of birth and people with the same cultural background (Knipscheer & Kleber, 2006).

Ahmed and colleagues interviewed ten immigrant new mothers with a score ≥10 on the EPDS at 12–18 months postpartum (Ahmed et al., 2008). Many of the women in this group attributed their depression to social isolation, physical changes, feeling overwhelmed, and financial worries. Some of the barriers these mothers encountered to receiving care included stigma, embarrassment, language, fear of being labeled unfit, and staff attitudes. Some of the factors that aided in their recovery included getting out of the house; getting support from friends, family, and community support groups; and personal psychological adjustment.

In a sample of Vietnamese and Hmong women living in the US ($N = 30$), 43 percent were clinically depressed or anxious. These rates were higher than in other samples, with less-acculturated mothers having the highest rates. Particularly disturbing was that one-third had contemplated suicide in the past week. On a more hopeful note, the author noted that even with high levels of depression and anxiety, these mothers were still responsive to their babies (Foss, 2001).

In a multifactorial model, Dennis and colleagues (2004) found that stressful life events, including immigration in the past five years, predicted depressive symptoms at 1 week postpartum. Stress-related factors included number of life events during the previous 12 months, mothers' dissatisfaction with their job, substance abuse, and family violence. Other predictors included history of non-postpartum depression, lack of perceived support, lack of readiness for hospital discharge, dissatisfaction with their infant feeding method, and pregnancy-induced hypertension. Their study included 594 mothers in Vancouver, British Columbia. Mothers with an EPDS score of ≥9 were considered to have depressive symptomatology. The percentages ranged from 29 percent at 1 week postpartum to 20 percent at 8 weeks. Recent immigrants had almost five times the rate of depression.

Not all studies have shown an effect of acculturation, however. In a study of Hispanic mothers, Beck et al. (2005) explored the relationship between acculturation and postpartum depressive symptoms among Hispanic subgroups. Data were collected in two locations: Connecticut ($N = 377$) and Texas ($N = 150$). Puerto Rican mothers showed more acculturation than mothers of Mexican or other Hispanic origin. Beck et al. found no consistent relationship between acculturation, postpartum depressive symptomatology, and diagnoses of postpartum depression. The two significant predictors of depression were Puerto Rican ethnicity and cesarean delivery. The Puerto Rican mothers were actually more acculturated, but were also younger, had more children, bottle-fed more, and were more likely to be single. The findings were limited in that language was the main measure of acculturation. Further, they noted that Hispanics are a heterogeneous group, and should not be treated as all the same.

Similarly, a study of 470 Hispanic women were recruited at 22–24 weeks gestation from community clinics (Ruiz et al., 2012). The authors noted that rates of preterm birth have increased by 10 percent among Hispanics, and the rate is related to their level of acculturation into US culture. Overall, acculturation has been associated with poorer health outcomes among Hispanics. Using a psychoneuroimmunology framework, they noted that depression could impact the estriol/progesterone balance, which maintains pregnancy. The researchers measured acculturation, depression by CES-D, serum estriol and progesterone, and preterm birth. They discovered that women born in the US, not immigrants, had the highest rates of depression. Acculturation predicted estriol/progesterone (E/P) ratio. The interaction of depression with E/P ratio predicted preterm birth.

Maternal age

Research on the relationship between postpartum depression and maternal age has yielded inconsistent results; mothers on the high and low ends of the age spectrum have the highest risk for depression. One recent prospective study of 901 women found that women under the age of 20 were at high risk for PPD (Webster et al., 2000b). The high-risk mothers were also significantly more likely to be unmarried and primiparous. Another study of 465 women found that women ages 20–24, *or* 30 and older, were significantly more likely to be depressed at 4 months postpartum (Chaudron et al., 2001). Adolescent mothers reported significantly lower self-esteem, more parenting stress, more child abuse potential, and a poorer quality of home environment than did mothers who were not adolescents in another study. While this study did not address depression, it does demonstrate that the younger mothers are more prone to risk factors for depression (Andreozzi et al., 2002). In a US sample ($N = 2,592$), Mirowsky and Ross (2002) compared three groups of young adults: non-parents, those who became parents before age 23, and those who became parents after age 23. They found that respondents who were younger than age 23 at first birth reported more depression than did non-parents. Non-parents were more depressed than were respondents whose first birth was after age 23. Women who had their babies at age 30 had the lowest levels of depression.

Mothers at either end of the age spectrum are vulnerable to depression. Young mothers may be more at risk for depression because they have a higher likelihood of single marital status, low SES, and possible past abuse (reflected in teen-mother status, and/or earlier age of consensual sexual activity). Older mothers may have been through infertility assessments, high-risk pregnancies, and possible pregnancy losses. They may have had multiples as a result of fertility treatments. In addition, older mothers have often attained a higher education level, and react with shock when mothering is difficult and overwhelming. These mothers often feel that they cannot "complain" because they went to such great lengths to become pregnant.

Socioeconomic status

Poverty also increases the likelihood of depression, and increases the difficulties new mothers experience because it limits support, access to medical care, and access to community resources. Poor mothers often face additional stresses as they deal with uncertain income, dangerous housing or neighborhoods, and the negative effects of being at the bottom of the social strata. The connection between poverty and depression has been found in both American samples and samples outside the US.

US samples

In a study of 114 Hispanic and African American women with low-risk pregnancies, 51 percent were depressed. The women's depression scores correlated to other health-related variables including bodily pain, general health, and emotional and physical functioning. Yonkers et al. (2001) found that 37 percent had depressive symptoms of a low-income minority sample, and 7–9 percent met criteria for major depression (McKee et al., 2001). In the National Maternal Health Survey ($N = 7,537$), a stratified nationally representative sample of births in 1988, 24 percent were depressed when their babies were approximately 17 months old. This study sampled from 48 states, the District of Columbia, and New York City. Blacks, and mothers of low and very low birthweight babies were oversampled, as were low-income mothers (McLennan & Kotelchuck, 2000; McLennan et al., 2001). Three years later, 17 percent were depressed, and 36 percent of those with elevated depression scores at Time 1 had elevated depression scores at Time 2 (McLennan et al., 2001).

Even within the group of poor mothers, there is variation. In a study of 191 low-income women (Ritter et al., 2000), women with a higher relative income, who had social support and higher self-esteem, had lower levels of depression. Another recent study of 509 postpartum teens found that none of the demographic factors they included were related to depression severity (Koleva & Stuart, 2014). These included age, week of pregnancy, years of education, income, number of children, marital status, living with a partner, head of household status, annual income <$20,000, and employment.

A recent program, MOMCare, was designed to address depression care in low-income, ethnic-minority women (Grote et al., 2015). This was a collaborative program that grew out of feedback obtained from a previous randomized trial of interpersonal psychotherapy for perinatal depression. It was designed to address barriers related to poverty and race/ethnicity. Patients were screened during pregnancy and approached to participate in the study if they screened positive for depression (PHQ-9 ≥10) and/or had a diagnosis of major depression on the MINI. The researchers excluded patients with substance abuse, schizophrenia or bipolar disorder, severe partner violence, multiple suicide attempts, or currently seeing a psychiatrist or psychologist. One hundred sixty-four women were randomized to either intensive maternity care for patients who screened positive for depression (longer and more frequent maternity visits) or with an add-on of MOMCare, specifically designed to provide depression-care management. The MOMCare intervention yielded a small but significant benefit. It improved depression severity and remission rates over the study period. It also improved PTSD severity and generalized anxiety. Most of the women had histories of childhood trauma and significant life stresses. The MOMCare program improved access and adherence to evidence-based care for low-income pregnant and postpartum women.

International studies

Low SES is a risk factor for depression around the world. In a study of 4,879 women, who were part of a longitudinal study of women from the first year postpartum to when their children were ages 6–7, 16 percent had persistently high symptoms of depression (Giallo et al., 2014). These symptoms started in the postpartum period and worsened over time. Several risk factors associated with SES were related to high symptoms: young maternal age, being from a non-English-speaking family, or not completing high school. In addition, history of depression, antidepressant use during pregnancy, child development problems, low parenting self-efficacy, poor quality of relationships, and stressful life events. History of depression was the strongest predictor overall.

Patel et al. (2002) noted that depression is common in developing countries, where there is often a vicious cycle of poverty, depression, and disability for women. In a sample from India, economic deprivation and a poor marital relationship were both important risk factors in the development of postpartum depression, and its continuing on past 6 months postpartum (Patel et al., 2002). Other poverty-related variables, such as hunger and low education, were also associated with depression. This entire sample was low-income. Even so, relative poverty made a difference. Similarly, in a sample of 257 Turkish women, living in a shanty was one predictor of depression (Danaci et al., 2002). In an Irish sample from a disadvantaged neighborhood, 28 percent of 377 women were depressed when contacted a year after birth. The four risk factors associated with their depression were lower age, lack of a confidant, previous miscarriage, and previous treatment for depression (Cryan et al., 2001).

Debt is one aspect of poverty that has been specifically related to depression. In a longitudinal study of 271 families with young children, worry about debt was the strongest predictor of depression in mothers at the initial and follow-up contacts (Reading &

Reynolds, 2001). Indeed, worrying about debt predicted depression 6 months later. Other economic factors associated with depression included overall family income, not being a homeowner, and lack of access to a car.

Although poverty is a risk factor, and depression occurs in low-income communities, we should not assume that all low-income populations have higher levels of depression. Indeed, as I'll describe in subsequent sections, there are populations with much lower incomes that are doing some very important things in terms of protecting new mothers. Even within a low-income population, higher relative income, social support, and high self-esteem buffer the effects of poverty.

Maternity leave and employment

Maternity leave and decisions mothers make about returning to work can also influence depression. During pregnancy, job strain was related to depression in a sample of 300 Thai women (Sanguanklin et al., 2014). The strength of this relationship was related to two types of coping strategies: social support, and wishful thinking. Family support reduced psychological distress in these mothers.

A prospective study of 817 employed mothers in Minnesota assessed women at 5 and 11 weeks (Dagher et al., 2009). Using hierarchical linear regression, they found that higher EPDS scores were associated with higher psychological demands, lower schedule autonomy, and lower perceived control over work and family. The prevalence of postpartum depression in this sample was 5 percent at 11 weeks postpartum. They found that women with demanding jobs, with little control over their schedules, had more depressive symptoms.

A Canadian study of 447 mothers examined the relationship between employment status and depressive symptoms at 6 months postpartum (des Rivieres-Pigeon et al., 2001). The authors found that women on maternity leave, or women who were employed, had the lowest levels of depression. Women home full-time were more likely to report a lack of social support, and to have an unwanted or mistimed pregnancy.

Women who have control over when (or if) they return to work have the lowest levels of depression. However, other psychosocial variables, such as previous depression and lack of social support, continue to have an influence. In the final section of this chapter, I describe the most influential of the social factors—social support.

Social support

> This was the first grandchild on my side. I thought everyone would come to see me. My mom did, but only after I called and asked her to come. My dad came the next day, but only for the day ... I was very isolated after the baby. I had no friends with babies. It was hard ... I thought my family would come and everyone would hold the baby. Everyone came to my house at Christmas and they spent six hours in the basement playing video games. I was really hurt by that. Nobody would help me. I've really never said anything. Maybe it would have been better if I had said something. [DeeDee]

Of the social factors considered, far and away the most influential factor is a woman's level of social support. As the research on non-postpartum depression has repeatedly demonstrated, lack of social support is related to depression. This is especially true when women are faced with stressful life events. Social support is also related to many of the factors described in the previous chapters. It increases self-esteem and self-efficacy, acts as a buffer when a woman is faced with a temperamentally difficult child, can alter a woman's attributional style, and even lower her inflammation levels (Runsten et al., 2014). Any effort to prevent postpartum depression must include a strong component of social support. The social-support literature has included general support, partner support, and the impact of the social network.

Types of support

Social support is usually divided into two main types: emotional, and instrumental. Emotional support includes love, support, empathy, and encouragement. It lets the person know that she is valuable. It includes talking over concerns and giving positive feedback. Instrumental support includes supplying assistance with responsibilities and problems, and offering practical help with tasks such as chores and babysitting. Support can be further divided into received support (what she actually gets) and perceived support (belief that support is available). Perceived support is usually more strongly related to mental health (Reid & Taylor, 2015).

General support

Social support helps prevent depression across the social strata. A study of 123 women at 2 weeks postpartum found that social support had a significant effect on depressive symptoms, functional status, and infant care, but did not moderate the effect of adverse birth events on these same outcomes (Hunker et al., 2009). In a study of 191 low-income women, Ritter et al. (2000) found that women with good social support were less likely to become depressed. Moreover, women who had high levels of support were more likely to have high levels of self-esteem. Joanne describes this reaction from most of her friends, but noted that one friend continued to reach out to her.

> I was usually an outgoing person, but I didn't have the energy to relate to others. My friends didn't know what to do. They thought I had had a nervous break-down. Many stayed away. Even now, many are surprised that I can still function. I had one friend who was very supportive and loving continually, even though she didn't understand. She brought meals, wrote little notes. She made no demands on my recovery. My mother-in-law and husband were helpful during that time too.

In a prospective hospital-based study, Webster and colleagues (2000b) found that low social support was strongly related to depression at 16 weeks postpartum. Several types of support were specifically related to depression including low support from friends and family, and feeling unloved by their partners. Fifty-one percent of the depressed women had a score of 25 or below on the Maternity Social Support Scale, while only 32 percent of the non-depressed women had a comparable score.

In another study, Webster et al. (2000) found that social support was related to both depression and physical health. Women with low support during pregnancy reported poorer health during pregnancy and postpartum. They were more likely to delay seeking prenatal care, but to seek medical care more frequently once they did, and they were more likely to be depressed after the baby was born.

An Australian study of 247 women (Haslam et al., 2006) found lower rates of PPD in women who had emotionally supportive parents and high self-efficacy. Mothers were assessed in their last trimester of pregnancy, and at 4 weeks postpartum. Surprisingly, partner support was not related to PPD. The authors hypothesized that support from women's parents likely increased mothers' sense of competence and self-efficacy in caring for their new babies. In addition, support from parents may have been more specific than partner support to the needs of new mothers.

A qualitative study of 41 Canadian mothers found that social support was important for women's recovery from postpartum depression (Letourneau et al., 2007). In this study, mothers identified two types of support that were most helpful: instrumental support (e.g., help with household chores) and informational support (e.g., information about PPD). Affirmation support was more helpful when it came from other mothers who had been depressed. Mothers also identified partners, friends, family, other mothers, and healthcare providers as important sources of support. The mothers in this study indicated that they preferred one-on-one to group or telephone support, especially in the beginning. However, once mothers started to recover, they found that group support was helpful.

A study of 344 pregnant women found that 23 mothers screened positive for moderate to severe anxiety (Mann et al., 2008a). Religiosity and social support were significantly associated with lower anxiety, whereas a history of psychiatric disorders was associated with a higher risk. Among the specific factors were self-rated religiosity, self-rated spirituality, and participation in religious activities. In another study with this same population, Mann et al. (2008b) found that women who participated in organized religious activities were markedly less likely to report depressive symptoms (EPDS ≥13). This finding was true even after controlling for the effects of social support and baseline depression scores. Religious attendance may have had a stress-buffering effect that specifically helps women as they make the transition to new motherhood.

A recent study sought to examine why support is helpful in terms of preventing postpartum depression (Reid & Taylor, 2015). They examined whether support directly impacts the risk for PPD, or indirectly impacts it by mediating the harmful effects of stressors. Data were from the Fragile Families and Child Well-being Study, a study of 4,900 births from 75 US hospitals. Life stress increased risk for PPD, while partner, friend, and family support lowered risk for all women regardless of family type. Social support did not reduce the effects of stress, contrary to their hypothesis. In other words, social support protects maternal mental health, and lowers the risk of depression, but it is not enough to protect against the harmful effects of stress. Further, the relationship between PPD and social support differs based on family type. For disadvantaged mothers, support is particularly important, as most of these mothers face significant life stress. Unfortunately, stress can erode the positive effects of support. The researchers suggested that clinicians explore possible ways to mitigate stress because it is a substantial risk factor for depression, and social support alone is not enough to govern its harmful effects.

Partner support

Partners are key sources of social support. Several studies have found that when that partner support is not available, mothers are more likely to be depressed. A survey of

396 mothers in Canada found that lack of partner support was significantly related to depressive symptoms (Dennis & Ross, 2006b). Women with depressive symptoms at 8 weeks had significantly lower perceptions of relation-specific and postpartum-specific partner support than had non-depressed women. In addition, depressed women reported conflict with their partners, and indicated that their partners made them angry, tried to change them, and made them work hard to avoid conflict. Multivariate analysis revealed three variables with regard to support that were important: perceived social integration, partner encouragement to obtain help when needed, and partner agreement with how the mother was handling infant care. The authors concluded that shared activities, problem-focused information and assistance, and positive feedback from the partner decreased a mother's likelihood of developing depression at 8 weeks postpartum.

Kathy describes a number of challenges she faced with each of her five children. Her first husband was uninvolved and absent much of the time, and that made a difference in terms of the difficulties she experienced.

> My first was 9 weeks premature, in the NICU for 9 weeks. I pumped faithfully every 3 hours that whole time, taking herbs and Reglan, only to bring a baby home that cried furiously at the breast. He was on an NG feeding tube. I gave up. My second was only 3 and a half weeks early, but was small for gestational age and cried like she was hungry and not getting enough, so after one month, I gave up. She was up every 90 minutes screaming with reflux. My husband was absent as much as possible from our lives. My third was full-term, and he nursed 3 months, but finished each feed with a bottle. He had colic. I bonded well with him, but I also bonded well with my fourth, who never breastfed because a lactation consultant told me he wouldn't latch well and had a short tongue. I remarried and had a full-term fifth child who had trouble moving one half of her face and latches and feeds well half the time. I pump and breastfeed and she gets a bottle. I'm in a much better marriage. I bonded well with her. She is fragile and scares me because she sleeps too long, and does not wake and cry for food. I wake her.

Another study examined social support with three samples of postpartum women: 105 middle-class White women, 37 middle-class mothers of premature babies, and 57 low-income African American mothers (Logsdon & Usui, 2001). Using structural equation modeling, the authors found that when women received support and reported that they felt close to their partners, they had higher self-esteem and lower risk of depression. This was true for all three groups of mothers.

In a study of 193 mothers and fathers, Dudley et al. (2001) found that fathers were even more influenced by the quality of the relationship than mothers. Mothers' depression was influenced primarily by their own personalities, and perinatal and infant-related factors. In contrast, fathers were more influenced by the mothers' personality difficulties, unresolved past events, the mothers' current mental health, infant difficulties, and the state of their marriage/relationship. Depression in one partner was moderately correlated with depression in the other.

A study of 107 husbands and wives after the birth of their first child had similar findings. Lutz and Hock (2002) found that men who were less satisfied with their marriages were more likely to be depressed. For both men and women, fear of abandonment and fear of loneliness were significantly related to depressive symptoms. These relationships were stronger for men than for women in the sample.

In a qualitative study of 9 mothers and 5 fathers, the mothers all had a EPDS >13 at 6–8 weeks postpartum (Tammentie et al., 2004). Support from partners, family members, and friends was important during the postpartum period. For depressed mothers, there was a great discrepancy between their expectations and the realities of parenting. More mothers than fathers strove for protection, perceived that the infant tied them down, and had high expectations of family life. Mothers and fathers felt overwhelmed by the amount of time and effort the baby took, and both felt exhausted and inadequate. Having a baby also changed their key relationships, and there was often no time for each other.

A related question is the impact of marriage on childbearing. Does marital status make any difference in maternal depression postpartum? Kiernan and Pickett (2006), using data from the UK Millennium Cohort Study ($N = 18,533$), compared four sets of parents: married parents, cohabiting parents, solo mothers with a closely involved father, and solo mothers without an active partner. They were assessing whether partnership status was related to maternal smoking during pregnancy, breastfeeding, and maternal depression. They found that all three were inversely related to parental connectedness. Cohabiting mothers had worse health outcomes than did the married mothers. Among mothers who were not married, smoking was more likely among the women without a regular partner. For breastfeeding, stronger parental bonds were associated with initiation of breastfeeding, with a significant difference between the cohabiting vs. solo mothers. Maternal depression was associated with looser parental bonding. Among non-married mothers, this difference was most striking among cohabiting vs. solo mothers. They found the worse outcomes among the cohabiting mothers.

Partner support also proved helpful in treatment of PPD. With a sample of 29 women with PPD, 13 were randomly assigned to receive psychoeducation for seven sessions. The second group had partners participate in four of the seven sessions. At the conclusion of the study, women whose partners were included in the intervention had significantly decreased depressive symptoms compared with the women whose partners were not included (Misri et al., 2000b). When partner support is absent, support from friends can protect women from depression. A study of social support among women with critically ill children sought to determine whether friend support would buffer the negative effect of low spousal support (Rini et al., 2008). This study included 163 mothers of critically ill children. All were married, and they were assessed at 3, 6, and 12 months after their children received stem-cell transplants. Women with low spouse and low friend/family support had the poorest function of all groups. Women with low spouse support, but high friend/family support fared much better. In fact, their functioning was comparable to the women with high spousal support.

The role of culture: social structures that protect new mothers

The above-cited studies focus on women's networks involving family or friends. Researchers have also examined the role of culture in supporting new mothers. In their classic paper, Stern and Kruckman (1983) found that depression, or even the postpartum blues, are virtually non-existent in many diverse cultures around the world. Although these cultures differed dramatically from one another, they had common elements. In a more recent review, Eberhard-Gran and colleagues noted that most cultures have special postnatal customs including special diet, isolation, rest, and assistance for the mothers (Eberhard-Gran et al., 2010), and there were many commonalities in these customs. Unfortunately, customs that included rest and assistance for the mother have been decreasing since the 1950s. Because these cultural structures help prevent depression, it is important for us to understand them, even though they have decreased. The characteristics of these social structures are listed below.

A distinct postpartum period

In almost all the societies Stern and Kruckman (1983) studied, the postpartum period was recognized as a time that is distinct from normal life, and is a time when mothers recuperate, their activities are limited, and they are taken care of by female relatives. This was also common practice in colonial America, and was referred to as the "lying-in" period. Forty days is commonly marked as the postpartum period in Judaism, Christianity, and Islam. Mothers are considered "unclean" until that time has passed, and they are no longer bleeding. This is similar to the 40-day period in Latin America, *la cuarantena* ("the quarantine"), and "doing the month" in China (Eberhard-Gran et al., 2010).

Protective measures reflecting the new mother's vulnerability

During the postpartum period, new mothers are recognized as being especially vulnerable. In some cultures, the postpartum period is considered a time of ritual uncleanness, while in others it is a time for mothers to rest, regain strength, and care for their babies. There were many rituals associated with vulnerability, for example, certain foods mothers must either eat or avoid. For example, in China, mothers must have a special hot postpartum tea and avoid cold foods and drinks. Postpartum porridge was common in the Middle Ages as something that guests would bring that would protect mother and child (Eberhard-Gran et al., 2010). Other examples are the wrapping of the mother's head or abdomen, and limitations on the amount of company they receive. All of these rituals protected the mother, and set aside the postpartum period as distinct from normal life.

Social seclusion and mandated rest

Related to the concept of vulnerability are the widespread practices of social seclusion for new mothers. During this time, she is supposed to rest and restrict normal activities. In the Punjab, women are secluded from everyone but female relatives and the midwife for five days. After the five days, there is a "stepping out" ceremony for the mother and baby. In other cultures, the time of seclusion can be for as long as 3 months. Seclusion and rest also allow mothers to recover, promote breastfeeding, and limit their normal activities. In Nigeria, women and infants are isolated in a "fattening room," where the mother's duty, for 2 or 3 months postpartum, is to gain weight, sleep, and care for her infant (Eberhard-Gran et al., 2010).

Functional assistance

In order to isolate women and ensure that they are getting the rest they need, they must be relieved of their normal workload. Functional assistance involves the care of older children, household help, and personal attendance during labor. As in the colonial period in the US, women often return to their families' homes to ensure that this type of assistance is available. In Germany, *Wochenbett* (weeks in bed) means that women should not only rest, but literally stay in bed during the postpartum period (Eberhard-Gran et al., 2010).

Social recognition of her new role and status

In cultures where there is a low incidence of the blues or depression, there is a great deal of personal attention given to the mother (i.e., "mothering the mother"). The status of the new mother is recognized through social rituals and gifts. For example, in Punjabi culture, there is the ritual stepping-out ceremony, ritual bathing and hair washing performed by the midwife, and a ceremonial meal prepared by a Brahmin. When she returns to her husband's family, she returns with many gifts she has been given for herself and the baby. Ritual bathing, washing of hair, massage, binding of the abdomen, and other types of personal care are also prominent in the postpartum rituals of rural Guatemala, Mayan women in the Yucatan, and Latina women both in the US and Mexico. Here is a description of one of these recognition rituals performed by the Chagga people of Uganda.

> Three months after the birth of her child, the Chagga woman's head is shaved and crowned with a bead tiara, she is robed in an ancient skin garment worked with beads, a staff such as the elders carry is put in her hand, and she emerges from her hut for her first public appearance with her baby. Proceeding slowly towards the market, they are greeted with songs such as are sung to warriors returning from battle. She and her baby have survived the weeks of danger. The child is no longer vulnerable, but a baby who has learned what love means, has smiled its first smiles, and is now ready to learn about the bright, loud world outside.
>
> (Dunham, 1992, p. 148)

Social capital

Societal support can also be studied by examining social capital. Social capital refers to resources that are embedded in social networks. It includes neighborhood and social network support, partner support, and internal resources. With high social capital, women give and receive support to people whom they trust.

A study of 383 pregnant Greek women found that women who reported low social capital had higher scores on the EPDS in the first year postpartum (Kritsotakis et al., 2013). In contrast, women with high social capital had lower scores and less PPD. Social capital can also be found in community relationships and by participating in community activities. In Kritsotakis et al.'s research, participating in community activities did not lower depressive symptoms. It could be that depressed women get little support when they participate in community activities, especially if the communities have low-quality support. In fact, participation may be a physical and emotional burden. Personal relationships may be a better type of support for some women in terms of reducing depressive symptoms than the weaker social ties accessed through participating in activities.

Social capital also protected mothers who experienced adverse birth outcomes (Wakeel et al., 2013). This study used data from the 2007 Los Angeles Mommy and Baby study ($N = 3,353$). The researchers examined the relationship between stress and personal capital during pregnancy, and the impact of both on adverse outcomes, such as low birthweight, preterm birth, and small for gestational age. They found that more stress relative to social capital is associated with more preterm birth and pregnancy complications, and lower gestational age.

What twenty-first-century mothers face

Since the 1950s, postpartum rituals have gradually died out in the US. Some of this support was originally provided in the hospital. However, once hospital stays shortened to 24 hours for a vaginal birth, mothers went home and immediately stepped right back into their lives. Unfortunately, no community support rituals rose up to take the place of the hospital-based lying-in period (Eberhard-Gran et al., 2010). Further, once a woman has had her baby, she is no longer the focus of attention. For example, after a baby is born in mainstream US culture, all the attention shifts from the mother to the baby (Eberhard-Gran et al., 2010). Many of the mothers interviewed for this book felt a profound sense of loss and abandonment by their medical caregivers and their families. In general, there was little acknowledgment of what these women had been through, both physically and emotionally, by giving birth. Below is what some of these mothers said.

> I really wanted someone to make me feel special. All the attention was on the baby. [Barbara]

> I feel a sense of anti-climax. I was used to being the center of attention. Then I had to go back to being a normal healthy person. I'm not begging for attention, but now everyone only pays attention to the baby. It would be nice to have some attention afterwards. While you're pregnant, you're feeling fat and slobby, and don't want it. After the baby, you want it. [Julie]

> I felt like I didn't matter. I felt like they weren't interested in me after I had my baby… My husband said "of course they are not interested. You've had your baby." The 6-week visit seemed like an eternity away. I wrote [my midwife] a note to thank her. She didn't even mention it when I saw her at 6 weeks … When I felt great, they treated me nicely. Now when I feel so awful with this baby, no one seems to be available to me. [Karen]

> My doctor thought her job was done after my daughter was born. It's ridiculous to think the job is done just because you've delivered the baby. I called her a couple of times after, and she told me to see a social worker. I eventually left my OB. There were many reasons, but mainly because she left me high and dry after delivery. [Jan]

> After the birth, I had several people tell me that the most important thing was that I had a healthy baby. Yes, that is important. But what about me? No one pays attention to the fact that you've had major surgery. They would have paid more attention if you had had your appendix out. [Sally]

Summary

Social factors have a significant role to play in the development of postpartum depression. Women who experience stressful life events during the childbearing year are at increased risk for depression, as are mothers at both ends of the age continuum. Low-income and immigrant status can also make mothers vulnerable to depression, but not in all cases. Control over when to return to work can be protective, but lack of control increases risk. Social support can be an important buffer against life stress. Beyond a woman's immediate circle of family and friends, an entire culture can determine whether mothers are supported or vulnerable to depression.

Part III

Treatment options

Chapter 14

Complementary and integrative treatments I

Omega-3s, SAMe, and exercise

Complementary and integrative modalities are widely used for a variety of conditions, including psychiatric disorders (Freeman, 2009). Werneke and colleagues (2006) noted that up to 57 percent of psychiatric patients have used integrative therapies to treat depression and anxiety. This chapter describes the efficacy of omega-3s, SAM-e, and exercise. The other complementary and integrative modalities are described in Chapter 15.

Omega-3 fatty acids

> Overall, omega-3 EFA [essential fatty acids] are exciting therapeutic agents to explore in the context of psychiatric disorders. They hold the potential for primary prevention and contribute to other health benefits as well.
>
> (Freeman et al., 2006)

Over the past 100 years, there has been a critical shift in the diets that Western populations consume: specifically, in the ratio of omega-6:omega-3 fatty acids, which has had a negative impact on our health. As a population, we have decreased the amount of anti-inflammatory omega-3s we consume while we increased our consumption of pro-inflammatory omega-6s. Omega-6s and omega-3s are both polyunsaturated fatty acids (PUFAs; see Figure 14.1). Omega-6 fatty acids are ubiquitous in our diets and are found in vegetable oils, such as corn and safflower oils. Omega-3s are found in fatty fish and some plant sources, and are not as readily available in our diets. While some omega-6s are necessary for good nutrition, they become harmful when the ratio of omega-6s to omega-3s is too high—as it is in modern diets. Kiecolt-Glaser and colleagues (2007) noted that the hunter–gatherer diet had an estimated ratio of omega-6s:omega-3s of 2:1 or 3:1. In contrast, the typical North American diet, with its high amounts of vegetable oils in processed foods, ranges from 15:1 to 17:1. There is a similar pattern in Australia and New Zealand, with a ratio of approximately 10:1 (Rees et al., 2005).

With regard to depression, the long-chain omega-3s are of interest. These are eicosapentaenoic acid (EPA) and docosahexaenoic acid (DHA). Alpha-linolenic acid (ALA) is the parent omega-3 fatty acid, and is found in flax and other plant sources (see Figure 14.1). ALA is the parent omega-3 fatty acid, and while important for good nutrition, it is too metabolically removed from the long-chain omega-3s to be sufficiently

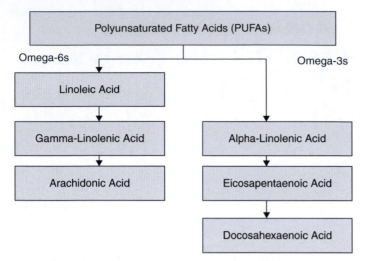

FIGURE 14.1 Polyunsaturated fatty acids: omega 6s and Omega3s (Wang et al., 2004). Used with permission

anti-inflammatory to have efficacy in the prevention or treatment of depression (Freeman et al., 2006a). Only about 10 percent of ALA that is consumed is metabolized into the long-chain omega-3s needed to prevent or treat depression and other perinatal mood disorders.

Much of the research on the mental health effects of omega-3s comes from studying populations who have high rates of fish consumption.

Omega-3s and depression in population studies

People who eat a lot of fish have lower rates of mood and anxiety disorders, including perinatal depression. The amount of fish necessary to achieve these protective effects was about 50 lbs of seafood a year (1–1.5 pounds per person per week) (Noaghiul & Hibbeln, 2003). Hibbeln (2002) found that postpartum depression was up to 50 times more common in countries with low fish consumption in his study of 14,000 women in 22 countries. For example, the rate of postpartum depression in Singapore was 0.5 percent, compared to 24.5 percent in South Africa. Similarly, Rees and colleagues (2005) observed that the rates for postpartum depression in North America and Europe are ten times those in Taiwan, Japan, Hong Kong, and some regions of China. A recent study of 55 women from Western Norway found that lower levels of EPA/DHA at 28 weeks gestation predicted higher levels of depression at 3 months postpartum (Markhus et al., 2013).

In contrast, a study of 865 pregnant Japanese women did not find lower rates of depression in women who ate more fish (Miyake et al., 2006). One possible explanation for their findings is a ceiling effect, because Japan has one of the rates of highest fish-consumption in the world. In addition, EPA/DHA levels were estimated from dietary questionnaires rather than measured directly from participant plasma.

A recent study from Singapore recruited 698 mothers at 26–28 weeks gestation, and measured their plasma levels of omega-3s and 6s (Chong et al., 2015). They measured depression and anxiety in pregnancy, and at 3 months postpartum. The overall rate of depression was low, 7 percent during pregnancy (EPDS ≥15) and 10 percent postpartum (EPDS ≥13). They found that lower omega-3s, and a higher omega-6:omega-3 ratio, were associated with higher anxiety during pregnancy. Lower omega-3s were not associated with depression in pregnancy or postpartum, or with postpartum anxiety. The researchers noted that low omega-3s, and a high ratio of omega-6s:omega-3s, were related to high levels of inflammation. Their findings are consistent with previous studies examining the link between inflammation and anxiety.

Another recent study found similarly mixed results. In this study, 118 women at risk for postpartum depression were given either EPA- or DHA-rich fish oil, or a soy placebo, and were assessed at 26–28 weeks gestation, 34–36 weeks gestation, and 6–8 weeks postpartum (Mozurkewich et al., 2013). Serum DHA was inversely related to depression at 34–36 weeks, but there were no other significant differences.

Treatment with EPA and DHA

In addition to its efficacy in prevention, EPA and DHA can also be used as a treatment for depression and other psychiatric conditions. EPA, in particular, has an antidepressant effect for all patients, but also for specific populations, including pregnant and breastfeeding women (Borja-Hart & Marino, 2010; Kendall-Tackett, 2010; Kiecolt-Glaser et al., 2015). A review from Australia found that EPA had efficacy in the treatment of depression in four of the six studies reviewed. One gram of EPA per day was the effective dose. Doses higher than 2 g were too much, and seemed to have the reverse effect. This suggests that there is an optimum dose, and exceeding it diminishes efficacy of the treatment (Rees et al., 2005). Similarly, in a meta-analysis of ten studies ($N = 329$), EPA with DHA had a significant antidepressant effect for patients with depression and with bipolar disorder (Lin & Su, 2007). However, Lin and Su did note some methodologic limitations of some of the studies they cited.

EPA and DHA were also used to treat major depression during pregnancy (Su et al., 2008). In this study, 36 pregnant women with major depression participated in a randomized clinical trial comparing a placebo to 3.4 g EPA/DHA (2.2 g DHA, 1.2 g EPA). Compared to the placebo group, subjects in the EPA/DHA group had significantly lower depression scores on the Hamilton Rating Scale for Depression at 6 and 8 weeks than the placebo group, and had a higher (although non-significant) remission rate. EPA and DHA were well tolerated and there were no adverse effects for either mother or baby. The authors noted that this treatment was likely effective because it halted the arachidonic acid cascade. Arachidonic acid is a long-chain, omega-6 fatty acid and is proinflammatory (see Figure 14.1). People with mood disorders often have higher levels of arachidonic acid in their plasma than do those without mood disorders.

Not all studies have found that EPA/DHA are effective treatments, however. An open-label trial with mothers with previous PPD found that fish-oil supplements did not prevent depression from reoccurring. In this study, women were recruited at 34–36 weeks gestation. The women were treated through 12 weeks postpartum, with dosages of 1,730 mg EPA and 1,230 mg DHA. Recruitment for the study ceased when four of the seven women in the study became depressed. The authors hypothesized that perhaps an inadequate dose of EPA or DHA, or wrong ratio, had been used, or administration that was too late in the pregnancy to prevent depression. The authors urged that, despite their negative findings, there continue to be studies of EPA and DHA in the treatment of postpartum mood disorders (Marangell, Martinez, Zboyan, Chong, & Puryear, 2004).

In a study of 59 women with perinatal major depressive disorder, women received either 1.9 g EPA and DHA/day or a corn-oil placebo (Freeman et al., 2008). Women in both groups also received supportive psychotherapy. The women in the study had an overall low level of omega-3s in their diet, with women eating less than half of a serving per month. Both groups had significantly lower depression scores after 8 weeks. There was no difference between the treatment and placebo groups. One possibility is that psychotherapy may have obscured the effects of the omega-3s.

EPA is also useful for other conditions, including depressive symptoms in bipolar disorder in a 12-week double-blind trial (Frangou et al., 2006). In this study, 75 patients were randomly assigned to one of three conditions for adjunctive therapy: placebo, 1 g or 2 g EPA. After 12 weeks, both EPA groups showed substantial improvement over the placebo. One gram was as effective as 2 g, and there was no advantage to 2 g over 1 g. The authors noted that EPA was well-tolerated, safe, and effective, and may prove more acceptable to patients than pharmacologic interventions.

Hallahan and colleagues (2007) tested the efficacy of EPA/DHA supplementation in patients recruited from London emergency departments who had made repeated suicide attempts. In this study, 49 patients with repeated suicide attempts were randomized to receive a placebo, or 1.2 g EPA and 900 mg DHA. After 12 weeks, the patients receiving EPA and DHA had significantly improved depressive symptoms and lower daily stresses. The authors noted that these were significant markers for suicidality, and that supplementation with EPA and DHA had lowered their risk.

A report by the American Psychiatric Association's Omega-3 Fatty Acids Subcommittee concluded that the preponderance of evidence points to a protective effect of EPA and DHA in mood disorders (Freeman et al., 2006a). EPA and DHA provided a significant benefit in unipolar and bipolar disorder, but the results were inconclusive for other psychiatric disorders. They further noted that supplementation with omega-3s could also help counter some of the metabolic and obesity effects of medications for psychiatric conditions.

Fish-oil capsules, the chief way to supplement with omega-3s, were found to be tolerable for pregnant and postpartum women (Freeman & Sinha, 2007). In a study of 59 pregnant and postpartum women with major depression, participants received four capsules daily with either 1.84 g EPA and DHA, or corn oil. Thirteen women reported side effects; the most common were unpleasant breath or heartburn/reflux. Six women reported side effects in the omega-3 group, and seven in the placebo group. No participant dropped out of the study due to tolerability of side effects.

Why they work: stress, inflammation, and EPA

EPA is a powerful anti-inflammatory that specifically lowers proinflammatory cytokines, and this likely explains its efficacy in treating depression. EPA mediates the inflammatory action of arachidonic acid by competing for the same metabolic pathways (Chong et al., 2015; Noorbakhshnia et al., 2015). In a large population study, high levels of omega-3s (ALA, EPA, and DHA) in participants' plasma were related to lower levels of the proinflammatory cytokines IL-1α, IL-1β, IL-6, and TNF-α, and higher levels of anti-inflammatory cytokines, such as IL-10. For people with low levels of omega-3s, the opposite was true: these people had high levels of proinflammatory cytokines and low levels of anti-inflammatory cytokines (Ferrucci et al., 2006).

Parker et al. (2006), in their review of the literature, noted that people with major depression had significantly higher ratios of arachidonic acid: EPA in both serum cholesteryl esters and phospholipids. If someone has a high proportion of omega-6 fatty acids in their diets, they have high levels of arachidonic acid, rather than EPA, in the cell membranes of both tissues. This, in turn, leads to a high proportion of inflammatory eicosanoids. Increased arachidonic acid also affects production of EPA and DHA because it competes for the metabolizing enzymes.

Researchers have examined the impact of EPA and DHA on the stress and inflammatory-response systems. Maes and colleagues measured omega-3s in college students, and found that students with deficient levels of EPA/DHA in their plasma had higher levels of inflammation when exposed to a lab-induced stressor compared to students who were not deficient. In other words, students with higher EPA/DHA levels had less of an inflammatory response to stress (Maes et al., 2000a). Similarly, Kiecolt-Glaser and colleagues (2007) found that a history of stress and depression appeared to "prime" the inflammatory response system in their study of 43 older adults. This priming effect made individuals more vulnerable to subsequent stress (Kiecolt-Glaser et al., 2015). However, even modest levels of supplementation with EPA and DHA caused norepinephrine levels to drop. A study from Japan had similar findings (Hamazaki et al., 2005). Participants took either a placebo or 762 mg of EPA/DHA for two months in this double-blind trial. The researchers noted that EPA concentrations increased in the red blood cell membranes in the supplemented group. The EPA/DHA group also had significantly decreased levels of plasma norepinephrine.

In summary, EPA and DHA downregulate the stress response, and by doing so, these fatty acids help mothers become more resilient to stress. This is especially valuable for women who are highly stressed, or who have experienced trauma, as EPA and DHA increase resilience to stress and can decrease risk for PPD (Kendall-Tackett, 2007).

Additional effects of DHA in the perinatal period

During the perinatal period, DHA may help prevent depression. In many Western countries, pregnant women's diets are often deficient in DHA. This is a problem because babies need high amounts of DHA in the last trimester of pregnancy for their brain and vision development. Any stores of DHA that mothers have are diverted to their babies, which may put the mothers at risk for depression. As Rees and colleagues (2005) describe for mothers in Australia, during the last trimester of pregnancy, babies accumulate an average of 67 mg/day of DHA. The average intake for Australian mothers is 15 mg/day. In contrast, DHA consumption from diet is about 1,000 mg/day for Japanese, Koreans, and Norwegians.

A double-blind, randomized trial that included 2,399 pregnant women in Australia found that DHA supplementation did not prevent PPD, nor did it improve child cognitive or language development (Makrides et al., 2010). The women were recruited at 21 weeks gestation. They received either 800 mg DHA and 100 mg EPA, or a vegetable oil placebo until birth. They were evaluated at 6 weeks and 6 months postpartum for postpartum depression (EPDS >12). The percentage of depressed women in both groups was relatively low (10 percent vs. 11 percent for treatment vs. placebo, respectively). Child development was measured at 18 months via Bayley Scales of Infant and Toddler Development. Interestingly, DHA increased gestation length. There were significantly fewer babies born at 34 weeks gestation in the DHA group, but significantly more women in the DHA group were either induced, or had cesareans because they were post-dates.

The current recommended minimum dose is 200–400 mg/day. This may prove to be too low a dose to prevent depression. According to McNamara (2009), in order to prevent affective disorders, you need a 7 percent erythrocyte DHA level, which can be achieved with an adult dose of 700–1000 mg. Interestingly, that amount is similar to the amount of DHA that women who eat a lot of fish consume through diet in countries such as Japan or Norway (Rees et al., 2005).

Safety during pregnancy and lactation

EPA and DHA supplements are generally safe for peripartum women (Makrides et al., 2010; Marangell et al., 2004; Shoji, 2006). A few studies have found very mild negative effects at high-dose levels, but in most studies, there are no adverse effects. These findings are summarized below.

Studies during pregnancy

Because of ethical considerations regarding testing substances on pregnant women, the majority of studies on the impact of EPA and DHA are population studies examining fish consumption. One study sampled 182 women from the Faroe Islands: a whaling, island community between the Shetland Islands and Iceland (Grandjean et al., 2001). Among Faroe Islanders, fish consumption was high: 72 g of fish, 12 g of whale muscle, and 7 g of whale blubber per day. In this sample, DHA level was the best predictor of gestational length, with a 1 percent increase in relative concentration related to a 1.5-day increase in gestation. An increase of 1 percent in relative EPA concentration was related to a 246 g decrease in birthweight. This decrease was not clinically significant, however, given the generally high birthweights of babies born in the Faroe Islands.

A study of 488 women in Iceland found that women who took cod liver oil were at increased risk for developing hypertension in pregnancy (Olafsdottir et al., 2006). That finding, as presented in the article abstract, is somewhat misleading. In the full article, the authors noted that when the data were divided into centiles, a U-shaped curve appeared, showing that women at highest risk for hypertension were at the highest and lowest levels of supplementation. Women with modest levels of supplementation were at the lowest risk for hypertension, demonstrating that there is an optimum dose of cod liver oil that was beneficial. Too much or too little increased the risk for hypertension. In addition, cod liver oil contains not only EPA and DHA, but three fat-soluble vitamins (A, D, and E) that can be toxic in large doses. Finally, the researchers estimated consumption of cod liver oil from questionnaire data, not directly from participant serum.

Modest levels of cod liver oil supplementation appeared safe in another randomized trial of 341 women, where mothers were supplemented from 18 weeks gestation to 3 months postpartum (803 mg EPA, 1,183 mg DHA) (Helland et al., 2003). There were no teratogenic effects noted. All the babies in this study breastfed for at least 3 months. At 4 years of age, children whose mothers had taken cod liver oil during pregnancy and lactation had a higher Mental Processing Composite score.

Another line of research examined the effect of fish consumption during pregnancy, and whether it protected offspring from allergic disease (Romieu et al., 2007). The rationale for the study was that the anti-inflammatory properties of omega-3s moderate the immune system. The sample was a cohort of 462 pregnant women and their infants, who were followed until age 6. After adjusting for potential confounding variables, they found that fish intake during pregnancy protected infants from eczema at 1 year, and allergy and wheeze at 6 years. An increase in weekly fish intake from once to 2.5 times a week decreased the risk of eczema by 37 percent, and risk of positive skin prick test at age 6 by 35 percent. Risk was significantly lowered for non-breastfed children. There was no additive protective effect of mothers' fish consumption for breastfed infants.

In a meta-analysis, Szajewska et al. (2006) found that supplementation with EPA and DHA significantly increased the length of pregnancy. Supplementation did not influence the rate of preterm deliveries, low birthweight infants, or eclampsia or pre-eclampsia. EPA/DHA may enhance gestation length, but the effect size was small. The incidence of adverse effects from supplementation was low, and most were mild (e.g., fish burps). One study included in the review reported an increase in blood loss at delivery among the fish oil group. None of the other studies reported increased bleeding. Overall, neonates, across studies, did not differ in rates of adverse effects from non-supplemented neonates.

Impact on breastfeeding

EPA and DHA also appear to have no negative impact on breastfeeding babies, even at high dosages. Freeman and colleagues (2006b) conducted a small, randomized trial using three different dosages of EPA/DHA with 16 mothers with postpartum major depression (300 mg EPA/200 mg DHA; 840 mg EPA/560 mg DHA; or 1,680 mg EPA/1,120 mg DHA). Depression significantly decreased in all three groups. The study was limited by a small sample and no control group (therefore, not ruling out a placebo effect). There were no adverse effects noted for mother or baby at any dosage level.

For 83 mothers, EPA and DHA did create some small changes in breast milk fatty acid composition when they were supplemented at very high doses from 20 weeks gestation to delivery. These changes appeared to be beneficial, however, not harmful. Fish-oil supplementation significantly increased EPA and DHA concentrations in breast milk (Dunstan et al., 2004b), and in the erythrocytes of mothers and babies in the fish oil group (Dunstan et al., 2004a). High EPA/DHA increased IgA and sCD14 in the milk. These are potentially protective changes. The dose used in this study was very high (2.2 g DHA, 1.5 g EPA): *11 times* the recommended minimum of DHA. Dunstan and colleagues did express some concerns about what the alterations in fatty acid composition might mean, but these concerns were more hypothetical than actually observed.

Sources of EPA and DHA

As described in previous sections of this chapter, women are often deficient in long-chain omega-3 fatty acids during pregnancy and postpartum. However, they may also be limiting a key source of omega-3s—fish—because they are rightly concerned about possible contaminants that are neurotoxins for their developing babies. One way out of this dilemma is to use fish-oil supplements. Fortunately, there are brands that are inexpensive, widely available, and tested for contaminants, making them more accessible to lower-income women (see the US Pharmacoepia website for a specific listing of brands that are tested for contaminants and that are USP verified: www.USP.org).

Summary

Evidence suggests that EPA and DHA are often deficient in childbearing women, but appear to protect mental health. The most recent evidence is somewhat mixed in terms of using EPA as a monotherapy, but it does appear to have an important role as an adjunct to other therapies. The role of DHA is less clear. It is not an effective monotherapy, but it, too, appears to have a role in prevention. Both EPA and DHA are present in fish and fish-oil products. As there are many additional health benefits from correcting deficiencies of EPA and DHA, and there is no apparent harm, the evidence supports their use as a possible preventive strategy and adjunctive treatment. A review in the *British Journal of Psychiatry* summarized these findings as follows:

> There is good evidence that psychiatric illness is associated with the depletion of EFAs [essential fatty acids] and, crucially, that supplementation can result in clinical amelioration ... The clinical trial data may herald a simple, safe and effective adjunct to our standard treatments.
>
> (Hallahan & Garland, 2005, p. 276)

S-Adenosyl-L-methionine (SAMe)

S-Adenosyl-L-methionine (SAMe) is another supplement that can be effective in treating depression. SAMe is crucial to cell metabolism and is a substance that naturally occurs in the body in all animals. It is derived from the amino acid methionine and adenosine triphosphate. Our bodies manufacture methionine from protein. SAMe contributes to a process known as methylation that regulates serotonin, melatonin, dopamine, and adrenaline. It also regulates neurotransmitter metabolism, membrane fluidity, and receptor activity (Bratman & Girman, 2003). If people have low levels of B6, B12, or folic acid, homocysteine increases. High homocysteine levels are harmful to cardiovascular health and have been related to depression.

Moreover, high levels of homocysteine during pregnancy raise the risk of spina bifida and other birth defects, which is why folic acid supplements are recommended for pregnant women. SAMe lowers homocysteine by helping the body metabolize it. So not being deficient in B6, B12, or folic acid naturally helps boost levels of SAMe. SAMe also regulates brain neurotrophic activity and proinflammatory cytokines (Papakostas et al., 2010).

A meta-analysis of 28 studies indicated that SAMe decreased depression significantly more than a placebo, and it was comparable to antidepressant medications in its effectiveness (Agency for Healthcare Research and Quality (AHRQ), 2002). The authors of this report noted that in placebo trials, SAMe provided an active treatment. Clinically, patients improved, but SAMe did not completely eradicate depression.

A recent randomized trial of 73 patients whose depression was not responding to SSRIs found that SAMe was a useful augmentation treatment (Papakostas et al., 2010). The patients all stayed on their medications and received either 1,600 mg SAMe or a placebo for the 6-week trial. Remission rates were significantly higher for those who received adjunctive SAMe than those who received a placebo. The authors concluded that SAMe was a safe, well-tolerated adjunctive treatment for non-responders with major depression.

To date, there have been no studies that treat pregnant women for depression with SAMe (Freeman, 2009). However, an AHRQ report summarized five studies on SAMe used antenatally for cholestasis in pregnancy with no adverse effects for either mother or baby. SAMe is generally very well tolerated. The standard dose is 200 mg/twice a day, with rapid titration up over the next one to two weeks. It may take as much as 1,600 mg/day to achieve an initial response in depression, but a maintenance dose can be as low as 200 mg/twice a day (Bratman & Girman, 2003).

There are two downsides to this supplement. First, it is expensive, and that can be prohibitive for many. Second, SAMe degrades easily. A consumer has no way of knowing whether the SAMe that they purchased was handled correctly. Consequently, consumers may pay top dollar for an inert substance.

At this time, its impact on breastfeeding is also unknown. Because it naturally occurs in the body, it is most likely safe, but there is no research to confirm this. However, no adverse effects have been reported via breastfeeding (Freeman, 2009). In summary, SAMe shows promise for treating PPD. It also appears to be safe for pregnancy and lactation, but there are still some unknowns, so mothers should be aware of these.

A similar line of research has examined whether folic acid, or folate, could be used to increase naturally occurring SAMe, rather than using a SAMe supplement. The current recommendation is that folate should not be used as a monotreatment for depression, but can be combined with SAMe. Supplementation with 400–1,000 mg of folate daily would likely prove a useful adjunct to treatment (Freeman, 2009; Papakostas et al., 2010).

Exercise

Exercise is another effective treatment for depression in general, and postpartum depression in particular (Daley et al., 2007). Traditionally, exercise has been recommended for people with mild to moderate depression. However, exercise can alleviate major depression as effectively as medications. Exercise can also be safely combined with other modalities.

Exercise as a treatment for depression

A number of studies have demonstrated the effectiveness of exercises a treatment for depression. A study from Duke University Medical Center was one of the first to conduct a randomized trial of patients with major depressive disorder (Babyak et al., 2000). Prior to this study, most studies of exercise had focused on mild to moderate depression. In this study, 156 patients with major depression (>50 years old) were randomized into one of three treatment groups: aerobic exercise alone, sertraline alone, and a combination of exercise and sertraline. After 4 months, exercise was as effective as sertraline in alleviating depression. The more striking findings, however, occurred at 10 months. At that time, the exercise-only group had a significantly lower rate of relapse than either medication alone or the medication/exercise groups. The authors speculated that this was because by learning to exercise, the exercise-only group had a coping tool that they could use when faced with life stressors.

In 2007, these same researchers replicated their findings (Blumenthal et al., 2007). Two-hundred twenty adults with major depression were randomized to one of four conditions: sertraline, exercise at home, supervised exercise, or a placebo control. After 4 months of treatment, 41 percent of the patients were in remission and no longer met the criteria for major depression. Efficacy rates by treatment were as follows: medication,

47 percent; supervised exercise, 45 percent; home-based exercise, 40 percent; and placebo, 31 percent. The exercise condition was 45 minutes of walking on a treadmill at 70–85 percent maximum heart rate capacity, three times a week, for 16 weeks. The home-exercise group received the same instructions, but was not supervised and had minimal contact with the research staff. The authors concluded that the efficacy of exercise was comparable to medications. The supervised program was especially effective, but the home program was also comparable to medications. All treatments were more effective than the placebo.

A recent Cochrane review of 37 studies found that exercise was an effective treatment for depression (Cooney et al., 2013). It was as effective as psychotherapy in seven trials, and as effective as medications in four trials.

Exercise for pregnant women

Similar positive results have been found in samples of pregnant women. A study of 230 pregnant women examined the relationships between depressive symptoms, body-image satisfaction, and exercise in the first, second, and third trimester of pregnancy, and at 6 weeks postpartum (Downs et al., 2008). Depressive symptoms and body image in early pregnancy predicted depression later in pregnancy. Exercise moderated these effects. In a sample of 80 women with PPD at 6 weeks, women were assigned to exercise three times a week, or receive standard care (Heh et al., 2008). Women who exercised were significantly less depressed at 5 months than the standard-care group.

A sample of 1,220 women from North Carolina were enrolled in a study in the third trimester of pregnancy (Demissie et al., 2011b). The researchers were investigating the impact of moderate to vigorous activity on depressive symptoms in pregnancy. They assessed past-week physical activity at 17–22 weeks gestation, and depressive symptoms at 24–29 weeks gestation, using the CES-D. They found that women with moderate to vigorous physical activity were half as likely to be depressed as women reporting lower levels of activity. They also found that women participating in adult or childcare, or indoor household activities, had higher depressive symptoms.

The mood-altering effects of exercise appear fairly quickly. In a study of 26 women, Lane and colleagues (2002) found that women's moods significantly improved after each exercise session. Depressed mood was especially sensitive to exercise, and decreased significantly after each session.

A recent meta-analysis of six trials with pregnant women found that exercise significantly reduced depression scores compared to women in the control conditions (Daley et al., 2015). The authors concluded that there was "some evidence" that exercise reduced depression in pregnancy, but the data were limited. Given exercise's many other benefits, it seems a low-risk intervention to offer to pregnant women who are depressed, or are at risk for depression.

Exercise for postpartum women

A study of 28 women from Taipei at 2–6 months postpartum enrolled participants in a program of yoga and pilates for 12 weeks (Ko et al., 2013). Women in the high-depression group showed a significant decrease in depression. Similarly, a study of 62 mothers were enrolled in an 8-week program of exercise and parenting education, and 73 mothers were enrolled in education only (Norman et al., 2010). Mothers in the exercise/education group had significantly lower depression and higher well-being than the education-only group. For those at risk for depression, it reduced the risk by 50 percent.

One way that exercise might reduce depressive symptoms is through its impact on self-efficacy. A randomized trial included 38 women with postpartum depression and found that there was no significant difference in exercise rates between the groups, and there was no significant decrease in depression (Daley et al., 2008). However, self-efficacy did increase in the exercise group.

Most previous studies of exercise and depression have used aerobic exercise. However, a recent study compared resistance training to flexibility training for a group of 60 postpartum women (LeCheminant et al., 2014). Resistance training twice a week significantly decreased depressive symptoms. There was no significant change for flexibility or wait-list conditions.

A review of 17 studies of PPD and exercise found that leisure-time physical activity decreased postpartum depressive symptoms (Teychenne & York, 2013). The fact that exercise is defined as "leisure-time activity" might be key to understanding these findings. The study of 550 women in North Carolina, who were part of the PINS study, found that if an activity is fun, it's associated with lower levels of inflammation. If the activity is not fun (such as exercise that takes place as part of a job or caregiving), it actually increases inflammation (Demissie et al., 2011a).

Exercise is also anti-inflammatory

One reason why exercise works as a treatment for depression is because it lowers inflammation. People who exercise have lower inflammatory biomarkers than people who are sedentary (Kiecolt-Glaser et al., 2015). Chronic inflammation affects the body's composition and metabolism in several ways, including the loss of body protein and the accretion of fat (Roubenoff, 2003). For example, cachexia, or loss of lean muscle mass, is at least partially mediated by the proinflammatory cytokines IL-1β, IL-6, and TNF-α. Exercise can reverse these inflammatory-mediated changes.

Initially, exercise acts as an acute physical stressor, and raises IL-6 and TNF-α. Over a longer period of time, however, exercise lowers inflammation. Older adults, for example, are one group with higher levels of proinflammatory cytokines because levels naturally increase as we age. Indeed, researchers hypothesize that this age-related rise in inflammation creates vulnerability to diseases, such as heart disease, cancer, and Alzheimer's (Kiecolt-Glaser et al., 2007). Because of this increased vulnerability of older adults, they are frequently the population of choice for studies on exercise, depression, and inflammation. The results of these studies are helpful for understanding the mechanism underlying exercise's impact on depression.

A study of adults, ages 60–90, tested the effects of physical activity on perceived stress, mood, and quality of life (Starkweather, 2007). The researchers also assessed serum IL-6 and cortisol. The patients ($N = 10$) assigned to the exercise group were instructed to walk for 30 minutes, five times a week for the 10-week study. The control group was ten older adults who were not engaging in physical activity. After the 10-week exercise intervention, the subjects had significantly lower stress on the Perceived Stress Scale, and improved mood and quality of life on the SF-36 Health Questionnaire. They reported better physical functioning, more vitality, better mental health, and less bodily pain. They also had a significant decrease in serum IL-6.

Exercise also had a positive effect on wound healing, and this is an indirect measure of systemic inflammation (Emery et al., 2005). In this study, participants were randomized into exercise and control conditions, and were then given a punch biopsy so that researchers could monitor participants' rate of wound healing. For the exercise group, wounds healed in 29 days. In the control group, it took 38 days. Exercise one hour a day, three days a week lowered perceived stress and improved wound healing. This study is of interest because we know from these researchers' other studies that wound healing is impaired when stress or hostility levels are high (Kiecolt-Glaser et al., 2005). Stress and hostility both increase systemic inflammation. When systemic inflammation is high, wound healing is impaired because proinflammatory cytokines are systemically in the plasma, and not at the wound site where they belong. The Emery et al. (2005) study indicates that exercise improves wound healing by lowering levels of circulating systemic cytokines and diverting them to the wound site.

Overall level of fitness is also related to inflammation (Hamer & Steptoe, 2007). The sample was 207 men and women from London. Participants who responded with higher systolic blood pressure to a lab-induced stress also had a higher IL-6 and TNF-α response. The TNF-α response to stress was five times greater in the low-fitness group compared to the high-fitness group. Participants who were physically fit had a lower inflammation response when under stress, which likely protected them from both depression and chronic disease.

Exercise and breastfeeding

As the previously cited studies indicate, exercise is helpful in lowering systemic inflammation and treating depression. Yet mothers may be concerned that it will negatively impact breastfeeding. Research studies have generally found that exercise had no negative effects on breastfeeding (Amorin et al., 2007). An Australian study of 587 new mothers (Su et al., 2007) examined the relationship between mothers' exercise, initiation and duration of breastfeeding, and exercise's effect on infant growth. Mothers were interviewed seven times over the first year. At 6–12 months, exercise had not decreased breastfeeding duration. At 12 months, exercise had no significant impact on infants' growth. Researchers concluded that exercise is safe for breastfeeding mothers, and important for maintaining health.

A more specific question regarding exercise and breastfeeding is whether exercise causes lactic acid to build up in mothers' milk. In a study of 12 women, milk and blood samples were taken after a non-exercise session, after maximal exercise, and after a session that was 20 percent below the maximal range (Quinn & Carey, 1999). They found that in women with an adequate caloric intake, moderate exercise neither increased lactic acid in breast milk nor caused babies to reject it. When women exercised in the "hard" range (using the perceived-exertion scale), lactic acid increased. The authors recommended exercise in a moderate range because it neither increases lactic acid accumulation in the breast milk nor alters babies' willingness to breastfeed.

In summary, exercise is a highly effective treatment for depression—alone or in combination with other treatments—and it has no negative effect on breastfeeding. Exercise can be a viable alternative treatment if mothers refuse medication. The one challenge with exercise is getting mothers to do it because it is often the last thing depressed people feel like doing. However, mothers may be motivated to try when they realize that it's an effective alternative to medications. Blumenthal et al.'s (2007) study found a slightly higher remission in the supervised vs. at-home exercise groups. This is likely due to compliance rates being higher because participants knew people expected them to show up to exercise. It's easier to skip exercise in an unsupervised home program. The supervised program also provided at least some social support. A similar approach, perhaps involving a mothers' exercise group, may be useful for mothers who want to give this modality a try.

Summary

Omega-3s, SAMe, and exercise are all effective treatments for depression—even major depression. All of these modalities can be safely combined with other treatments and have no negative impact on breastfeeding.

In the next chapter, other complementary and alternative treatments for depression are described, including bright light therapy, Vitamin D, St. John's wort, and some emerging treatment modalities.

Chapter 15   **Complementary and integrative therapies II**

Bright light therapy, vitamin D, St. John's wort, and emerging therapies

As described in the previous chapter, there is a range of effective, evidence-based, complementary and integrative treatments for depression in new mothers. In this chapter, bright light therapy, vitamin D, St. John's wort, and some emerging therapies are described. Most of these treatment modalities are effective for even major depression.

Bright light therapy

Some people dread the change of seasons. Shorter, darker days mean fatigue, oversleeping, overeating, and having a general sense of malaise: a pattern known as seasonal affective disorder (SAD) (Sullivan & Payne, 2007). Symptoms include depression, lethargy, difficulty waking, impaired concentration, lack of interest in social activities, and craving carbohydrates, which can lead to winter weight gain (National Alliance on Mental Illness [NAMI], 2007). In industrialized countries, the average amount of time that most people are exposed to bright light (>1000 lux) is about an hour a day. If a person is not susceptible to seasonal depression, this does not pose a problem. If, however, someone is susceptible, it can be (Crowley & Youngstedt, 2012).

Bright light therapy effectively treats seasonal affective disorder, and the response is often within days (NAMI, 2007). Light therapy can also treat other affective disorders, including perinatal depression, offering an alternative to medications for pregnant or breastfeeding mothers (Oren et al., 2002; Terman & Terman, 2005). An expert panel for the American Psychiatric Association concluded that bright light therapy was an effective treatment for both seasonal and non-seasonal depression, with results comparable to antidepressants (Golden et al., 2005).

Light therapy in pregnant and postpartum women

According to Crowley and Youngstedt (2012), perinatal women may be particularly vulnerable to the lack of light exposure. At the end of pregnancy, they may be restricted in their mobility, and therefore not spend as much time outside. After the baby is born, they may also spend more time indoors, in addition to sleeping during the day. Both of these can desynchronize circadian rhythms, increasing the risk for depression.

To date, only a few studies of bright light therapy have included pregnant and postpartum women, with mixed findings in terms of effectiveness. The larger literature on light therapy in general, however, suggests that this modality is worth investigating further. For example, in a clinical trial, patients were randomized to receive light therapy at 10,000 lux, 30 minutes a day and a placebo medication; or 100 lux (placebo light) with 20 mg fluoxetine (Lam et al., 2006). A total of 96 patients with seasonal major depression participated for 8 weeks. The researchers found that light therapy was as effective as fluoxetine in relieving symptoms, with an identical clinical response rate for even severe depression. By one week, patients in the light therapy group had a greater response to treatment, but this difference disappeared at subsequent assessment points. There were more side effects with fluoxetine, but both treatments were generally well-tolerated, with no overall difference in adverse effects.

Bright light alleviated depression in two case studies of new mothers who suddenly became depressed after the birth of their babies (Corral et al., 2000). These mothers refused antidepressants, but agreed to a trial of bright light therapy. Both of these women responded to bright light therapy, and had significantly lower rates of depressive symptoms after treatment.

In a study of 15 women with PPD, ten were assigned to receive light at 10,000 lux for 6 weeks, and five were assigned to dim red light (600 lux). After 6 weeks, both groups improved, and there was no significant difference between the groups (Corral et al., 2007).

An open-label trial with 16 pregnant women with major depression found that there was a 49 percent improvement in depressive symptoms after 3 weeks of treatment with bright light (10,000 lux). Based on their results, the authors recommended a randomized trial to further test the efficacy of this intervention with depressed pregnant women (Oren et al., 2002).

Bright light therapy was also an intervention in a recent study of mothers with babies in the NICU (Lee et al., 2012). They noted that in addition to the normal stresses associated with having a baby in the NICU, being in the NICU, with its low level of light, desynchronizes circadian rhythms. With that in mind, they conducted a pilot study with 30 mothers, randomizing 15 mothers to receive 3 weeks of bright light therapy. Seventy-three percent of the mothers were African American, with a mean age of 26. The light in the NICU was <10 lux bedside, and 100 lux in the lobby. The design called for mothers using a light visor, and the adherence rate was approximately 88 percent. They found that the mothers in the experimental group had lower levels of depression and nighttime and morning fatigue, and improved physical health-related quality of life. Self-reported sleep quality was better. The authors noted that none of the between-group differences were statistically significant due to the small sample size, but they were clinically significant. Further, the effect sizes ranged from small to large.

Light intensity, duration, and timing of light exposure

There are several characteristics of light related to its effectiveness as a treatment. These characteristics include light intensity, duration, and timing of light exposure. Researchers have investigated a wide range of light intensities and several appear effective. Light intensity is measured in lux, which is brightness by proximity. Lights at closer distances have a higher lux than the same light that is further away.

Lights with intensities of 10,000 lux appear to be most effective. At this level of intensity, 30–40 minutes of exposure is sufficient. Two studies with light exposures of 30–40 minutes at 10,000 lux achieved a 75 percent remission rate in depression. It took 2 hours to achieve similar remission rates at 2,500 lux, and in some cases, even with longer exposure, lower-intensity lights were not as effective (Terman & Terman, 2005). Another potential problem with longer exposure times is that patients are less likely to comply. This may particularly be true for mothers of young children, who probably won't find it practical to sit in front of a light box for 2 or 3 hours.

Another study used a Litebook LED (1,350 lux) for 30 minutes, and found that amount light significantly lowered depression scores compared to a placebo light (Desan et al., 2007). This was a small trial ($N = 23$), and patients were assessed after 1, 2, 3, and 4 weeks of treatment. By 4 weeks, 57 percent of patients in the LED condition were in remission compared to 11 percent of patients in the control condition. The authors speculated that this lower intensity light worked because it was in the 450–480 nm range, and that melatonin rhythms were best shifted by those wavelengths. Because of this concentration in short wavelengths, even lower-intensity light might prove as effective as brighter light boxes, while using smaller, more convenient devices.

Timing

Timing of light exposure also makes a difference. Morning exposure to bright light is generally more successful than light exposure later in the day. In their review of 25 studies, Terman and Terman (2005) found significantly higher remission rates with morning exposure (53 percent), compared with midday (32 percent) and evening (38 percent).

One exception to the use of morning light is in patients with bipolar disorder. Morning light exposure can increase the risk of a manic episode. This problem can be addressed by timing light exposure to later in the day and having patients continue on their medications during light treatment (NAMI, 2007; Terman & Terman, 2005).

Dawn simulation

Because of the effectiveness of morning light exposure, a variant to standard light therapy has been added to the repertoire of possible treatments: dawn simulation. As the name implies, dawn simulation refers to a light that comes on before a patient is awake, and gradually increases in intensity over a period of 15–90 minutes (the length can be tailored to individual preference). The advantage to this treatment is that it does not require sitting in front of a light box for an extended time, making it a more practical alternative for new mothers or mothers of young children. Although a relatively new technique, it is showing promise as a treatment for seasonal depression (Golden et al., 2005). Some newer lighting devices are both light boxes and dawn simulators.

One theory about why dawn simulation is effective is because of its impact on the early dawn interval, when melatonin levels wane and core body temperature rises. The early dawn interval is when circadian rhythms are most susceptible to light-elicited phase advances. According to this theory, depression is more likely to be triggered when it is still dark outdoors in the early dawn interval. To test this theory, Terman and Terman (2006) randomly assigned 99 adults with seasonal major depression to one of five treatment conditions. These included dawn simulation, dawn light pulse, post-awakening bright light therapy (30 minutes at 10,000 lux), negative air ionization at high flow rate, and ionization at low flow rate. After 3 weeks of treatment, patients who received bright light therapy (57 percent) and dawn simulation (50 percent) had the greatest improvement in symptoms. They concluded that bright light therapy still appeared to be the most effective. However, if there are problems with non-compliance or non-response, dawn simulation or dawn pulse are viable alternatives.

Why light is effective

Researchers have proposed a number of possible mechanisms for why bright light alleviates depression. Most explanations have to do with modifying the internal circadian clock. Our circadian rhythms, or daily patterns of sleep and arousal, are regulated by the pineal gland, which secretes melatonin. The suprachiasmatic nucleus of the hypothalamus regulates synthesis of melatonin (Erman, 2007). The pineal gland responds to light via light receptors in the retina. The superiority of exposure to morning light is likely due to the diurnal variations in retinal photoreceptor sensitivity, with greater sensitivity to morning light. Indeed, exposure to evening light can lead to insomnia and hyperactivation in some people (NAMI, 2007; Terman & Terman, 2005).

Preliminary evidence indicates that there is an inflammatory component to seasonal depression as well. Lam and colleagues (2004) hypothesized that during winter, proinflammatory cytokines increase for patients with seasonal depression. In a study of 15 patients, and a matched group of normal controls, those with seasonal affective disorder had significantly higher levels of IL-6. After 2 weeks of bright light therapy, symptoms improved, and 64 percent of patients had at least a 50 percent reduction in depressive symptoms. However, light therapy did not lower inflammation after 2 weeks. The authors concluded that seasonal depression involves activation of the immune–inflammatory system, which is not immediately altered by light therapy (Leu et al., 2001).

Safety issues

Because light boxes can be relatively expensive (about $60 USD), and appear to be simple, patients often consider assembling a unit themselves. Just because they can, doesn't mean they should. Clinicians generally recommend that patients don't use homemade devices for several reasons. First, it is difficult for consumers to find lights that are sufficiently bright enough to generate a therapeutic effect. Second, some patients have experienced excessive irradiation, and corneal or eyelid burns with homemade devices. Finally, homemade devices often use incandescent lights, which are not recommended because 90 percent of light output from incandescent bulbs is on the infrared, or heat, end of the spectrum. Not only can infrared exposure at high intensity burn the lens, cornea, and retina, but it is on the wrong end of the color spectrum for a therapeutic effect (Terman & Terman, 2005). The NAMI (2007) recommends bulbs with a color temperature between 3000 and 6500 degrees Kelvin, and are in the white to blue range of the color spectrum. These do not harm patients' eyes.

Light boxes with high levels of exposure to UV can also cause eye damage. The NAMI recommends lights that are encased in a box with a diffusing lens that filters out UV radiation (NAMI, 2007). Patients wanting to try light therapy should use a lighting apparatus from a reputable dealer. Because price may be an issue, many hospitals, and some manufacturers, have loaner programs that allow patients to try the lighting device in their homes before buying them. Many are also now available on Amazon.com.

Summary

Bright light therapy is a generally safe, well-tolerated treatment option for seasonal depression, and it's useful for non-seasonal depression as well. Bright light therapy is also breastfeeding-friendly and can be used during pregnancy. Although therapeutic light boxes can be costly at first, a single purchase will last for years. For patients who dread the change of seasons, or who want an alternative to antidepressant medication, this investment is often well worth the price.

Vitamin D

Vitamin D is a preprohormone that influences metabolism and immune function, and a deficiency of vitamin D has been related to a number of inflammatory diseases, such as rheumatoid arthritis, cardiovascular disease, and diabetes (Wagner, 2011). Vitamin D deficiency reduces intestinal calcium absorption by more than 50 percent, causing the parathyroid to correct the calcium imbalance by releasing calcium from the bones. Hyperparathyroidism has been linked to cardiovascular disease (Lee et al., 2008).

Vitamin D protects beta cell function from inflammatory cytokines, particularly IL-6 and TNF-α (Penckofer et al., 2008). When it is deficient, IL-6 inhibits insulin receptor signal transduction. IL-6 is associated with hyperglycemia and hyperinsulinemia. Given that a deficiency in vitamin D increases inflammation, it is not surprising that it has a role in depression (Berk et al., 2013).

Vitamin D deficiency is rampant worldwide among pregnant and postpartum women, partly because so much of our day is spent indoors, and because of our efforts to prevent skin cancer. A prospective study of 796 pregnant women from Perth, Australia (a very sunny place), measured vitamin D levels at 18 weeks gestation, and measured depression at 3 days postpartum (Robinson et al., 2014). The researchers used six items from the EPDS that measured mood fluctuations, sadness, anxiety, appetite changes, and sleep disturbances. They measured these with a 4-point Likert scale instead of the standard response categories. As hypothesized, women in the lowest quartile for vitamin D status had the highest levels of depressive symptoms, even after accounting for potentially confounding variables, such as BMI and demographic factors.

Vitamin D is measured via serum: 25-hydroxyvitamin D (ng/ml). Severe deficiency is ≤10, deficient = 10–20, insufficient = 21–29, and sufficient ≥30. Toxic levels are >150 (Lee et al., 2008). Standard recommended supplements are 400 IU per day for adults. However, newer guidelines are emerging with the recommended dosage for pregnant women being 4000 IU/day, and 6400 IU for lactating women (Wagner, 2011). These recommendations follow from Wagner et al.'s earlier clinical trials demonstrating that these high levels are safe, and not toxic, for pregnant and postpartum women (Wagner et al., 2006).

Summary

These findings suggest that pregnant women be screened for vitamin D deficiency, as many women around the world are deficient. Vitamin D deficiency increases susceptibility to a wide range of chronic health conditions because it increases inflammation. Deficiency has also been linked to perinatal depression. Addressing vitamin D deficiency can prevent depression, or help women heal once it has occurred.

St. John's wort

Herbal medications have a long history of use around the world. Despite their increasing popularity in the US, many healthcare providers are uncomfortable with patients medicating themselves for something as serious as depression. To make matters worse, patients often do not tell their doctors that they are taking herbs for fear of censure. This can be dangerous because of the potential for herb–drug interactions. It is important for healthcare providers to know if patients are taking herbs.

Why patients take herbs

From the patient's perspective, herbs offer a number of advantages. If you understand why women might prefer these modalities, you can talk more comfortably with them about their choices. And women are more likely to be forthcoming about using them.

- **Control:** One reason patients prefer herbs is that they can control their own healthcare. Instead of having to wait for a doctor's appointment, they can address their depression right away. They also have control over when they start treatment and when they stop.
- **Privacy:** Patients may be ashamed to admit that they are depressed, and are frightened by the possibility that their employers or others will find out that they are taking antidepressants. Unfortunately, on occasion, medication information *does* get released to employers via insurance forms or just plain gossip—even with confidentiality regulations in place. Further, antidepressant use can influence hiring and promotion decisions in some types of jobs. Antidepressant use can even be used against mothers in custody evaluations. Even if mothers do not encounter these difficulties, patients may still not want others to know.
- **Costs:** Newer and name-brand antidepressants can be expensive, especially if not covered by insurance. In contrast, herbs are generally reasonably priced, and can be purchased at discount and warehouse stores. The savings each month can be substantial compared with name-brand non-generic prescription drugs. This is becoming less of an issue, as many frequently used antidepressants are available in generic form, but cost can still be a concern for some mothers.
- **Side effects and safety:** The side-effect and safety profiles of herbs are significantly better than those associated with medications (Klier et al., 2006; Schultz, 2006). For some, the side effects of antidepressants prove intolerable and are a common reason why patients stop taking them. Most herbs have very low incidence of adverse effects. For example, according to one review, the risk of adverse events associated with St. John's wort was ten times lower than with standard antidepressants (Schultz, 2006). Along these same lines, although antidepressant use during pregnancy is likely safe, many women fear teratogenic effects of medications taken during pregnancy, and therefore may be reluctant to take antidepressants at that time (Dennis & Allen, 2008).
- **Patient compliance:** Patient compliance is an important issue. Just because women are prescribed antidepressants doesn't mean they will take them. In one study of depressed men and women in New York City ($N = 829$), only 28 percent were still taking their antidepressants 3 months later (Olfson et al., 2006). In this study, patients were more likely to stop taking them if they were Hispanic, had less than 12 years of education, or were lower-income. They were more likely to continue taking their

medications if they had more than 12 years of education, had participated in psychotherapy at some point, and had private health insurance. A study of PPD showed a similar trend (Boath et al., 2004). This study included 35 women with PPD who had been prescribed antidepressant medication. Of the 35, 20 found the medication helpful, 4 chose not to take it because they were breastfeeding, and 9 women likely had poor compliance (based on comments they made on their surveys). The results of this study suggest that many self-manage medication, and end up taking a dosage that is likely ineffective.

St. John's wort (*Hypericum perforatum*) is the most widely used herbal antidepressant in the world (Dugoua et al., 2006). Herbalists have used St. John's wort since the Middle Ages. At that time, it was used to treat insanity resulting from "attacks of the devil." It derives its name from St. John's Day (June 24) because it blooms near this day on the medieval church calendar. "Wort" is the old English word for a medicinal plant. It is native to Great Britain, Wales, and northern Europe, and since settlers brought it to North America in the 1700s, it is now a common wildflower in the Northeastern and North Central US.

Efficacy of St. John's wort

A large body of evidence indicates that St. John's wort effectively treats depression (Sarris, 2007; Werneke et al., 2006). A number of clinical trials have compared the efficacy of various St. John's wort extracts to either a placebo or an antidepressant. In one trial, 375 patients were randomized to receive either St. John's wort (*Hypericum perforatum* Extract WS 5570) or a placebo for 6 weeks to treat mild to moderate depression (Lecrubier et al., 2002). At the end of 6 weeks, patients receiving St. John's wort had significantly lower scores on the Hamilton Depression Rating Scale. Significantly more patients were in remission than were patients receiving the placebo. Both groups had similar rates of adverse effects. Fifty-three percent of the patients in the St. John's wort group responded to treatment, compared with 42 percent of the placebo group.

One trial compared St. John's wort to the tricyclic antidepressant imipramine. The first randomized trial compared St. John's wort (*Hypericum* extract ZE 117) to imipramine for 324 outpatients with mild to moderate depression (Woelk, 2000). After 6 weeks of treatment, St. John's wort was as effective as imipramine in lowering depressive symptoms. Adverse effects were significantly more likely in the imipramine group, with 63 percent reporting adverse effects compared with 39 percent reporting adverse effects in the St. John's wort group. In addition, only 3 percent in the St. John's wort group dropped out of the study due to adverse effects vs. 16 percent of the imipramine group. The author concluded that St. John's wort is therapeutically equivalent to imipramine, but better tolerated by patients.

Two clinical trials compared St. John's wort to sertraline for major depression. In the first study, 340 adults with major depression were randomly assigned to receive *H. perforatum*, a placebo, or sertraline for 8 weeks (Hypericum Depression Trial Study Group, 2002). Subjects responding to the medication could opt to receive still-blinded treatment for another 18 weeks. Depression was assessed at baseline, and again at 8 weeks. The rate of full response was low and almost identical for both the St. John's wort and sertraline groups (24 percent vs. 25 percent). The low response rates for both medications suggest limitations to the study. Eight weeks may not have been sufficient for patients with severe depression to recover, or the dosages may have been too low. The authors noted that their findings were not unusual in that approximately 35 percent of studies of standard antidepressants show no greater efficacy than the placebo.

Another study that same year had opposite findings (Van Gurp et al., 2002). This study included 87 patients with major depression recruited from Canadian family practice physicians. Patients were randomly assigned to receive either St. John's wort or sertraline. At the end of the 12-week trial, both groups improved, and there was no difference between the two groups. There were significantly more side effects in the sertraline group at 2 and 4 weeks. The authors concluded that St. John's wort, because of its effectiveness and benign side effects, was a good *first choice* for a primary-care population.

St. John's wort was also compared to paroxetine in a study of 251 patients with moderate to severe major depression (Szegedi et al., 2005). In this study, patients were randomly assigned to receive 20 mg paroxetine or 900 mg St. John's wort (*Hypericum* extract WS 5570). After 2 weeks, dosages for non-responders were doubled: 1,800 mg St. John's wort or 40 mg paroxetine. After 6 weeks of treatment, the response rates were 70 percent for St. John's wort and 60 percent for paroxetine. The remission rates for St. John's wort were 50 percent vs. 35 percent for paroxetine. The authors concluded that St. John's wort was as effective as paroxetine, and better tolerated.

Anghelescu and colleagues (2006) also compared the efficacy and safety of *Hypericum* extract WS 5570 to paroxetine for patients with moderate to severe depression. The acute phase of treatment lasted for 6 weeks, with another 4 months of follow-up to prevent relapse. The patients improved on both treatments with no significant difference in efficacy between paroxetine and St. John's wort. The authors noted that St. John's wort was an important alternative to standard antidepressants for depressed patients.

Mechanism for efficacy

Researchers still do not understand the exact mechanism for St. John's wort's antidepressant effect. Researchers have recognized hyperforin as the possible antidepressant constituent (Lawvere & Mahoney, 2005; Wurglies & Schubert-Zsilavecz, 2006). Hyperforin appears to inhibit the reuptake of the monoamines and GABAergic activity (Deligiannidis & Freeman, 2014). It may relieve depression by preventing the reuptake of serotonin, the same mechanism as the selective serotonin reuptake inhibitors (SSRIs, e.g. fluoxetine, sertraline). Indeed, only hyperforin (and its structural analogue, adhyperforin) inhibit neurotransmitter reuptake (Muller, 2003).

St. John's wort, and particularly hyperforin, also appears to be anti-inflammatory (Dell'Aica et al., 2007; Wurglies & Schubert-Zsilavecz, 2006), and it modulates cytokine production (Werneke et al., 2006). Hyperforin has had antinociceptive (anti-pain) and anti-inflammatory effects in animal studies (Abdel-Salam, 2005). It inhibits the expression of another inflammatory marker—intercellular adhesion molecule (Zhou et al., 2004). *In vitro* effects show that St. John's wort is antioxidant, anticyclooxygenase-1, and anticarcinogenic (Zanoli, 2004). Only recently has St. John's wort been shown to specifically lower levels of the proinflammatory cytokines involved in depression (Hu et al., 2006). The study used an animal model to test whether St. John's wort could counter the toxic side effects of chemotherapy. The investigators specifically investigated whether St. John's wort had an impact on the levels of proinflammatory cytokines, including IL-1β, IL-2, IL-6, IFN-γ, and TNF-α. They found that St. John's wort did inhibit proinflammatory cytokines and intestinal epithelium apoptosis. Although not a study of depression, it was the first to demonstrate that St. John's wort inhibits the cytokines that are high in depression.

Dosage

The dosage of St. John's wort is 900 mg per day (300 mg/three times per day), standardized to 0.3 percent hypericin and/or 2–4 percent hyperforin (Lawvere & Mahoney, 2005). It generally takes 4–6 weeks to take effect (Ernst, 2002). St. John's wort reaches peak level in the plasma in 5 hours, with a half-life of 24–48 hours. Herbalists often combine it with other herbs to address the range of symptoms that depressed people have. Some of these herbs include lemon balm, kava, schisandra, rosemary, black cohosh, and lavender (Humphrey, 2007; Kuhn & Winston, 2000). Unfortunately, it can be challenging for women to know if a brand of herbs they purchase is of good quality. As of this writing, the US Pharmacoepia does not verify brands of St. John's wort. However, ConsumerLabs.com does rate brands of herbs. For a small subscription fee, women can access this resource, and read the rating of specific brands of herbal products.

Safety concerns

Taken by itself, St. John's wort has an excellent safety record, with a very low frequency of adverse reactions (Humphrey, 2007; Muller, 2003). Approximately 2 percent of patients who take St. John's wort develop side effects. The most common are mild stomach discomfort, allergic reactions, skin rashes, tiredness, and restlessness. Like other antidepressants, St. John's wort can trigger an episode of mania in vulnerable patients or patients with bipolar disorder (Bratman & Girman, 2003). St. John's wort can also cause photosensitivity. A review of 38 controlled clinical trials, and two meta-analyses on St. John's wort, found its safety and side-effect profile to be better than standard antidepressants. The incidence of adverse events ranged from 0 percent to 6 percent (Schultz, 2006). There is also a significantly lower dropout rate in studies due to side effects in St. John's wort trials vs. studies of standard antidepressants.

Some have expressed concern that St. John's wort functions as a monoamine oxidase (MAO) inhibitor. It has been shown to function in this way in mice, but not in rats or humans (Bratman & Girman, 2003). As I describe in Chapter 18, patients who take MAO inhibitors cannot eat or drink anything with tyramine, a substance found in aged foods. Yet, St. John's wort is widely used in countries such as France without dietary restrictions, and people in these countries regularly consume cheese and red wine (both of which contain large amounts of tyramine).

More concerning is St. John's wort's interactions with several classes of medications. Studies suggest that the mechanism likely involves the drug-metabolizing enzyme CYP3A4 and the transport protein P-glycoprotein (Schultz, 2006). This enzyme accelerates the metabolism of anticoagulants, anticonvulsants, cyclosporins, birth control pills, protease and reverse transcriptase inhibitors used in anti-HIV treatments, and others, leading to lower serum levels of the medication than prescribed (Ernst, 2002; Schultz, 2006). It can also interact with prescription antidepressants, causing a potentially fatal episode of serotonin syndrome (Deligiannidis & Freeman, 2014; Looper, 2007; Schultz, 2006). Prescription antidepressants should not be taken while taking St. John's wort (Harkness & Bratman, 2003). Mothers who are taking St. John's wort need to tell their healthcare providers that they are taking it.

St. John's wort and breastfeeding

St. John's wort is generally safe to take while breastfeeding (Dugoua et al., 2006; Hale & Rowe, 2014). In a case study, Klier and colleagues (2002) examined the pharmacokinetics of St. John's wort in four breast milk samples from a mother taking the standard dose of St. John's wort (300 mg/three times per day). They tested the samples for both hypericin and hyperforin, and found that only hyperforin was excreted into breast milk at a low level. Both hyperforin and hypericin were below the level of quantification in the infant's plasma.

Klier and colleagues (2006) tested 36 breast milk samples from five mothers taking 300 mg of St. John's wort, three times a day. They also tested the plasma of the five mothers and two infants. As with their earlier case study, they found that only hyperforin was excreted into breast milk, at low levels. The relative infant dose of hyperforin was 1–3 percent of the mother's dose, a level of infant exposure comparable to antidepressants. No side effects were noted in either mothers or babies.

There is good evidence to support use of St. John's wort while breastfeeding (Dugoua et al., 2006). The authors found that St. John's wort neither affects milk supply nor infant weight. They noted that it could cause infant colic, drowsiness, or lethargy, although only a few cases have been reported. The authors concluded that common and traditional use of St. John's wort caused minimal risk for breastfeeding women and their babies. They did express some concern about use of St. John's wort during pregnancy, however.

Summary

St. John's wort is another effective alternative to antidepressants that may be more acceptable for some women. Its standard use is for mild to moderate depression, but it has also been used for major depression. However, some cautions are in order. Even though St. John's wort is a "natural" alternative to medications, it too is a medication and should be treated as such. It should never be used with commercial antidepressants. Mothers should tell their healthcare providers that they are taking it as it can interact with a number of different medications. If used with safety concerns in mind, normal use of this medication does not appear to be harmful for mothers or babies. Although hyperforin is excreted into breast milk, it appears in very low levels in infant plasma, and in some cases was undetectable (Hale & Rowe, 2014).

Emerging therapies

At this point, there is not a large empirical base on the efficacy of other alternative treatments for postpartum depression. However, some of these approaches are promising, and could be considered as possibilities for treating depressed mothers. These modalities include acupuncture, yoga, and aromatherapy (Deligiannidis & Freeman, 2014).

Acupuncture

Acupuncture has been used to treat major depression and PTSD in a number of studies (Kim et al., 2013; Wu et al., 2012). A recent review indicated that it is a beneficial, well-tolerated, and safe monotherapy for major depression (Wu et al., 2012). Another review of 52 systematic reviews or meta-analyses found that acupuncture was effective for treating headaches, and appears promising for anxiety, sleep disturbances, depression, and chronic pain (Lee et al., 2012). A review from the US Veterans' Administration noted that acupuncture shows promise as a treatment for depression, and that for major depression, there were greater effects of acupuncture vs. sham acupuncture. However, acupuncture did not improve response or remission rates, and did not differ from short-term use of antidepressants (Williams et al., 2011). Acupuncture has also been effective in treating symptoms of PTSD, with results comparable to those of antidepressants (Ruglass & Kendall-Tackett, 2015; Wang et al., 2012).

Acupuncture was helpful in alleviating symptoms in two studies of major depression in pregnant women (Manber et al., 2004, 2010). The response rate in the first study over 10 weeks was 69 percent for acupuncture, 47 percent for sham acupuncture, and 32 percent for massage, with 20 pregnant women in each group. Sham acupuncture involves using small, metal "needles" that look like acupuncture needles, and appear to puncture the skin, but do not.

In the second study, 150 pregnant women with major depression were also randomized to treatment to acupuncture specific for depression, not specific for depression, and massage groups (Manber et al., 2010). In both acupuncture groups, the practitioners avoided acupuncture points that should not be used with pregnant women because they could start labor contractions. The remission rates were 63 percent for acupuncture specific for depression, 44 percent for acupuncture not specific for depression, and 38 percent for massage.

Freeman (2009) also cautioned against using certain acupuncture points during pregnancy, as they may cause uterine stimulation and could potentially trigger premature labor and delivery.

Yoga

One recent study examined yoga as a possible treatment for postpartum depression (Buttner et al., 2015). The researchers randomized 57 depressed women (Hamilton Depression Rating Scale ≥12) to either yoga or wait-list conditions. The women in the yoga group attended classes twice a week for 8 weeks. At the end of the trial, women in both groups had improved, but women in the yoga group had significantly improved depression, anxiety, and health-related quality of life than women in the wait-list condition, with large effect sizes. They noted that yoga is a promising integrative treatment for perinatal depression.

Aromatherapy

Another interesting integrative modality is aromatherapy. In a recent pilot study, 28 mothers who were at risk for depression were randomized to either one of two aromatherapy conditions, or a control group where they received standard care (Conrad & Adams, 2012). All the mothers were 0–18 months postpartum. The essential oil blend of *rose otto* and *lavandula angustifolia* at 2 percent dilution was used in all treatments. Treatment was twice a week for 4 weeks, 15 minutes for each treatment. At baseline, there was no difference between the aromatherapy groups and the control groups on depression or anxiety. However, by both 2 and 4 weeks, there was significant improvement in both depression and anxiety scores.

Conclusion

Bright light therapy, St. John's wort, and vitamin D are effective treatments for depression. Some emerging techniques also appear promising. These modalities are generally low-cost, not harmful, and with some, mothers can initiate them themselves. These modalities also have the advantage of having a minimal impact on breastfeeding. They can be offered as an alternative to mothers who refuse to take medications. As with other treatments for depression, mothers should be monitored to determine whether these techniques are reducing their depression. If not, other options should be added, or used instead.

Chapter 16   **Community interventions**

In a wide variety of cultures, mothers with depression often indicate that they prefer having someone to talk with vs. being treated with medications (Dennis & Chung-Lee, 2006). Having someone to talk to can take place in more informal community interventions, or as part of psychotherapy. In this chapter, I describe the efficacy of community support. These modalities have been effective in both preventing and treating depression.

Community-based care and peer support is an important way for mothers to interpret, negotiate, and experience social norms of motherhood (Dennis & Chung-Lee, 2006). This can be administered in a wide range of ways. One review found that proactive telephone support, where providers initiated the contact, was helpful in at least four areas related to maternal/child health: preventing smoking relapse; preventing low birthweight; increasing breastfeeding duration and exclusivity; and decreasing the risk of postpartum depression (Dennis & Kingston, 2008). The authors indicated that telephone support, delivered by professionals or laypeople, is a flexible, efficient, cost-effective, and accessible form of healthcare. Telephone support can be the primary intervention, or it can be a component of a multimodal form of intervention.

Peer support

Peer support was helpful in preventing postpartum depression in a Canadian study (Dennis et al., 2009). In this study, 701 women were identified as being high-risk for depression via an online screening system. They were randomized to either standard care, or to receive telephone support from another mother who had previously experienced, and recovered from, postpartum depression. The peer volunteers were matched to the mothers based on ethnicity and area where they lived. The volunteers initiated contact 48–72 hours after randomization, and were asked to make a minimum of four contacts with mothers, and then as many as they deemed necessary. Women received, on average, eight contacts. The retention rate among the volunteers was high, suggesting that it was a rewarding activity for them as well. At 12 and 24 weeks postpartum, a research nurse blinded to treatment conditions followed up by telephone. The incidence of depression was 14 percent in the intervention group, and 25 percent in the control group at 12 weeks. Over 80 percent of women in the intervention group were satisfied with intervention and would recommend it to a friend. The authors concluded that this was an accessible intervention, and effective for mothers from diverse cultures. They also noted that lay people who have experienced similar problems could have a positive effect on maternal psychological well-being.

Mothers can also receive peer support online. A content analysis of 512 messages mothers posted in an online postpartum depression forum revealed that mothers were receiving emotional and instrumental support by participating in this forum (Evans et al., 2012). The researchers concluded that women did receive information, encouragement, and hope from online support groups. Emotional support was the most common. They recommended that clinicians vet sites before referring mothers to them.

Healthcare provider support

Healthcare providers can also provide support to new mothers. In a study of 2,064 women, half were assigned to an intervention of flexible care provided by midwives, and the other half were assigned to standard care. At 4 months postpartum, women in the flexible-care group had significantly better mental health than women in the standard-care group. The authors concluded that midwife-led, flexible care tailored to individual needs significantly improved new mothers' mental health and reduced the risk of postpartum depression (MacArthur et al., 2002).

Home visiting

A study of 623 women from England sought to determine whether additional support in the first month postpartum increased breastfeeding rates and decreased risk of postpartum depression (Morrell et al., 2000). Half of the mothers were assigned to receive home visits, and the others received standard care. At 6 weeks postpartum, there were no significant differences in health status, use of social services, depression, or breastfeeding rates. The mothers were very satisfied with the health visits, however.

A study from South Africa found that home visiting improved mother–infant interaction, but did not decrease depression (Cooper et al., 2002). In this study, 32 women were randomly assigned to receive home visits by trained community volunteers or usual care. The home visitors provided emotional support, and taught mothers to be more responsive to their babies using items from the Neonatal Behavioral Assessment Scale. This intervention had no significant impact on maternal mood (although it was better for mothers in the intervention group). However, it was significantly associated with mothers being more positive with their babies.

Skin-to-skin contact immediately after birth, and for the first month postpartum, has been used to prevent depressive symptoms (Bigelow et al., 2012). This intervention was administered by home visitors, and mothers recorded their times. With skin-to-skin contact, mothers hold their babies between their breasts, with the infants wearing only their diapers. Thirty women were randomized to the skin-to-skin group, and 60 mothers in the control group. Mothers in the skin-to-skin group held their babies skin to skin approximately 5 hours a day during the first week, and 2 hours a day until the end of the first month. The mothers in the skin-to-skin group had lower depression scores at the end of the first week, but after that the effects diminished, with no differences between the two groups at 2 and 3 months. The mothers in the skin-to-skin group did have lower salivary cortisol during the first month, however. Surprisingly, the researchers did not control for breastfeeding, and that is a significant potential confound as previous studies have demonstrated that breastfeeding also lowers cortisol (Heinrichs et al., 2001). Is it the skin-to-skin contact that lowered cortisol, or was it because skin-to-skin contact facilitated breastfeeding? There is no way to answer that question with this study design.

Another study used teams of nurses and community health workers, who were peers from the community, in a sample of 613 low-income, Medicaid-eligible women (Roman et al., 2009). Women were randomized to either usual-care or nurse/community health-worker conditions. The nurses made two prenatal visits, one post-delivery, and at least two additional visits in the first year. The community health-workers provided relationship-based support via phone and face-to-face contacts. They saw mothers every other week during pregnancy, and every week for the first month postpartum. They went to every other week from 2 to 6 months postpartum, and after 6 months evaluated the situation, and then continued to see the mothers either every other week or once a month, as needed. Mothers in the intervention received, on average, 24 visits, compared with 8.5 visits in the control group. The results indicated that the women who received support from the nurse community health-worker teams had significantly lower depressive symptoms. This was especially true for women with low resources, high stress, or a combination of low resources and high stress. There were no differences between the groups for social support or self-esteem.

Education

Education is a key component of many community-based programs that aim to reduce the risk of depression, and help mothers have more positive interactions with their babies. The results on the effectiveness of these programs, however, have been mixed. In one education program (Elliot et al., 2000), women identified during pregnancy as being vulnerable to depression were randomly assigned to a preventive intervention or a control group. At 3 months postpartum, 19 percent of the women in the "Preparation for Parenthood" group had scores in the depressed or borderline depressed ranges, compared with 39 percent of the mothers who received standard care. These findings were only for first-time mothers.

In contrast, a study from Denmark found that a short antenatal education program for first-time mothers did not prevent postpartum depression (Maimburg & Vaeth, 2015). This study compared 603 pregnant women who participated in the Ready for Child program for first-time mothers with 590 mothers who received standard care. The Ready for Child was a 9-hour education program that prepared women for labor, and discussed issues related to infant care and postpartum adjustment, including postpartum depression. They did find that lack of breastfeeding increased the risk for postpartum depression, but they concluded that the antenatal program did not change women's risk for depression.

Another recent study used an education and motivational interviewing technique to encourage mothers who screen positive for depression in a pediatric practice to contact community resources that can help (Fernandez y Garcia et al., 2015). In this sample from California, 104 mothers of children 0–12 years old were randomized to either Motivating Our Mothers (MOMS) intervention or the control group. Mothers in both conditions received a list of resources. The primary outcome measure was whether the mother contacted any of the resources to seek help. The MOMS intervention was a pamphlet and structured 5-minute interview meant to motivate mothers to seek assistance via free and accessible parenting and depression resources. The second part of this was a 15-minute semi-structured interaction by phone reviewing the same content 2 days later. At the end of the intervention, 74 percent of mothers in the MOMS intervention, compared with

54 percent in the control group, attempted to contact resources for follow-up for depression and parenting issues.

Dennis (2005) found no preventive effect of antenatal and postnatal classes, lay home visits, or early postpartum follow-up in her review of the literature. Home visiting by a professional was beneficial, and there was a positive trend for debriefing. She concluded that there was no clear evidence to recommend antenatal and postnatal classes, early postpartum follow-up, continuity-of-care models, psychological debriefing in the hospital, or interpersonal psychotherapy. Interventions that target at-risk women, are individually based, or initiated in the postpartum period are more likely to be beneficial.

Another study found that education during pregnancy was not helpful in reducing postpartum depression (Hayes et al., 2001). In this study, women were randomly assigned to either an education condition or normal care. Depression was assessed during pregnancy, and at two points postpartum. There were no differences between the control and intervention groups. Further, there was no relevant influence of social support or demographic variables. There was an improvement in depressive symptoms for both groups over time: mothers were more likely to be depressed during pregnancy than at either point postpartum. The authors concluded that their findings challenge two strongly held beliefs by professionals in the perinatal health field. First, that depression can be reduced through education, and second, that interventions done during pregnancy can endure into the postpartum period.

Similarly, a study of 540 predominantly White, high-income mothers participated in a two-step intervention that educated them on modifiable risk factors for depression, improved their level of social support, and enhanced their overall management skills (Howell et al., 2014). Mothers were randomized into the treatment or control conditions. Mothers in the control condition received usual care. The researchers assessed depression at 3 weeks, 3 months, and 6 months postpartum, and there was no difference between the groups, mainly because depression was low at all time periods, and in both groups, ranging from 3 percent to 6 percent.

A study on depression, in general, compared a problem-solving treatment, and eight sessions on prevention of depression, with a control comparison group in a European community sample (Dowrick et al., 2000). The participants were 452 participants, ages 18–65, who were identified through a community survey as having depressive disorders. The prevention group had 14 percent less depression than control group 6 months after the intervention. The authors concluded that problem-solving and psychoeducation reduced severity and duration of depressive disorders, and improved mental and social functioning. The problem-solving course was more acceptable than the prevention-of-depression course. Both were effective in reducing depression among participants.

Summary

Community-based programs show promise in helping women make a smooth transition to motherhood. Education programs appear to have only limited effectiveness, but can be effective for high-risk women. To be most effective, community-based programs must take place alongside more traditional, individually focused interventions for depression. Moreover, we need research that demonstrates the effectiveness of these programs in preventing or ameliorating postpartum depression.

Chapter 17   **Psychotherapy**

Another way mothers can increase support is through psychotherapy. In clinical trials, psychotherapy has proven as effective as medications in treating depression, with lower rates of relapse (Claridge, 2014; Rupke et al., 2006). A recent meta-analysis of 24 studies found a large effect size for one-group, pre/posttest studies of the effectiveness of psychotherapy for perinatal depression (Claridge, 2014). There was a positive, medium effect size when treatment was compared to a control group. The effect sizes were the same whether the study was conducted during pregnancy or postpartum, showing that the treatments were effective in reducing depression in both time periods.

Researchers have found two types of psychotherapy to be highly effective for treating for depression in new mothers: cognitive-behavioral therapy and interpersonal psychotherapy. The most commonly used modalities in research studies are interpersonal psychotherapy, followed closely by cognitive-behavioral therapy (Claridge, 2014). These studies are described below.

Cognitive-behavioral therapy

In numerous clinical trials, cognitive-behavioral therapy (CBT) has proven as effective as medications for treating depression and a whole range of co-occurring conditions, such as anxiety, chronic pain, and obsessive compulsive disorder (Marchesi, 2008; Marchesi et al., 2016; Rupke et al., 2006; Speisman et al., 2011). Moreover, patients who received cognitive therapy were less likely to relapse and drop out of treatment than those who received medications alone.

Cognitive therapy is based on the premise that distortions in thinking cause depression. It teaches patients to recognize and counter these thoughts (Rupke et al., 2006). The goal is to help patients identify distorted beliefs and replace them with more rational ones. Cognitive therapy is *not* simply learning to think "happy" thoughts. It is powerful enough to change the brain, although the mechanism by which this change occurs differs for medication vs. cognitive therapy (Barsaglini et al., 2014).

Cognitive therapy has been used to treat postpartum depression. A study from Australia compared standard care, group cognitive therapy, or individual counseling for women with postpartum depression. After 12 weeks, both types of psychological treatment were superior to standard care, and the researchers concluded that individual counseling was as effective as group cognitive therapy (Milgrom et al., 2005).

Researchers added cognitive therapy to medications to treat moderate to severe postpartum depression in another study (Misri et al., 2004). In this study, depressed, anxious mothers were assigned to receive paroxetine alone, or paroxetine with group cognitive therapy. Mothers in both groups improved after treatment, and there was no significant difference between the groups. From these results, there appeared to be no additional benefit of adding cognitive therapy to medications.

A small trial of 23 mothers with postpartum depression tested whether reducing depressive symptoms would also lower parenting stress (Misri et al., 2006). In this study, mothers were randomized to receive either medication or CBT. All of the mothers in the study were experiencing clinically significant levels of parenting stress before treatment. At the end of the study, both cognitive therapy and medication monotherapy decreased maternal stress. Rather than targeting stress directly, the treatments lowered postpartum depression, which led to a corresponding drop in parenting stress.

A study from Korea randomly assigned 27 pregnant women with depression to either a CBT intervention, or a control condition (Cho et al., 2008). The CBT intervention took place during pregnancy, and consisted of nine bi-weekly, one-on-one, one-hour sessions. The components included educating patients about depression, scheduling pleasant events, and changing negative thoughts to positive ones. Regarding marital relationships, the intervention consisted of promoting understanding of their spouses. In the control group, patients were educated about depression in one prenatal session. The authors found that CBT administered during pregnancy was an effective preventive measure for postpartum depression, and that it also improved marital satisfaction. The intervention used standard CBT techniques, but focused on behavioral techniques to improve marital relationships.

However, cognitive therapy was not effective in preventing depression in mothers of very preterm babies (Hagan et al., 2004). In this study, 101 mothers of babies of very preterm babies received six sessions of cognitive therapy. They were compared with 98 mothers who received standard care. There were no differences in onset or duration of depression between the two groups, and 37 percent of mothers were depressed. The authors indicated that mothers of very preterm infants had high rates of stress and depression, and that a 6-week intervention did not alter the prevalence of depression in this group.

A recent review of 18 studies also found that CBT was effective for treating perinatal anxiety disorders, including obsessive compulsive disorder, panic disorder, and specific phobias (Marchesi et al., 2016). The authors recommended cognitive therapy as a first-line treatment due to its safety and efficacy. They also noted that SSRIs are effective treatments, but can be problematic during pregnancy because they have been associated with an increased risk of prematurity and low birthweight. In late pregnancy, SSRI use has been associated with poor neonatal adaptation and persistent pulmonary hypertension (although this complication is rare).

A study from Quebec raises one limitation to CBT. In their study of CBT as a treatment for PTSD, Belleville and colleagues (2011) assessed 55 patients with PTSD before treatment, and 6 months after. The researchers found that many of the sleep parameters improved after treatment, but these improvements were not maintained after 6 months. Of the people who had sleep problems at baseline, 70 percent still had significant sleep problems after treatment, and sleep problems were associated with more depression, anxiety, and poorer health. Although cognitive therapy does improve sleep, there were still residual sleep difficulties, and this may be a particular issue for perinatal women.

Mindfulness-based cognitive therapy

A recent variant of cognitive therapy incorporates mindfulness as part of therapy, and is known as mindfulness-based cognitive therapy (MBCT). Mindfulness is a secular application of a technique originally derived from Buddhism. It involves paying attention to everyday experiences that people might usually ignore: the taste of coffee, the sensation of walking down the stairs, or the sound of rain on the roof. Practicing mindfulness has two key components:

- being *aware* in the present moment, and
- *accepting* thoughts and feelings without judging them.

The theory behind MBCT is that life stress leads to dysphoria, which leads to negative thinking and negative affect, which leads to depression. MBCT interrupts this cycle and decreases emotional reactivity. It contains the same elements as traditional cognitive therapy, but also incorporates practices of mindfulness. It teaches participants to hold negative thoughts in awareness, and accept them with a non-judgmental and compassionate attitude. It incorporates yoga, body awareness, daily homework, and targeted CBT to "harness the wandering mind" (Britton et al., 2012). MBCT has been used in numerous studies of depression, anxiety, and chronic pain. In a meta-analysis of 41 trials, involving 2,993 participants, MBCT lowered anxiety, depression, and pain (Goyal et al., 2014).

A study from Glasgow, with a non-postpartum sample, combined cognitive therapy with mindfulness meditation in an 8-week course for people with relapsing, recurring depression (Finucane & Mercer, 2006). With a sample of 13 patients, the mean pre-course depression score was 35.7. After the course, it was 17.8. Anxiety had a similar decline. Mindfulness was added to treatment to address the ruminative thinking style that increases vulnerability to relapsing depression. Ruminative thinking involves rehashing personal shortcomings and problematic situations. This style of thinking perpetuates, rather than relieves, stress. Mindfulness teaches patients to let go of negative thinking, and to be open to what is there without aversion or attachment. Patients in this trial found that the addition of mindfulness was helpful in preventing subsequent episodes of depression.

Recent studies have also examined its effectiveness with pregnant and postpartum women. For example, a pilot study from South Australia included ten pregnant women in the treatment group, and nine in the control group (Dunn et al., 2012). The treatment involved an 8-week program. The researchers found that 75 percent of the mothers in the treatment group experienced a decrease in stress symptoms at 6 weeks postpartum, but there was little change for mothers in the control group. Fifty percent of mothers in the mindfulness group experienced a positive change in their depression scores on the EPDS.

A qualitative study of 24 pregnant women with generalized anxiety disorder found that women who completed the program (23 out of 24) had significant improvements in anxiety, worry, and depression (Goodman et al., 2014). They also had significant increases in self-compassion and mindfulness. The authors concluded that MBCT was an effective, non-pharmacologic treatment for anxiety during pregnancy.

Another small randomized trial with 26 breastfeeding mothers from Spain found that mothers who participated in the mindfulness-based intervention had significantly higher self-efficacy, and were higher on some components of mindfulness (acting with awareness, non-judging, and non-reactivity), and self-compassion than mothers in the control group (Perez-Blasco et al., 2013). Mothers participated in eight sessions where they learned skills, such as mindfulness vs. autopilot, overcoming obstacles, acceptance, emotional debt, self-compassion and compassion, and forgiveness and conscious care. Mothers in the control group received no intervention. The authors concluded that their pilot demonstrated that a mindfulness-based intervention can improve mothers' well-being and self-efficacy, and reduce psychological distress in postpartum women.

Summary

What we think, and how we frame the world, has a substantial impact on our mental health. Cognitive therapy is a powerful way to treat even major depression. Not only does it treat depression, but it can also produce measurable changes in the brain that are comparable to those produced by antidepressants. It also has no impact on breastfeeding, and is a viable, effective alternative to medications for the treatment of depression.

Interpersonal psychotherapy

Interpersonal psychotherapy (IPT) is another type of psychotherapy that has also proven effective in the treatment of postpartum depression (Miniati et al., 2014), and for prevention of depression in high-risk, perinatal women (Zlotnick et al., 2016). For example, in an NIMH-collaborative research study, interpersonal psychotherapy was as effective as tricyclic antidepressants and cognitive therapy (Tolman, 2001). In addition, it was effective for almost 70 percent of the patients.

IPT is based on attachment theory, and the interpersonal theory of Harry Stack Sullivan. It is time-limited and focuses on the client's interpersonal relationships. Disturbances in the key relationships are hypothesized as being responsible for depression (Miniati et al., 2014). IPT addresses four problem areas: role transitions, interpersonal disputes, grief, and interpersonal deficits.

On a client's first visit, a specific problem is identified, and the client and therapist begin work on that issue. Mothers complete an interpersonal inventory and review information about key relationships, the nature of current communications, and how having a baby has changed those relationships (Grigoriadis & Ravitz, 2007). With postpartum women, the goal of interpersonal psychotherapy is to help them with role transitions and changes in roles they have already established. A related goal is to assist women in building, or making better use of, existing support (Grigoriadis & Ravitz, 2007).

A recent systematic review of 11 studies examined the efficacy of interpersonal psychotherapy for treating postpartum depression. The researchers found that IPT was effective for shortening recovery time for postpartum depression, and prolonging time in clinical remission (Miniati et al., 2014). Miniati et al. noted that IPT was a promising intervention for postpartum depression, perhaps even more effective than cognitive therapies. They suggested it as a first-line treatment for postpartum depression.

Similarly, two review articles indicated that interpersonal psychotherapy is effective and well-suited to the treatment of postpartum depression. In a review of four clinical trials, Weissman (2007) found that women who received 12–16 weeks of IPT showed a significant reduction of symptoms compared with women who received standard care. Weissman also indicated that IPT can be provided by mental health professionals, healthcare providers, or trained laypeople. Grigoriadis and Ravitz (2007) also concluded that IPT is an effective treatment for postpartum depression. They indicated that this approach can be easily integrated into primary care settings, and that it is short-term, highly effective, and ideally suited to the needs of postpartum women.

Clinical trials

Interpersonal psychotherapy was used to treat low-income, depressed adolescents in five school-based mental health clinics in New York City (Mufson et al., 2004). In this study, 63 teens with depression or dysthymia were randomly assigned to receive 16 weeks of interpersonal psychotherapy, or 16 weeks of treatment as usual. "Treatment as usual" included whatever individual psychotherapy the teens would have received if the program were not in place. The sample was 84 percent female, and 71 percent Hispanic. By the end of the intervention, teens receiving IPT had significantly fewer depressive symptoms, had better social functioning, greater clinical improvement, and a greater decrease in clinical severity on the Clinical Global Impressions Scale. The authors noted that the largest treatment effects occurred for the older and more severely depressed adolescents. They also noted that although medications are often seen as frontline treatment for depressed teens, these were difficult to access through school clinics. Moreover, minority families were reluctant to accept antidepressants. Of the four teens in the study that were prescribed antidepressants, all had poor compliance with their taking them. The authors concluded that this school-based program was a viable alternative to medications for depressed, low-income adolescents.

Perinatal samples

Another study compared IPT to parenting education for 50 low-income, pregnant women with major depression (Spinelli & Endicott, 2003). Both the IPT and education conditions were administered over 16 weeks. Women in their sample had a number of severe risk factors for depression: 47 percent had a history of childhood abuse (28 percent sexual abuse, 25 percent physical abuse, 6 percent both), and 73 percent had a history of major depression. In addition, many had chaotic home environments, unstable relationships, or partners involved in criminal activity. At the end of 16 weeks, significantly more women in the treatment group had reduced depressive symptoms by 50 percent or more on the Hamilton Depression Scale and the Beck Depression Inventory. The authors concluded that interpersonal psychotherapy was an effective first-line treatment for depression during pregnancy.

In a study of 120 women with postpartum major depression (O'Hara et al., 2000), women were assigned to either IPT or wait-list conditions for 12 weeks. The therapists were trained in IPT, and they followed a standardized treatment manual. O'Hara et al. found that women in the therapy group had significantly lower depression scores than did women in the wait-list group at 4, 8, and 12 weeks after treatment. The rate of recovery from depression was also significantly higher for women in the therapy group, and they scored better on postpartum adjustment and social support. The authors noted that IPT was effective for women with postpartum depression. It reduced depressive symptoms and improved social adjustment. The authors felt that IPT represents a viable alternative to pharmacotherapy, especially for women who are breastfeeding.

Klier et al. (2001) also found IPT effective for 17 women with postpartum depression. In this study, IPT was used in a group setting. Women had significantly decreased depression after attending the group, and this was still true at the 6-month follow-up. The authors noted some limitations in their study, such as small sample size, lack of a control group, and possible bias in the therapist's assessment of the women.

Reay and colleagues (2006) had similar findings in their preliminary study of 18 mothers with postpartum depression. In this study, mothers participated in a program of IPT with two individual sessions and eight group sessions. Mothers' depression decreased significantly after treatment. However, 67 percent of the mothers were also on antidepressants, and there was no control group.

Involving partners in treatment is another variation of IPT for postpartum depression. An open-label pilot study of Partner-Assisted IPT included ten couples for eight acute-phase sessions, and a 6-week follow up (Brandon et al., 2012). Involving the partner stems from the theory that partners derive comfort and security from each other. When one partner is depressed, it puts an extra burden on the non-depressed partner to maintain positive interactions. If the non-depressed partner does not understand depression, this relationship can turn into withdrawal, anger, and recrimination. The goal is to help the partner understand depression, and how to best support the depressed mother. The sessions specifically help partners understand the experience of the depressed mother, and teach them how to best respond in language that mothers perceive as supportive. They found that 90 percent of the women met criteria for clinical response during the acute phase, and 89 percent met criteria for symptomatic recovery at 6 weeks. They concluded that involving partners in treatment was safe, acceptable, and feasible, and was a useful component of both treatment and prevention of relapse.

Long-term effects

The effects of IPT appear to be long-lasting. In an 18-month follow-up of mothers who received IPT, different trajectories of recovery appeared (Nylen et al., 2010). One-hundred twenty women were randomized to a 12-week IPT treatment group or a wait-list condition. Of the 35 women who recovered in the acute phase, 57 percent sustained that recovery during follow up. More than 80 percent of women who did not recover in the initial phase did recover at some point during follow up. The authors concluded that IPT lead to long-term benefits even for women who did not initially recover. They noted that the women who did not recover during the acute phase might benefit from continued treatment. They also suggested offering maintenance treatment to women who have achieved stable remission.

Another study examined the long-term impact of group IPT at 2 years post-treatment for 50 mothers who had postpartum EPDS >13 in the first year postpartum (Reay et al., 2012). The mothers were randomized to IPT, or treatment as usual conditions. The IPT group received two individual sessions, eight 2-hour group sessions, and a 2-hour partners' evening. The researchers found that those who participated in group IPT improved more rapidly, were significantly less likely to develop persistent depressive symptoms, and were significantly more likely to maintain their recovery.

Prevention of depression

Another study also found interpersonal psychotherapy helpful in preventing postpartum depression in high-risk women (Zlotnick et al., 2006, 2016). In the first study, 99 low-income pregnant women were randomly assigned to receive standard antenatal care, or standard care plus an intervention based on IPT (Zlotnick et al., 2006). The goal of the intervention was to improve women's close, personal relationships; change their expectations about these relationships; build their social networks; and help them master their transition to motherhood. The intervention was four 60-minute group sessions during pregnancy, with one "booster" session after delivery. At 3 months postpartum, 4 percent of the intervention group became depressed compared to 20 percent of the control group.

The second study had a similar design. In this study, 205 women were randomized to receive IPT or treatment as usual (Zlotnick et al., 2016). The women were all on public assistance, with a mean age of 23. They were 38 percent Hispanic and 23 percent Black, and were all at high-risk for postpartum depression. The intervention was four 90-minute group sessions during pregnancy, and one 50-minute individual "booster" at 2 weeks postpartum. At 6 months postpartum, 16 percent of the women in the intervention group were depressed compared to 31 percent of the control group. The researchers concluded that paraprofessionals can deliver a group intervention to at-risk women and reduce the risk of postpartum depression.

Anti-inflammatory effects of psychotherapy

Although evidence is quite preliminary, both cognitive therapy and IPT likely have an anti-inflammatory effect (Kiecolt-Glaser et al., 2015). IPT's effect is due to increasing the amount and quality of support, which lowers inflammation and was described in Chapter 13.

With regards to the effects of cognitive therapy, it is helpful to examine the literature on the health effects of hostility. Hostility is of interest because it is a particular way of looking at the world. People high in hostility tend to attribute negative motives to others, have difficulty trusting others and establishing close relationships. Hostility also specifically raises inflammation. In one study, hostility was associated with higher levels of circulating proinflammatory cytokines (IL-1α, IL-1β, and IL-8) in 44 healthy, non-smoking, premenopausal women. The combination of depression and hostility led to the highest levels of IL-1β, IL-8, and TNF-α (Suarez et al., 2004). There was a dose–response effect: the more severe the depression and hostility, the greater the production of cytokines.

In another study, Suarez (2006) studied 135 healthy patients (75 men, 60 women) with no symptoms of diabetes. He found that women with higher levels of depression and hostility had higher levels of fasting insulin, glucose, and insulin resistance. These findings were not true for men, and they were independent of other risk factors for metabolic syndrome, including body mass index, age, fasting triglycerides, exercise regularity, or ethnicity. These findings were significant because pre-study glucose levels were in the non-diabetic range. The author noted that inflammation, particularly elevated IL-6 and C-reactive protein, may mediate the relationship between depression and hostility, and risk of type 2 diabetes and cardiovascular disease, possibly because they increase insulin resistance.

Kiecolt-Glaser et al. (2005) found that couples who were high in hostility had higher levels of circulating proinflammatory cytokines. As a result, the rate of wound healing for the high-hostility couples was 60 percent slower than in low-hostility couples. High-hostility couples had high levels of cytokines circulating systemically, where they were more likely to impair health and increase the risk of age-related diseases.

Cognitive therapy specifically addresses beliefs, such as hostility. Because negative cognitions increase inflammation, we could predict that reducing their occurrence would lower inflammation. That is indeed what Doering and colleagues (2007) found in their study of women after coronary bypass surgery. They found that clinically depressed women had a higher incidence of in-hospital fevers and infections in the 6 months after surgery, due, in part, to decreases in natural killer cell cytotoxicity. An 8-week program of CBT reduced depression, improved natural killer cell cytotoxicity, and decreased IL-6 and C-reaction protein. Because the immune system was functioning more effectively, this intervention decreased postoperative infectious diseases. Another study by these same authors found that depressed women were more susceptible to systemic infections after coronary bypass surgery due to depression's impact on natural killer cell cytoxicity (Doering et al., 2008). Major depression increased their risk of infections, such as pneumonia and upper respiratory infections.

In another study, CBT lowered C-reactive protein in a sample of 123 older adults with sleep difficulties (Irwin et al., 2014). The adults in the cognitive-behavioral group also improved in all their sleep parameters. Sleep parameters improved at 4 months, and C-reactive protein dropped at 16 months. Sleep improvements likely lowered C-reactive protein, but the mechanism is unclear.

Summary

Cognitive therapy and interpersonal therapy are both effective treatments for postpartum depression. At this time, there is more empirical support for cognitive therapy. Mothers may have an easier time locating a practitioner who can provide it. However, interpersonal psychotherapy shows a lot of promise for both preventing and treating postpartum depression. Indeed, at some point in the near future, IPT may supplant cognitive therapy as the frontline psychotherapy for postpartum depression.

Trauma-focused treatment

As described in Chapters 8, 10, and 12, women may come into the postpartum period with significant histories of psychological trauma. Trauma may be due to previous or current events, or both. Trauma treatment involves a combination of patient education, peer counseling, and psychotherapy. Medications can also be used and are described in Chapter 18. All of these modalities can be combined.

Patient education

Women who have been traumatized by birth events, past abuse, or other events are often frightened by posttraumatic reactions. Education is the first component of a treatment plan. It can reassure women that they are not going "crazy," which many actually fear, and lets them know that they are not alone in their reactions. Patient education contains four key elements: normalization, removing self-blame and doubt, correcting misunderstandings, and establishing clinician credibility (Friedman, 2001; Kendall-Tackett, 2014b). Patient education is always used as an adjunct to other treatment modalities. However, most clinicians agree that it is an important component of any type of therapeutic approach.

A quasi-experimental study examined the impact of a psychoeducation intervention for pregnant women with a history of abuse-related PTSD (Rowe et al., 2014). The program was a self-study program with a weekly phone tutoring session. There were 17 pregnant women in the experimental group, and 43 matched women in the control group. Women in the education group had better scores than did women in the control group on all measures: dissociation during labor, rating of labor experience, and perception of care in labor. They had better scores on measures of PTSD, postpartum depression, and mother–infant bonding. The authors noted that their preliminary findings indicated that this trauma-specific prenatal intervention improved the labor experience, resulted in less PTSD, improved mother–infant bonding, and slightly attenuated postpartum depression.

Normalization

Normalization lets women know that their symptoms are similar to those experienced by millions of people who have been through traumatic events. This can create a profound sense of relief. Women learn that there is no stigma attached to their reactions, nor is it a result of their "weakness." Rather, normalization communicates that symptoms of PTSD are a common human response to trauma.

Removing self-blame and self-doubt

Many survivors of traumatic events blame themselves for being in harm's way, and are ashamed that they did not take some kind of heroic steps to avoid the trauma or get out of the dangerous circumstance. Education can help patients realize that they did the best they could under the circumstances. Patient education can also help women evaluate how realistic their heroic fantasies are. It can communicate that their "failure" to act was due to the overwhelming nature of the event itself, and is part of the experience of trauma.

Correcting misunderstandings

Patient education, and education of family members and friends, can help people understand the woman's behaviors in terms of trauma symptoms. Behaviors that seem strange or upsetting can be explained when seen through the woman's experiences. This can help those in a woman's support network work with, rather than against, treatment goals.

Clinician credibility

Finally, patient education can help establish clinicians as knowledgeable about psychological trauma, and that they understand what patients are experiencing. This enlists patients' cooperation in treatment and can facilitate the development of trust.

Peer counseling

Peer counseling uses an approach similar to that of Alcoholic Anonymous, in that everyone involved in the group has had personal experience of trauma. Examples of postpartum peer counseling includes groups for women who had cesarean or other difficult births, mothers of premature or ill infants, mothers who have experienced previous childbearing loss, and mothers who are abuse survivors. The relationships in the peer group are equalitarian, and there is no authority figure or professional who leads the group. These groups can also take place online. Peer counselors often serve as role models for new clients, and demonstrate that it is possible to move beyond traumatic experiences (Friedman, 2001; Kendall-Tackett, 2014b).

Trauma-focused psychotherapy

When people are traumatized, they develop a conditioned response that pairs the traumatic event with certain environment cues (e.g., sights, sounds, smells) and bodily sensations (e.g., pain): a process known as fear conditioning. In trauma-focused psychotherapy, there are two specific goals. The first is to unlearn the conditioned response that triggers PTSD symptoms. The second is to address PTSD-related cognitions about themselves and others.

Psychotherapy is generally the treatment of choice for people with PTSD (Friedman et al., 2009). Two of the most effective individual treatments are cognitive-behavioral therapy and Eye Movement Desensitization and Reprocessing (EMDR). These techniques are described below.

CBT

CBT in trauma treatment is designed to counteract conditioned fear responses, and to normalize abnormal thoughts, behaviors, and feelings of patients with PTSD. CBT was effective in reducing trauma, anxiety, and depression symptoms in 105 mothers of preterm infants (Shaw et al., 2014). Mothers were randomly assigned to an either six- or nine-session intervention based on CBT, or one session comprised of education about the NICU and parenting a preterm baby. The treatment was a manualized program of trauma-focused CBT, along with education about possible trauma triggers and parenting a preterm baby (including learning about vulnerable child syndrome). It contained psychoeducation, cognitive restructuring, and trauma exposure. The mothers were assessed at 4–5 weeks, and 6 months postpartum. They found that the six-session intervention reduced trauma, anxiety, and depression symptoms compared to the control group. The mothers showed increased benefit of the intervention at 6 months. There was no difference between the six- and nine-session interventions.

Three common forms of CBT are exposure therapy, cognitive therapy, and stress-inoculation training (National Center for PTSD, 2014b).

Exposure therapy

Exposure therapy is specifically designed to alleviate the conditioned emotional response of the traumatic event to traumatic stimuli. After a traumatic event, patients naturally tend to avoid any memories of it, or any stimuli that reminds them of their trauma. When patients avoid processing their trauma, however, it inhibits their recovery. Exposure therapy helps patients master their fears, and counters the belief that they are weak or incompetent (National Center for PTSD, 2014b).

Exposure therapy begins when patients are asked to imagine the traumatic event. In a single session, patients are asked to repeatedly describe what happened, and their thoughts and feelings that occurred during the trauma (Foa & Cahill, 2002). During their narratives, patients are asked to report their level of distress every 10 minutes. If treatment has been successful, patients can confront their traumatic pasts without triggering PTSD symptoms, especially intrusive thoughts or hyperarousal. This form of treatment is highly effective. However, van der Kolk (2002) cautions that too much exposure to traumatic memories can backfire, and actually precipitate PTSD symptoms, such as hyperarousal and sensitization.

According to recent findings, exposure-based cognitive therapy also appears safe to use for anxiety disorders during pregnancy (Arch et al., 2012). Pregnant women have been excluded from previous studies because of the possible impact of the therapy on fetal programming. This risk has proven more hypothetical than actual, and the current state of knowledge is that the benefits (and risk associated with not treating, or treating with medications) far outweigh possible risks of using exposure therapies during pregnancy. Arch et al. recommended that research on physiological markers during and after treatment with exposure therapies be conducted before recommending exposure treatments for all pregnant women with anxiety disorders. These include measures of cortisol, sympathetic functioning, and inflammatory response.

Cognitive therapy

As described earlier, cognitive therapy addresses distortions in thinking. Women who've been traumatized often see the world as a dangerous place and see themselves as helpless (Friedman et al., 2009). The goal of cognitive therapy is to help patients identify these automatic thoughts, and to replace them with more accurate ones. This form of therapy is also highly effective in reducing symptoms of PTSD.

Stress-inoculation training (SIT)

SIT uses a combination of methods to help survivors cope with anxiety, trauma-related stimuli, and threatening situations. SIT is based on social learning theory, which states that traumatic events create behavioral, social, and cognitive fear responses. SIT includes relaxation techniques, biofeedback, cognitive restructuring, and assertiveness training to help patients deal more effectively in social relationships. Stress inoculation training is as effective as exposure therapy for reducing PTSD symptoms, and these improvements last over time (National Center for PTSD, 2014b).

Eye movement desensitization and reprocessing (EMDR)

EMDR is another treatment that has proven effective for many people who have experienced traumatic events. It is based on hypothesis that saccadic eye movements can reprogram the brain, and therefore can be used to help alleviate the emotional impact of trauma. (Saccadic eye movements are the quick eye movements that jump from one fixation point to another.)

During EMDR, women imagine a traumatic memory, or any negative emotions associated with that memory. Then women are asked to articulate a belief that is incompatible with their previous memory (e.g., on their personal worth). While women are remembering this event, they are asked to use their eyes to follow the clinician's fingers that are making rapid movements. During treatment, women are asked to rate the strength of both the traumatic memory and the counteracting positive beliefs (Friedman et al., 2009).

Studies have demonstrated that this method of treatment is effective; 50–70 percent of patients no longer met criteria for PTSD after receiving EMDR treatment. In contrast, only 20–50 percent of women who received supportive therapy no longer met PTSD criteria (Friedman, 2001).

A case study of three women who suffered from posttraumatic stress symptoms after their first births all underwent EMDR during a subsequent pregnancy (Stramrood et al., 2012). Following EMDR, all three patients had fewer PTS symptoms and felt more confident about their pregnancies and upcoming deliveries compared with before treatment. Despite the fact that all three women had complicated deliveries the second time, they looked back positively on their second deliveries. In addition, all three women were sufficiently confident following EMDR that they attempted a vaginal birth for their second delivery, rather than requesting an elective cesarean.

Complementary and integrative treatments for trauma

The use of complementary and integrative treatments for PTSD is relatively new. These treatments have been incorporated into trauma treatment because patients have demanded more holistic methods (Kim et al., 2013). Even organizations that are relatively conservative with regard to treatment, such as the US Veterans Administration, have recognized the demand for these modalities, and are beginning to incorporate them into treatment for PTSD (Williams et al., 2011). The following is a brief summary of some of these recent findings on these techniques as trauma treatments.

Acupuncture

Recent studies have found acupuncture that is effective in lessening PTSD symptoms. For example, in a randomized trial of 138 Chinese participants following the Wenchuan earthquake, researchers compared the effectiveness of electroacupuncture to paroxetine, treating participants for 12 weeks (Wang et al., 2012). After treatment, participants in the acupuncture group had lower levels of PTSD, depression, and anxiety than those in the paroxetine group at every assessment point (6 and 12 weeks, 3 and 6 months).

Mindfulness

Mindfulness can help trauma survivors develop more compassion toward themselves and others, and become less critical of themselves. It reduced symptoms and changed behavior. It also changed cognitions, and improved self-management, relaxation, and acceptance (Dutton et al., 2013; National Center for PTSD, 2010). Mindfulness also reduced rumination over traumatic events, which increases PTSD symptoms (Kearney et al., 2013). Mindfulness could be used by itself, or together with standard treatments (National Center for PTSD, 2010).

Expressive writing

Expressive writing is another complementary and integrative treatment for trauma and PTSD. Expressive writing is based on the work of James Pennebaker, who found that writing about stressful and traumatic life events for a brief period, even as little as 20 minutes per day over several days, resulted in significant reductions in depression, anxiety, PTSD symptoms, and health problems. Expressive writing is thought to be helpful because it helps trauma survivors understand their experiences in a broader perspective, and derive some meaning from them (Koopman et al., 2005). A recent review also noted that expressive writing was effective for treating postpartum PTSD (Peeler et al., 2013).

Expressive writing has been helpful for those who have experienced combat or interpersonal violence. For example, one study included 47 women who had experienced severe intimate partner violence 5 years prior to the study. The women were randomly assigned to either expressive- or neutral-writing conditions (Koopman et al., 2005). The expressive-writing group was asked to write about their most stressful or traumatic life experience. The neutral-writing group was instructed to write about their daily schedules. There were four writing sessions that were 20 minutes each. The effects of expressive writing were strongest for women who were depressed and it reduced the symptoms of depression in these women.

Conclusions

Research on treatment confirms that there are many effective, non-pharmacologic treatments for perinatal depression. All treatments for depression are anti-inflammatory, and many involve some type of social support. When mothers can talk with others about their postpartum experiences, it alleviates their symptoms and eases their transition to motherhood. This research demonstrates that social relationships are vital to mothers' mental health, and that psychotherapy is an essential part of the treatment arsenal.

In the next chapter, I summarize the final treatment option: the use of antidepressant medications.

Chapter 18   Antidepressants in pregnant and breastfeeding women

For many practitioners, antidepressants are front-line treatment for depressed mothers (Geddes et al., 2007). While not all women are willing to take them, they do have their place in the repertoire of treatments for depression. It is also important to know both the risks and benefits of antidepressant use in perinatal women.

Helping mothers weigh their options

When you help mothers weigh their options about whether to take medications, consider the severity of their depression. A mother who is severely impaired will likely benefit from medications (Chaudron, 2007; Chaudron et al., 2007). Another consideration is the type of symptoms they have. Medications are especially helpful in treating sleep disturbance, including early-morning awakening, decreased sleep efficiency, frequent awakenings through the night, and possibly hypersomnia; appetite disturbance, eating too much or too little; fatigue; decreased sex drive; diurnal variations in mood (e.g., feeling worse in the morning); restlessness or agitation; impaired concentration; and "pronounced anhedonia"—or the inability to experience pleasure (Preston & Johnson, 2009).

Another factor is the mother's feelings about being on medications. Some mothers do not want them. In a review of 40 studies, Dennis and Chung-Lee (2006) found that women were often reluctant to take antidepressants, even after education about their relative safety. Mothers were afraid that they would become addicted, that they would have negative side effects or harm their infants, and they worried about the stigma associated with taking antidepressants. In a study from France (Chabrol et al., 2004), 405 new mothers were asked about the acceptability of treatments for depression including psychotherapy by consultation, psychotherapy by home visit, and antidepressants. They found that both forms of psychotherapy were more acceptable than antidepressants— even after they learned that about the relatively small amount of antidepressant in their breast milk. However, the information the researchers gave to the mothers may be why the mothers were reluctant to use them. Below is a partial account of what they told mothers with regard to antidepressants.

> However, the effects of the antidepressants on the developing brain of the child and the long-term consequences are unknown. In the case of breastfeeding it is therefore recommended not to prescribe antidepressants except in the cases where the advantages can clearly be shown to outweigh the potential risks.
>
> (p. 7)

223

Physicians often have the same misgivings, and may avoid prescribing antidepressants to pregnant or lactating women. A study of 61 Australian general practitioners and Canadian family practice physicians found that physicians from both countries said they were confused about whether antidepressants during pregnancy were safe to prescribe because of the many conflicting reports (Bilszta et al., 2011). The family practitioners differed from the general practitioners regarding beliefs about the safety of antidepressants: 42 percent of general practitioners believed that they were safe for the mothers during pregnancy vs. 83 percent of family practitioners. The family practitioners were more likely than the GPs to believe that antidepressants were safe for the fetus (10 percent vs. 48 percent), and they had more confidence about using them during pregnancy (33 percent vs. 57 percent).

A study analyzing Tennesee Medicaid data, which included 228,876 singleton pregnancies, found that prescriptions for depressed, pregnant women decreased following US and Canadian public health advisory warnings about the risk of perinatal complications related to the use of antidepressants in pregnancy (Bobo et al., 2014). Rates dropped more quickly for SSRIs than other types of antidepressants. Pre-warning, the rate of prescribing increased steadily. After the advisories, the prescribing rate dropped quickly.

Factors to consider in medication use

Medications present four specific challenges when treating pregnant and postpartum women including complications: (1) during pregnancy of untreated depression (including preterm birth), (2) associated with exposing a developing fetus to medication, (3) to the newborn of maternal depression, and (4) of medication exposure via breast milk (Kendall-Tackett & Hale, 2010).

Making decisions about which antidepressant to use can be complex (Chaudron, 2007). Newport and colleagues (2002) stated that no decision is risk-free when treating pregnant and breastfeeding women. Practitioners should balance the risk of medication exposure against the negative effects of maternal depression on the developing fetus and infant.

To further complicate matters, a mother's history may predict whether she will even respond to medication. In a recent study, 22 mothers who were treated with antidepressants were asked to record biopsychosocial variables for 8 months (Misri et al., 2012). During that time, depression scores decreased by 58 percent, and anxiety scores decreased by 35 percent. For depression, women had a smaller decrease in symptoms if they had a family and personal history of psychiatric illness. For anxiety, women had a smaller decrease in symptoms if they had a personal history of psychiatric illness, and a history of sexual abuse. The results of this study suggest that biological and psychosocial variables predict outcomes for pharmacological treatment for women with postpartum depression and anxiety.

In selecting an antidepressant, Remick (2002) recommended the following considerations. First, has the patient been on a particular antidepressant before and did she have a positive response to it? Second, if a patient is possibly suicidal, a tricyclic or MAOI would not be a good choice because these medications are potentially lethal in overdose, or in combination with certain foods. Third, the side-effect profile of the medications should also be considered. These side effects include sedation, weight gain, orthostatic hypotension, and sexual dysfunction, and can be more or less troubling for individual patients. Fourth, another consideration is other medications a patient is currently taking; possible drug–drug interactions should also guide the choice. Finally, the costs of a medication need to be considered. The newer medications are considerably more expensive than the older antidepressants that are available in generic form. For patients without prescription coverage this can be a deciding factor.

Types of antidepressants

There are four major types of antidepressants. All work to increase the amount of neurotransmitters (serotonin, norepinephrine, or dopamine) available in the brain. These categories are described below.

Tricyclics

Tricyclic antidepressants (TCAs) are the oldest, and least expensive, of the antidepressants. They have a solid track record of effectiveness and include medications, such as Pamelor (nortiptyline) and Elavil (amitriptyline) (Osborne et al., 2014). They are effective, but tend to have side effects that people do not like, so patient compliance is often a problem with TCAs. Once patients start to feel better, they may choose to discontinue the medications, and this can negatively affect their treatment. One recent article urges psychiatrists to still consider using these medications, especially during pregnancy, because of their long track record of safe use without any significant risk of congenital anomalies (Osborne et al., 2014).

TCAs have another serious drawback: the risk of suicide. Tricyclics can be lethal in too large a dose. If these medications are used, patients must be closely monitored, and not given sufficient medication in each prescription period to provide the means for patients to kill themselves. (MAOIs should also be avoided if there is a suicide risk.) Preston and Johnson (2009) recommend the following medications as alternatives to TCAs for suicidal patients, or those at high-risk for suicide: fluoxetine (Prozac), sertraline (Zoloft), paroxetine (Paxil) or bupropion (Wellbutrin).

Selective serotonin reuptake inhibitors (SSRIs)

SSRIs include such commonly used medications as fluoxetine (Prozac), sertraline (Zoloft), paroxetine (Paxil), citalopram (Celexa), and escitalopram (Lexapro). As their name implies, they work specifically on serotonin receptors. While these medications have side effects, they are fewer than the other antidepressants, and their dosing schedule is less complex. SSRIs are effective for approximately 80 percent of patients (Preston & Johnson, 2009).

One of the major complaints of patients using SSRIs are their sexual side effects, in the general population, and in postpartum women (di Scalea et al., 2009). A study of 70 postpartum women examined these effects and compared two antidepressants: nortriptyline (a TCA) or sertraline (an SSRI). The women were randomly assigned to receive one of these medications for major depression in an 8-week clinical trial. At the beginning of the trial, 73 percent complained of three or more sexual concerns. By 8 weeks, only 37 percent mentioned sexual concerns. Those whose depression remitted were significantly less likely to report sexual concerns than those women whose depression did not remit. This finding was independent of the medication type that they were on. The authors concluded that sexual concerns are more a function of depression rather than a side effect of a particular medication. What this might mean is that mothers who continue to report sexual side effects may still be depressed, and this bears further scrutiny.

Because SSRIs have the potential for interacting with other medications, a careful history of other medications (prescription, other-the-counter, and herbal) should always be taken. SSRIs can be dangerous if taken with MAOIs, non-sedating antihistamines (e.g., Hismanal), TCAs, and lithium because they may increase the levels of each. There can also be problems if they are taken with carbamazepine and St. John's wort (Preston & Johnson, 2009). If switching from an SSRI to St. John's wort, the wash-out period is 5 days.

Mixed-function antidepressants

Some of the newer types of antidepressants include venlafaxine (Effexor) and mirtazapine (Remeron). Venlafaxine is a selective norepinephrine reuptake inhibitor (SNRI), and is a frontline treatment for depression and PTSD. Mirtazapine is a tetracyclic antidepressant, and is classified as a noradrenergic and specific serotonergic antidepressant. It is most useful as an add-on medication to enhance the effectiveness of other antidepressants, such as buproprion and venlafaxine, in cases of severe or treatment-resistant depression.

Desvenlafaxine (Pristiq) is the synthetic form of the major active metabolite of venlafaxine. A study of the milk and plasma of ten depressed, breastfeeding mothers revealed a level of infant exposure of 4.8 percent for all ten mothers, and 5.3 percent for the exclusively breastfeeding mothers (Rampono et al., 2011). The authors noted that the data for safety are encouraging, but they urge further studies before recommending it as a monotherapy for mothers.

Monoamine oxidase inhibitors

MAOIs are also very effective antidepressants, but they have fallen out of favor because of the strict dietary restrictions associated with their use. MAOIs include phenelzine (Nardil), isocarboxazid (Marplan), and tranylcypromine (Parnate). When taking these medications, patients cannot eat or drink anything with tyramine, a byproduct of bacterial fermentation, common in foods such as red wine and cheese. When these foods are consumed with an MAOI, hypertensive crisis, or even death, can occur. They are not widely used in the US, but may be prescribed for refractory or atypical depressions. These medications are enjoying a renaissance of use, however, because if the dietary restrictions are observed, some feel they are safer than TCAs, and have fewer side effects (Kiecolt-Glaser et al., 2010).

These medications are the only antidepressants that are contraindicated for breastfeeding mothers. There is some concern that the medications may cause permanent changes in the baby, and the risk does not outweigh the benefits.

Dilemmas in treating pregnant women

In a recent study in the US, 15 percent of reproductive-aged women (aged 15–44 years) with employer-sponsored insurance filled a prescription for antidepressants (Dawson et al., 2016). The dilemma to treat pregnant women for depression is not new, but the array of treatment choices, and spectrum of mood and anxiety disorders, is. This often leaves clinicians in a "gray zone" of whether to treat or not (Chaudron, 2007). The benefits likely outweigh the risks, but we should not be glib because there *are* some risks associated with using medications during pregnancy (Malm et al., 2015).

In utero *effects of antidepressants*

In treating depression, the most difficult choices involve using a medication during pregnancy. Prenatal exposure carries risk of fetal complications, although statistically rare, that need to be thoroughly discussed with the mother. In short, providers need to be able to decide which medication best fits with a particular patient, and to help the patient accept it without stigma or guilt (Chaudron, 2007). Potential complications must be balanced with the impact of untreated depression, which also increases the risk of complications (see Chapters 3 and 4).

Antidepressants and preterm birth

One possible risk of antidepressant use in pregnancy is the increased risk of preterm birth. In a study of depressed, pregnant women, more than 20 percent of infants with continuous exposure to selective serotonin reuptake inhibitors (SSRIs) during pregnancy were delivered preterm (Wisner et al., 2009). This study included 238 women who were assessed at 20, 30, and 36 weeks gestation. The patients were divided into three groups: depression with no SSRI exposure; SSRIs with either continuous or partial exposure; and untreated major depression with either continuous or partial depression exposure. Women were on the following medications: 34 percent sertraline, 25 percent fluoxetine, 23 percent citalopram or escitalopram, and 18 percent other medications. At study end, 20 percent of the infants with continuous SSRI exposure were preterm. However, the rate of preterm birth among the mothers with continuous *untreated depression* was also 20 percent. The rate of preterm birth among the non-exposed or partially exposed groups ranged from 4 percent to 9 percent. All other outcomes did not differ between the groups.

Suri and colleagues (2007) also examined the impact of prenatal antidepressant exposure on 90 women, 49 of whom had major depression and were treated with antidepressants while pregnant. There were 22 women with major depression who were not treated with antidepressants, and 19 healthy comparison women. The primary outcomes were infants' gestational age at birth, birthweight, 1- and 5-minute Apgar scores, and admission to special care nursery. The rates of preterm birth were 14 percent for women taking antidepressants, 0 percent for women who were depressed, but not on medications, and 5 percent for the healthy controls. The rates of admission into special care were 21 percent, 9 percent, and 0 percent for the three groups, respectively. Medication dose was also significantly related to preterm birth, with higher doses leading to shorter gestational ages; preterm was 20 percent in the high-dose group, 9 percent in the low-dose group, and 0 percent in the no antidepressant group. Birthweight and Apgar scores did not differ significantly based on medication exposure. The authors concluded that medication status, not depression, was related to gestational age at birth.

Similarly, a study from the Netherlands of 7,696 pregnant women found that the offspring of mothers with untreated depression had reduced body and head growth *in utero* (El Marroun et al., 2012). Mothers taking SSRIs during pregnancy had fewer depressive symptoms, but their offspring had reduced head size, and the mothers had double the odds of preterm birth. There were no reductions in body size for offspring of mothers taking SSRIs. They had two sources of data on SSRI use: self-report and prescription records. Small head size in neonates predicts behavioral problems, and internalizing problems, such as anxiety and ADHD. They noted that their data did not allow them to compare whether untreated depression or SSRI use had the most deleterious effects, and noted that for some women the benefits of SSRI use outweighed the risk.

A population study included all singleton births in Finland between 1996 and 2000 (Malm et al., 2015). The researchers compared pregnancies exposed to SSRIs ($n = 15,729$), women with psychiatric illness who did not take SSRIs ($n = 9,652$), and women with no SSRI exposure and no psychiatric illness ($n = 31,394$). Mothers who received SSRIs had lower risk of late preterm birth, very preterm birth, and cesarean section. The risk of preterm birth was 16 percent lower, and the risk of very preterm birth was 50 percent lower for women using SSRIs during pregnancy. The risk of cesarean section dropped by 30 percent. However, SSRI-exposed offspring had more neonatal complications and mal-adaptation, such as low Apgar scores, and were more likely to be monitored in the NICU.

In a large population study in British Columbia, Canada ($N = 119,547$), infants exposed to SSRIs *in utero* were compared with infants whose mothers were depressed and not treated, and with infants of non-depressed mothers. The percentage of SSRI exposure ranged from 2 percent to 5 percent over the 39-month recruitment period. Birthweight and gestational age were significantly less for the SSRI-exposed infants compared with untreated infants of depressed mothers. The most commonly used medications were paroxetine (44.7 percent), fluoxetine (27.2 percent), sertraline (25.6 percent), fluvoxamine (4.6 percent), and citalopram (3.3 percent) (Oberlander et al., 2006).

The timing of medication exposure influences the complications associated with their use. First- and third-trimester exposure are the times of greatest concern.

First-trimester exposure

A recent review found that the overall risk of major congenital malformations related to exposure in the first trimester did not seem greatly increased (Sie et al., 2012). Several studies have had similar findings. For example, a prospective study collected data from women whose babies were born between 1995 and 2003. There were 200 neonates exposed to antidepressants *in utero*, and 1,200 controls (Maschi et al., 2008). There were three groups that differed in the timing of when they took antidepressants: before conception and during first trimester; during the second and third trimesters; and before conception and during the entire pregnancy. The most commonly used medications were paroxetine (58 cases), fluoxetine (32 cases), and amitriptyline (26 cases). As with previous studies, there was significantly increased risk of preterm birth for exposed- vs. non-exposed infants. This was particularly true for the chronically exposed group.

Of 200 exposed infants, 14 experienced adverse events, and three required NICU/SCN admission. No statistically significant difference was found after adjusting for prematurity, birthweight, and sex of the infant. There were no significant effects found by medication type. Three cases (5 percent) of neonatal complications were reported with paroxetine exposure, one of which required admission to the NICU. In contrast, in a subgroup of the non-exposed group, there were 17 complications (5 percent), six of which required NICU admission. One case of cardiac malformation was reported following paroxetine exposure in the first trimester, and a total of 2 percent of the control group had malformations, none of which were cardiac malformations. A major limitation of these findings is that data were collected via maternal interview, and therefore may have underreported, especially the minor effects (Maschi et al., 2008).

The results of the Sloane Epidemiology Center Birth Defects Study also confirmed that SSRIs do not significantly increase the risk of birth defects overall. They included three birth defects in their study: craniosynostosis, omphalocele, and heart defects (Louik et al., 2007). Sertraline increased the risk of omphalocele and septal defects, and paroxetine increased the risk of the heart defect, right ventricular outflow tract obstruction. It should be noted that even with these odds ratios, only 2–5 percent of infants with these defects were exposed to SSRIs in the first trimester. The authors concluded that the overall risk of having a child affected by SSRI use was only 0.2 percent.

First-trimester exposure may also increase the risk of miscarriage. In a sample of 937 pregnant women exposed to antidepressants prior to, and during early pregnancy, there were 122 spontaneous abortions, including three ectopic pregnancies (Einarson et al., 2009). In their comparison group of 937 non-exposed pregnant women, there were 75 spontaneous abortions, and no ectopic pregnancies. Logistic regression analysis indicated that antidepressant exposure, and prior spontaneous abortion, were the risk factors for current spontaneous abortion. The authors concluded that antidepressant exposure in the first trimester is associated with a small, but statistically significant, risk of miscarriage. It also increased the risk of mothers' decision to terminate the pregnancy. They urged caution in interpreting these results because it is important to consider the effects of underlying depression.

Third-trimester exposure and discontinuation syndrome

In neonates, third-trimester exposure is related to SSRI withdrawal or "discontinuation" syndrome (Hale et al., 2010). Discontinuation syndrome includes tremors, jitteriness, excessive crying, sleep disturbances, acrocynaosis, tachypnea, temperature instability, and irritability (Sie et al., 2012). When comparing exposed and non-exposed infants, the rates of complications were 14 percent for neonatal respiratory distress (vs. 8 percent), 9 percent for jaundice (vs. 8 percent), and 4 percent for feeding problems (vs. 2 percent). The length of hospital stay was significantly longer for exposed infants, suggesting that SSRI exposure created an independent effect. The authors concluded that exposure to prenatal SSRIs increased risk of low birthweight and respiratory distress, even when maternal illness severity was accounted for (Oberlander et al., 2006). These findings were contrary to what they predicted. They hypothesized that reducing depression would lessen adverse neonatal complications associated with maternal depression. They also noted that both exposure to SSRIs, and depressed maternal mood, had an additive negative effect of exposure to depression alone for these outcomes.

A convenience sample of 930 women who had taken antidepressants while breastfeeding responded to an advertisement on a breastfeeding and medication forum on a website (Hale et al., 2010). Five-hundred twenty-seven of these women had also taken antidepressants while pregnant. The women completed an online survey reporting on symptoms their infants experienced in the immediate postpartum period. The majority of the women reported that their infants never experienced symptoms of discontinuation syndrome. Twenty-five percent reported that their infants were irritable, 17 percent reported inconsolable crying, 14 percent had low body temperature, and 15 percent had trouble eating and sleeping. Mothers who took antidepressants both during pregnancy, and while breastfeeding, were 2–8 times more likely to report symptoms of discontinuation syndrome than women who took them only while breastfeeding. In addition, if mothers took antidepressants with shorter half-lives (meaning that the level dropped more quickly after delivery), they were more likely to have symptoms of discontinuation syndrome.

A large prospective study ($N = 997$ infants, 987 mothers) sought to prospectively investigate the effects of exposure to tricyclic and SSRI antidepressants on neonates during the third trimester (Kallen, 2004). The medications used included TCAs, such as clomipramine and amitriptyline, and SSRIs, including citalopram, paroxetine, fluoxetine, and sertraline. Following exposure, there was an increased risk for preterm birth and low birthweight. After exposure to antidepressants, especially TCAs, there was an increased risk for low Apgar scores, respiratory distress, neonatal convulsions, and hypoglycemia. Infant outcomes after exposure to paroxetine were not worse than exposure to other SSRIs. The author concluded by noting that there were neonatal effects of antidepressants used in late pregnancy, and that the SSRIs may be the drugs of choice during pregnancy.

A prospective study of neonates compared two groups of infants: babies exposed to medication in the second and third trimester of pregnancy ($N = 46$), and non-exposed babies ($N = 23$). Among babies exposed to medications, some were exposed to SSRIs alone. The SSRIs used in the study included fluoxetine, sertraline, and paroxetine. The second group was exposed to an SSRI and clonazepam (Oberlander et al., 2004). Maternal drug levels were assessed during pregnancy and at delivery. Infant drug levels were assessed via cord blood and at Day 2 postpartum. All but one of the babies was born healthy and at full term.

Thirty percent of the exposed infants showed symptoms of discontinuation syndrome. These symptoms were more common in the SSRI/clonazepam group (39 percent) than in the SSRI group alone (25 percent). The most common symptoms were mild respiratory distress, and in some rare cases, hyptonia. Indeed, all symptomatic infants had respiratory distress. The symptoms were self-limiting, and when these infants were assessed at 2 and 8 months on the Bayley Scales of Infant Development, there were no significant differences between the exposed and non-exposed groups. Discontinuation symptoms were especially likely when paroxetine was combined with clonazepam, as clonazepam appeared to change metabolism of paroxetine (Oberlander et al., 2004).

In a study of 2-month-olds, Oberlander and colleagues (2005) compared three groups of infants: those who had prenatal SSRI exposure, those with pre- and postnatal SSRI exposure, and unexposed infants. They found that 30 percent of the breastfeeding infants had detectable drug levels. When they were present, the infant medication levels were substantially lower than milk and maternal levels. The developmental effects of postnatal SSRI exposure have not been found, and that the effects of exposure via breast milk seem to be minimal (Oberlander et al., 2005).

In a review of 13 published articles, Moses-Kolko and Roth (2004) noted that exposure to SSRIs in late pregnancy increased overall risk of neonatal behavior syndrome compared to infants with early or no exposure, suggesting medication withdrawal. Tapering these medications in the third trimester may be advisable. Most of the studies they reviewed reported on the effects of fluoxetine and paroxetine. Neonates exposed to SSRIs primarily displayed central nervous system, motor, respiratory, and gastrointestinal symptoms. These symptoms are generally mild and self-limiting, and can be managed with supportive care. Severe symptoms are rare, and no reported neonatal deaths have occurred that are attributable to SSRI exposure.

Childhood effects of pre- and postnatal SSRI exposure

Two studies examined longer-term effects of pre- and postnatal exposure to SSRIs. Both studies included the same cohort of patients, and were designed to assess "behavioral teratogenecity" that may have occurred in the wake of SSRI exposure *in utero* and via breast milk. Behavioral teratogenecity included internalizing and externalizing behaviors as indicated on the Child Behavior Checklist. Internalizing behaviors included emotional reactivity, depression, anxiety, irritability, and withdrawal (Misri et al., 2006). Externalizing behaviors included hyperactivity, impulsiveness, noncompliance, verbal and physical aggression, task persistence, problem solving, disruptive acts, and emotional outbursts (Oberlander et al., 2007).

In these studies, 22 mother–infant dyads who were exposed prenatally to SSRIs were compared to 14 non-exposed mother–infant dyads. Of the 22 depressed mothers, 5 were taking fluoxetine, 14 paroxetine, and 3 sertraline. Nine of these women were also taking olanzapine. The exposure to the medication was substantial, averaging 181 days of prenatal exposure, 60 days postnatal for SSRIs, and 41 days postnatal for olanzapine (Misri et al., 2006; Oberlander et al., 2007). Amazingly, mothers in this study remained symptomatic even after being treated for depression: 64 percent still had anxiety symptoms, and 73 percent had depressive symptoms. At the 4-year visit, 59 percent had anxiety symptoms and 50 percent had depressive symptoms (Misri et al., 2006).

With regard to medication exposure, there were no significant differences in either parent or caregiver ratings of internalizing behaviors. Independent raters also rated the child's behavior in a laboratory setting where they were blind to their medication status, and there were no differences between exposed and non-exposed groups. When the entire cohort was measured, mothers were more likely to report symptoms in their children when they were anxious or depressed. This was not true for teacher ratings and the relationship remained, even after prenatal exposure was added to the model. Maternal mood was a better predictor of mother-reported internalizing behaviors than prenatal medication exposure (Misri et al., 2006).

Similarly, there was no difference at age 4 between the exposed and non-exposed groups in externalizing behaviors (Oberlander et al., 2007). Current maternal depression and anxiety were more predictive of externalizing at age 4 than prenatal medication exposure. Umbilical cord blood levels were associated with externalizing behaviors at 4 years, but once current maternal depression was added to the model, it only accounted for 11 percent of the variance in behavioral outcome. Exposure was related to the child's lower persistence in the laboratory observation. Poor neonatal adaptation predicted increased aggression at age 4. Current maternal stress and depression were better predictors of externalizing behaviors, regardless of prenatal depressed mood or medication exposure. This study was the first to consider the dual role of prenatal SSRI exposure and current maternal mood.

A more recent study of 166 mother–infant dyads compared mothers with major depression who took SSRIs during pregnancy ($n = 68$) and non-exposed controls ($n = 98$) (Santucci et al., 2014). They found no impact of prenatal SSRI exposure on the Psychomotor Development Index, Mental Development Index, or Behavioral Rating Scale. They did observe a significant difference in Psychomotor Development scores at 26 weeks for babies exposed to SSRIs *in utero*. However, this difference disappeared by 52 weeks. They concluded that the effects of SSRIs on psychomotor development may be transitory.

In contrast, a more recent study found that prolonged use of SSRIs during pregnancy was related to a delay in fine and gross motor development, even after adjusting for symptoms of depression and anxiety (Handal et al., 2015). Their findings were based on a population-based prospective pregnancy cohort study from Norway. There were 381 women who reported SSRI use during pregnancy (only 0.7 percent of the total study population), and 159 reported SSRI use on at least two questionnaires indicating "prolonged use." The delay in motor development was only weakly associated with prolonged SSRI use, and the authors concluded that the delay was not of clinical importance.

In another analysis from the same data set, Skurtveit and colleagues (2014) found that prolonged use of SSRIs during pregnancy was associated with lower language competence for the infants at age 3. These findings were independent of maternal depression and anxiety during pregnancy. Depression postpartum did not influence the results. Although a statistically significant result, very few of the children had clinically impaired language development.

A birth cohort study from Denmark found there was no increase in behavioral problems in children who had been exposed to SSRIs *in utero* (Grzeskowiak et al., 2015). Their sample included 210 pregnant women who took SSRIs, 231 depressed women who did not take antidepressants, and healthy controls who were neither depressed nor took SSRIs (n = 48,737). The researchers found no association between prenatal antidepressant use and overall problem behavior, hyperactivity, or peer problems at age 7. They did find an association between emotional symptoms, conduct problems, and antidepressant exposure. However, these associations attenuated when the mother's antenatal mood was taken into account. Untreated prenatal depression was associated with increased risk for all of the behavior problems that were included in this study, but there was also significant attenuation when antenatal mood was included in the analysis. The authors concluded that prenatal antidepressant exposure was not associated with behavior problems at age 7.

Breastfeeding and medications

Breastfeeding is another route by which babies can be exposed to medications. There are two key questions we need to ask about antidepressant use in breastfeeding mothers: do medications pass into breast milk, and do medications affect infants (Kendall-Tackett & Hale, 2010)?

With regard to breastfeeding, some have argued that we don't know the clinical significance of medications transferred via breast milk, nor do we know the long-term effects (Cipriani et al., 2007; Sie et al., 2012). Medication exposure via breast milk includes these commonly cited effects: infant irritability, poor-quality or uneasy sleep, and poor feeding. However, most of these effects have been documented in case studies where there may have also been prenatal exposure. In contrast, studies with larger samples generally find no adverse effects. Any risk/benefit analysis must also weigh the risks of infant exposure to mothers' medications *with the risks of not breastfeeding*, which is associated with considerable morbidity. In most cases, the risks associated with breastfeeding on medication are still less than the risk of not breastfeeding (Hale & Rowe, 2014). As described in Chapters 3 and 4, not treating depression is never an appropriate option.

Does medication cross into breast milk?

Of all antidepressants studied, sertraline has been studied the most, and these studies consistently reveal that levels are virtually undetectable in infant plasma the majority of the time. Similarly, studies of paroxetine indicate that transfer is quite minimal. In contrast, fluoxetine does transfer to infants, and because of its long half-life, could accumulate in them. Because of these characteristics, it is less preferable and should be avoided if other choices are available, particularly with newborns (Kendall-Tackett & Hale, 2010; Sie et al., 2012).

A study of 14 breastfeeding mother–infant dyads assessed maternal and infant platelet levels of 5-HT as an indication of medication transfer before and after 6–16 weeks of treatment for postpartum major depression (Epperson et al., 2001). The infants' plasma showed little to no change in platelet 5-HT levels after breastfeeding. Sertraline, and its major metabolite desmethylsertraline, were at or below the lower limit of quantification. When sertraline is administered in typical clinical dosages, it usually has a neglible effect on platelet 5-HT transport even in young, exclusively breastfed infants.

Paroxetine has also been studied with regard to breastfeeding in a study of 25 mother–infant pairs. The researchers found detectable levels of paroxetine in all maternal serum samples, and in 24 of 25 breast milk samples. However, in the infant serum samples, paroxetine was below the lower limit of detection. The mean infant dose of paroxetine was 1.1 percent of the maternal dose (Misri et al., 2000a). There were no adverse effects in any infants.

A recent meta-analysis of 67 studies of antidepressant levels in breastfeeding infants pooled data from 337 research cases, including 238 infants (Weissman et al., 2004). The researchers analyzed data on 15 different antidepressants and their major metabolites, and found that antidepressants were detectable in the breast milk for all the antidepressants they studied. Fluoxetine produced the highest proportion of elevated infant levels, and the highest mean infant level. Citalopram was also relatively high. Only one infant across studies had an elevated paroxetine level, and that infant had also been exposed prenatally. All other infant paroxetine levels were zero, and this included three infants with prenatal exposure.

The authors indicated that there are many factors that influence transfer of medication to infants via breast milk. They noted that some potentially serious short-term effects have been noted in case reports of infants exposed to antidepressants via breastfeeding. However, those symptoms could be due to withdrawal and re-exposure via breast milk. Compared with other antidepressants, fluoxetine was more likely to accumulate in breastfeeding infants. There was also a case report of an infant with no prenatal exposure having symptoms following exposure to citalopram via breastfeeding. This infant's level was 13 percent of the average maternal dose (Weissman et al., 2004).

With regard to long-term effects, Weissman et al. noted that low or undetectable infant plasma concentrations alone cannot reassure us that the antidepressant will have no effect on the rapidly developing brain, or whether chronic, low-dose exposure poses a risk. However, studies with asymptomatic infants are reassuring. Moreover, although antenatal exposure differs from exposure via breastfeeding, prenatal exposure provides a "loading dose" that far exceeds any exposure from breast milk, and can thus distort findings regarding exposure via breast milk. In addition, studies often fail to account for other confounds, such as maternal smoking or alcohol use, both of which can affect infant metabolism (Weissman et al., 2004).

Summary

Breastfeeding infants' exposure to paroxetine, sertraline, and nortriptyline are unlikely to have detectable or elevated plasma drug levels. In contrast, infants exposed to fluoxetine had higher levels of exposure, especially if they had been exposed prenatally. Citalopram may lead to elevated levels in some infants, but more data are needed. Although these appear safe for the majority of babies, some adverse effects have been identified through case studies. Therefore, breastfeeding mothers should be advised to watch for any possible signs of adverse reactions including irritability, poor feeding, or uneasy sleep. Premature babies, or others with impaired metabolism efficiency, should especially be monitored for adverse effects (Weissman et al., 2004). Similarly, Sie et al. (2012) indicate that there is "no evidence that breast feeding [*sic*] should be actively discouraged in maternal use of sertraline and paroxetine" (p. 475). They recommend avoiding fluoxetine because of its long half-life and the risk of accumulation in the infant.

Escitalopram, as a newer antidepressant, was not included in the Weissman et al. review, but it too has a favorable profile for breastfeeding mothers. A recent study examined the transfer of escitalopram and its metabolite into breast milk from eight women who were taking escitalopram for postpartum depression (Rampono et al., 2006). Mothers had been taking the medication for an average of 55 days. The total relative infant dose for escitalopram and its metabolite was 5.3 percent of the maternal weight-adjusted dose (3.9 percent for escitalopram; 1.7 percent for desmethylescitalopram). The levels were undetectable in four infants, and at very low levels in two others. Based on the infant dose calculations, the authors concluded that escitalopram is preferred to citalopram for the treatment of depression during breastfeeding, and is safe for breastfeeding women.

With regards to medications and breastfeeding, Yonkers (2007) makes the following observation.

> The take-home messages are that breastfeeding has many benefits, the amount of medication in breast milk varies according to when the drug is taken and what part of breast milk is assayed, but usually maternal use does not lead to substantial levels in the neonate. However, it is best that neonates be monitored for difficulty feeding, weight gain, sleep or state changes, etc … if the mother is undergoing antidepressant treatment while breastfeeding.
>
> (p. 1458)

The anti-inflammatory effects of antidepressants

Until recently, researchers believed that antidepressants' efficacy was due to their effects on the monoamine neurotransmitters, such as serotonin and norepinephrine. That conceptualization is accurate, but incomplete (Leonard, 2010; Maes et al., 2009). In a review of the literature, Maes (2001a) noted that most major classes of antidepressants, including TCAs, SSRIs, SNRIs, heterocyclics (e.g. trazodone), and MAOIs downregulate proinflammatory cytokines, including IL-1β and TNF-α, and increase glucocorticoid receptor functioning. Long-term therapy normalizes the inflammatory response system, including downregulating IL-6 and acute-phase proteins (such as C-reactive protein). He concluded that antidepressants may have their effect because of their immunoregulatory effects, an effect noted by several others (Kubera et al., 2004; Leonard, 2010; Pace et al., 2007; Roumestan et al., 2007; Vollmar et al., 2008). In addition, anti-inflammatory

COX-2 inhibitors, such as Celebrex, boost the effects of the antidepressant reboxetine (Kiecolt-Glaser et al., 2015; Pace et al., 2007). COX-2 is a signaling molecule that can contribute to glucocorticoid resistance. Blocking it with a COX-2 inhibitor increases glucocorticoid resistance.

Antidepressants also decrease levels of acute-phase proteins, such as C-reactive protein (Berk et al., 2013). A study compared C-reactive protein levels in cardiac patients with major depression before and after treatment with one of the SSRIs: sertraline, fluoxetine, or paroxetine. In these patients, C-reactive protein dropped significantly after treatment, independent of whether depression resolved (O'Brien et al., 2006). Another study tested the anti-inflammatory effects of the antidepressants, fluoxetine, and desipramine, in two animal models of human disease (Roumestan et al., 2007). In their model of septic shock, both antidepressants decreased TNF-α levels. In the model of allergic asthma, fluoxetine and the steroid prednisolone reduced several types of leukocytes, including macrophages, lymphocytes, neutrophils, and eosinophils. The authors concluded that antidepressants had a direct peripheral anti-inflammatory effect. They noted that antidepressants can be useful in treating inflammatory conditions—especially those with comorbid depression—noting that antidepressants may allow patients to cut down on steroid use.

An *in-vitro* study of inflammation was designed to test whether the antidepressant venlafaxine would modulate the inflammatory response (Vollmar et al., 2008). Venlafaxine is a norepinephrine–serotonin reuptake inhibitor. In an astroglia–microglia co-culture, they demonstrated that venlafaxine was anti-inflammatory, and decreased IL-6 and IL-8.

Another study compared the antidepressants venlafaxine, fluoxetine, and imipramine in three groups: older adults with treatment-resistant depression, age-matched adults without depression, and young, healthy control volunteers (Kubera et al., 2004). The researchers found that imipramine, venlafaxine, and a combination of fluoxetine and 5-HTP lowered IL-6. None of the medications lowered TNF-α. They speculated that the therapeutic activity of antidepressants is at least partly due to their impact on IL-6. They also found that tricyclic antidepressants, SSRIs, serotonin norepinephrine reuptake inhibitors, and 5-HTP, have all downregulated the immunoregulatory system by suppressing the IFN-gamma/IL-10 production ratio (Kubera et al., 2001).

In a review of the literature, O'Brien and colleagues (2004) noted that antidepressants have immunoregulatory effects, particularly by increasing production of IL-10, an anti-inflammatory cytokine. They proposed that future antidepressants target immunoparameters by either blocking the actions of pro-inflammatory cytokines or increasing the production of anti-inflammatory cytokines.

Summary

Several recent studies have demonstrated that antidepressants have action beyond their impact on the monoamine neurotransmitters. They downregulated inflammation and at least part of their efficacy is likely due to their immunoregulatory effects.

Phases of depression management with medications

In this final section, the phases of depression management with medication are described. Management of depression with medication has three main phases: acute, continuation, and maintenance (Preston & Johnson, 2009). Knowing about the phases of management can help you communicate a treatment plan, chart any discussion of medications with mothers, as well as discussions about weaning, attempting non-drug treatments, and the mother's competence to consent to treatment.

Acute phase

The acute phase occurs during the first 6–12 weeks of the depressive episode. It begins with the first dose and lasts until the patient is asymptomatic (Preston & Johnson, 2009). The objectives during this stage are to rapidly reduce symptoms of depression, and monitor patients for suicide risk. It is important to evaluate whether the antidepressant you prescribed is effective. If it is not, there are two possible explanations that may account for the effect: the dose is inadequate, or treatment has not been sufficiently lengthy for an adequate response. Assessments should include an evaluation of symptoms, work or school productivity, and whether interpersonal relationships have improved.

In this phase, it is also important to talk to patients about what they should expect from medications. Patients who are adequately educated are more likely to comply with treatments when they understand side effects, and have realistic expectations about what medications will do. Preston and Johnson (2009) recommend that the following be part of educating patients about medication use.

(1) Medications may take 10–21 days before patients notice a difference in symptoms.
(2) When symptoms do improve, it is likely that they will be the ones with a biological basis, such as sleep disturbance. They may not help with more psychologically based symptoms, such as self-esteem.
(3) Treatment is working when patients are sleeping better, have less daytime fatigue, and have some improvement in emotional control.
(4) There may be side effects, but these can be managed.
(5) The total length of time to be on antidepressants varies for each individual.
(6) Antidepressants are not addictive.

Continuation phase

The continuation phase lasts from 4 to 9 months. The objective during this phase is to prevent a relapse of symptoms, which can occur if treatment is terminated during this time (Lesperance & Frasure-Smith, 2000). If symptoms have not improved, or if the patient has relapsed, it is appropriate to re-evaluate both the diagnosis and patient compliance. Are there comorbid conditions (especially substance abuse) that are keeping treatments from being effective? Is the medication effective for the patient, or should another be tried? Is the patient complying with treatment and taking the medications at the appropriate intervals?

A larger dose may be needed in some cases, or the patient may need to be on the medication for a longer period of time. Preston and Johnson (2009) noted that the most common mistake that family physicians make is to undermedicate their depressed patients. This is also true for patients with anxiety, who often require substantially higher dosages for symptoms to remit. Generally, the length of an adequate trial is 4–6 weeks. If the medication is not effective after that time, another medication should be considered, or an additional medication could be added to the regimen.

Maintenance phase

This phase should be initiated for patients who have had multiple episodes of depression or who have particularly severe or difficult to treat episodes, and are therefore at high risk of recurrence. This phase may be for life in some patients, particularly those who have had three or more episodes of major depression.

Conclusions

Antidepressants are an important part of the treatment arsenal for women with postpartum depression and related conditions. These medications can treat even severe depression, and all but one type are compatible with breastfeeding. They can be combined with other modalities described in the previous chapters (except for St. John's wort) to give mothers additional tools to reduce inflammation, improve their sleep, cope with future life stresses, and increase their sense of competence and self-efficacy.

Epilogue   **Some final thoughts**

There is much you can do to help new mothers suffering from perinatal depression. I have a few final thoughts to help you on your way.

Listen to mothers

This suggestion is for people like me. I'm a teacher, and I like to teach and tell people what I know. I have to remind myself to listen first. Just letting a mother tell her story can be therapeutic in and of itself. It will also allow you time to figure out what the mother's real concerns might be. Sometimes mothers know and can articulate what is bothering them. They just need someone to hear them, and validate what they are saying. Other mothers may not fully understand why they feel so bad. They just need to tell their story. I always know that I need to listen more when I start getting "Yeah, but …" in response to a suggestion. If we listen, and the mother feels we've truly heard her, she'll be more likely to follow our suggestions.

Let mothers know about factors that might be influencing their emotional state

After listening carefully, it is then time to share what you know. Sometimes mothers really do not know why they feel bad. This can be true, even years later. Dozens of times, I've been teaching a seminar and had participants come up and say that they never realized that a crying baby (or some other factor they identified with) could have caused their emotional distress. These women are generally healthcare providers with grown children. Having someone simply name the factors involved can be validating to mothers, and lets them know that they are not the only ones that have experienced what they are going through.

Offer specific suggestions that can help

Once you have narrowed down the cause (or causes) of a mother's distress, offer her some strategies to alleviate the problem. For example, if she is in pain, teach her some ways to alleviate it. If she is having breast pain, address the problem, or make an immediate referral to a lactation specialist. If a mother is highly fatigued, brainstorm with her about how she can get more rest. Also be sure to rule out physical problems. If she has a baby with a difficult temperament or was premature, put her in contact with other mothers you know who have similar issues. This can include online support.

Help her mobilize her own support system, including offering referrals to people or organizations that can offer long-term support

Your role is pivotal in terms of helping mothers identify depression and referring them to the sources of help they need, but you cannot be a mother's long-term source of support. It's not practical, and in the long run, it's not best for the mother. What you can do is help mothers find support among their own network, and in their own communities.

One of the most helpful things you can do is give mothers "permission" to get help and support. So often, mothers labor under the belief that they must tough things out themselves. Over the years, I've had many mothers relate to me the apocryphal tale of the mother in the field who gives birth, and gets right back to work. Yes, unfortunately, this does happen—especially in impoverished communities. However, it is far from ideal, and as I described in Chapter 13, does not happen in many of the non-Western cultures with low rates of depression. In fact, I've found that just telling mothers about what happens in cultures that support new mothers can be very liberating, and encourages them to seek out support for themselves postpartum.

You might also have to refer mothers for other types of help. That means finding online and community resources. Resources can include support groups on various topics (breastfeeding, depression, difficult birth, premature babies, childbearing loss, mothering multiples, or single mothering). In rural communities, websites can be very helpful as specialized groups may not exist. Mothers may also need referrals for therapy and/or medications. Organizations, such as Postpartum Support International (www.postpartum.net), keep a list of professionals who specialize in the needs of postpartum women. Your state psychological or medical association can also provide you names of professionals in your community who can help depressed mothers. You may want to speak with these individuals before referring mothers, however. Also, be sure to find out what their payment policy is—especially for your low-income mothers.

Conclusions

Intervention with new mothers can make a significant difference in their lives, and the lives of their families. In closing, I'd like to share the words of Salle Webber, a postpartum doula who understands the pivotal role you can have in young families.

> Incredible as it seems, our culture, with its emphasis on education, has left young adults entirely unprepared to face the practical realities of parenting. And this may be the most important job they will ever hold. So, for those of us who are comfortable and happy in the work of parenting, we can serve the future of humanity through our humble sharing of our skills and our love for children and families.
>
> (Webber, 1992, p. 17)

I wish you great success in this important work.

References

Abdel-Salam, O. M. (2005). Anti-inflammatory, antinociceptive, and gastric effects of *Hypericum perforatum* in rats. *Scientific World Journal*, 5, 586–595.

Abraham, S., Taylor, A., & Conti, J. (2001). Postnatal depression, eating, exercise, and vomiting before and during pregnancy. *International Journal of Eating Disorders*, 29, 482–487.

Abramowitz, J. S., Meltzer-Brody, S., Leserman, J., Killenberg, S., Rinaldi, K., Mahaffey, B. L., & Pedersen, C. (2010). Obsessional thoughts and compulsive behaviors in a sample of women with postpartum mood symptoms. *Archives of Women's Mental Health*, 13, 523–530. doi:10.1007/s00737-010-0172-4

Abramowitz, J. S., Moore, K., Carmin, C., Wiegartz, P. S., & Purdon, C. (2001). Acute onset of obsessive–compulsive disorder in males following childbirth. *Psychosomatics*, 42, 429–431.

Abramowitz, J. S., Schwartz, S. A., Moore, K., Carmin, C., Wiegartz, P. S., & Purdon, C. (2002). Obsessive–compulsive symptoms in pregnancy and the puerperium: A review of the literature. *Anxiety Disorders*, 87, 49–74.

Adewuya, A. O., Ologun, Y. A., & Ibigbami, O. S. (2006). Post-traumatic stress disorder after childbirth in Nigerian women: Prevalence and risk factors. *British Journal of Obstetrics & Gynecology*, 113, 284–288.

Affonso, D. D., De, A. K., Horowitz, J. A., & Mayberry, L. J. (2000). An international study exploring levels of postpartum depressive symptomatology. *Journal of Psychosomatic Research*, 49, 207–216.

Agency for Healthcare Research and Quality. (2002). *S-Adenosyl-L-methionine for treatment of depression, osteoarthritis, and live disease*. Rockville, MD: US Department of Health and Human Services.

Ahlund, S., Clarke, P., Hill, J., & Thalange, N. K. S. (2009). Post-traumatic stress symptoms in mothers of very low birth weight infants 2–3 years postpartum. *Archives of Women's Mental Health*, 12, 261–264.

Ahmed, A., Stewart, D. E., Teng, L., Wahoush, O., & Gagnon, A. J. (2008). Experience of immigrant new mothers with symptoms of depression. *Archives of Women's Mental Health*, 11, 295–303.

Ahn, S., & Corwin, E. J. (2015). The association between breastfeeding, the stress response, inflammation, and postpartum depression during the postpartum period: Prospective cohort study. *International Journal of Nursing Studies*, 52, 1582–1590.

Ahokas, A., Aito, M., & Rimon, R. (2000). Positive treatment effect of estradiol in postpartum psychosis: A pilot study. *Journal of Clinical Psychiatry*, 61, 166–169.

Ahokas, A., Kaukoranta, J., Wahlbeck, K., & Aito, M. (2001). Estrogen deficiency in severe postpartum depression: Successful treatment with sublingual physiologic 17-beta estradiol: A preliminary study. *Journal of Clinical Psychiatry*, 62, 332–336.

REFERENCES

Akman, I., Kuscu, K., Ozdemir, N., Yurdakul, Z., Solakoglu, M., Orhan, L., & Karabekiroglu, A. (2008a). Mothers' postpartum psychological adjustment and infantile colic. *Archives of Diseases of Childhood*, 91, 417–419.

Akman, I., Kuscu, K., Yurdakul, Z., Ozdemir, N., Solakoglu, M., Orhon, L., Karabekiroglu, A., & Ozek, E. (2008b). Breastfeeding duration and postpartum psychological adjustments: Role of maternal attachment styles. *Journal of Paediatrics and Child Health*, 44, 369–373.

Alcorn, K. L., O'Donovan, A., Patrick, J. C., Creedy, D., & Devilly, G. J. (2010). A prospective longitudinal study of the prevalence of post-traumatic stress disorder resulting from childbirth events. *Psychological Medicine*, 40, 1849–1859.

Alder, J., Stadlmayr, W., Tschudin, S., & Bitzer, J. (2006). Post-traumatic symptoms after childbirth: What should we offer? *Journal of Psychosomatic Obstetrics & Gynecology*, 27, 107–112.

Alexander, J. L. (2007). Quest for timely detection and treatment of women with depression. *Journal of Managed Care Pharmacy*, 13(9), S3–S11.

Alton, M. E., Zeng, Y., Tough, S. C., Mandhane, P. J., & Kozyrskyj, A. L. (2016). Postpartum depression, a direct and mediating risk factor for preschool wheeze in girls. *Pediatric Pulmonology*, 51(4), 349–357. doi:10.1002/ppul.23308

Alvarez-Segura, M., Garcia-Esteve, L., Torres, A., Plaza, A., Imaz, M. L., Hermida-Barros, L., San, L., & Burtchen, N. (2014). Are women with a history of abuse more vulnerable to perinatal depressive symptoms? A systematic review. *Archives of Women's Mental Health*, 17, 343–357.

American College of Obstetricians and Gynecologists. (2015). The American College of Obstetricians and Gynecologists Committee Opinion no. 630 screening for perinatal depression. *Obstetrics & Gynecology*, 125, 1268–1271.

American Psychiatric Association. (2013). *Diagnostic and statistical manual V.* Washington, DC: American Psychiatric Association.

Amorin, A. R., Linne, Y. M., & Lourenco, P. M. (2007). Diet or exercise, or both, for weight reduction in women after childbirth. *Cochrane Database Systematic Review*, July 18. doi:CD005627.

Anderson, L. N., Campbell, M. K., daSilva, O., Freeman, T., & Xie, B. (2008). Effect of maternal depression and anxiety on use of health services for infants. *Canadian Family Physician*, 54, 1718–1719.e1711-1715.

Andreozzi, L., Flanagan, P., Seifer, R., Brunner, S., & Lester, B. (2002). Attachment classifications among 18-month-old children of adolescent mothers. *Archives of Pediatric & Adolescent Medicine*, 156, 20–26.

Anghelescu, I. G., Kohnen, R., Szegedi, A., Klement, S., & Kieser, M. (2006). Comparison of *Hypericum* extract WS 5570 and paroxetine in ongoing treatment after recovery from an episode of moderate to severe depression: Results from a randomized multicenter study. *Pharmacopsychiatry*, 39, 213–219.

Ansara, D., Cohen, M. M., Gallop, R., Kung, R., Kung, R., & Schei, B. (2005). Predictors of women's physical health problems after childbirth. *Journal of Psychosomatic Obstetrics & Gynecology*, 26, 115–125.

Arch, J. J., Dimidjian, S., & Chessick, C. (2012). Are exposure-based cognitive behavioral therapies safe during pregnancy? *Archives of Women's Mental Health*, 15, 445–457.

Arinfunhera, J. H., Srinivasaraghavan, R., Sarkar, S., Kattimani, S., Adhisivam, B., & Bhat, B. V. (2015). Is maternal anxiety a barrier to exclusive breastfeeding? *Journal of Maternal, Fetal, and Neonatal Medicine*, 1–4, early online. doi:10.3109/14767058.2015.1104662

Armstrong, D. S., Hutti, M. H., & Myers, J. (2009). The influence of prior perinatal loss on parents' psychological distress after the birth of a subsequent health infant. *Journal of Gynecologic and Neonatal Nursing*, 38, 654–666.

Ashman, S. B., Dawson, G., Panagiotides, H., Yamada, E., & Wilkins, C. W. (2002). Stress hormone levels of children of depressed mothers. *Development & Psychopathology*, 14, 333–349.

Aswathi, A., Rajendiren, S., Nimesh, A., Philip, R. R., Kattimani, S., Jayalakshmi, D., Ananthanarayanan, P. H., & Dhiman, P. (2015). High serum testosterone levels during postpartum period are associated with postpartum depression. *Asian Journal of Psychiatry*, 17, 85–88. Retrieved from http://dx.doi.org/10.1016/j.ajp2015.08.008

Austin, M.-P., Hadzi-Pavlovic, D., Priest, S. R., Reilly, N., Wilhelm, K., Saint, K., & Parker, G. (2010). Depressive and anxiety disorders in the postpartum period: How prevalent are they and can we improve their detection? *Archives of Women's Mental Health*, 13, 395–401.

Ayers, S., Eagle, A., & Waring, H. (2006). The effects of childbirth-related post-traumatic stress disorder on women and their relationships: A qualitative study. *Psychology, Health & Medicine*, 11, 389–398.

Ayers, S., Harris, R., Sawyer, A., Parfitt, Y., & Ford, E. (2009). Posttraumatic stress disorder after childbirth: Analysis of symptom presentation and sampling. *Journal of Affective Disorders*, 119, 200–204.

Ayers, S., Wright, D. B., & Wells, N. (2007). Symptoms of post-traumatic stress disorder in couples after birth: Association with the couple's relationship and parent–baby bond. *Journal of Reproductive and Infant Psychology*, 25, 40–50.

Babyak, M., Blumenthal, J. A., Herman, S., Khatri, P., Doraiswamy, M., Moore, K., Craighead, W. E., Baldewicz, T. T., & Krishnan, R. R. (2000). Exercise treatment for major depression: Maintenance of therapeutic benefit at 10 months. *Psychosomatic Medicine*, 62, 633–638.

Badenhorst, W., Riches, S., Turton, P., & Hughes, P. (2006). The psychological effects of stillbirth and neonatal death on fathers: Systematic review. *Journal of Psychosomatic Obstetrics & Gynecology*, 27, 245–256.

Bagner, D. M., Sheinkopf, S. J., Vohr, B. R., & Lester, B. M. (2010). A preliminary study of cortisol reactivity and behavior problems in young children born premature. *Developmental Psychobiology*, 52, 574–582.

Baker, D. G., Nievergelt, C. M., & O'Connor, D. T. (2012). Biomarkers of PTSD: Neuropeptides and immune signaling. *Neuropharmacology*, 62, 663–673.

Bandelow, B., Sojka, F., Broocks, A., Hajak, G., Bleich, S., & Ruther, E. (2006). Panic disorder during pregnancy and postpartum period. *European Psychiatry*, 21, 495–500.

Banhidy, F., Acs, N., Puho, E., & Czeizel, A. E. (2006). Association between maternal panic disorders and pregnancy complication and delivery outcomes. *European Journal of Obstetrics & Gynecology*, 124, 47–52.

Barr, J. A., & Beck, C. T. (2008). Infanticide secrets: Qualitative study on postpartum depression. *Canadian Family Physician*, 54, 1716–1717.

Barrios, Y. V., Gelaye, B., Zhong, Q., Nicolaidis, C., Rondon, M. B., Garcia, P. J., Sanchez, P. A., Sanchez, S. E., & Williams, M. A. (2015). Association of childhood physical and sexual abuse with intimate partner violence, poor general health, and depressive symptoms. *PLoS ONE*. doi:10.1371/journal.pone.0116609

Barroso, N. E., Hartley, C. M., Bagner, D. M., & Pettit, J. W. (2015). The effect of preterm birth on infant negative affect and maternal postpartum depressive symptoms: A preliminary examination in an underrepresented minority sample. *Infant Behavior & Development*, 39, 159–165.

Barry, T. J., Murray, L., Pasco Fearon, R. M., Moutsiana, C., Cooper, P., Goodyer, I. M., Herbert, J., & Halligan, S. L. (2015). Maternal postnatal depression predicts altered offspring biological stress reactivity in adulthood. *Psychoneuroendocrinology*, 52, 251–260.

Barsaglini, A., Sartori, G., Benetti, S., Pettersson-Yeo, W., & Mechelli, A. (2014). The effects of psychotherapy on brain function: A systematic and critical review. *Progress in Neurobiology*, 114, 1–14.

Bascom, E. M., & Napolitano, M. A. (2016). Breastfeeding duration and primary reasons for breastfeeding cessation among women with postpartum depressive symptoms. *Journal of Human Lactation*, 32, 282–291.

Baumeister, D., Akhtar, R., Ciufolini, S., Pariante, C. M., & Mondelli, V. (2016). Childhood trauma and adulthood inflammation: A meta-analysis of peripheral C-reactive protein, interleukin-6, and tumour necrosis factor-alpha. *Molecular Psychiatry*, 21, 642–649. doi:10.1038/m-.2015.67

REFERENCES

Beck, C. T. (2001). Predictors of postpartum depression: An update. *Nursing Research*, 50, 275–285.

Beck, C. T. (2002). Postpartum depression: A metasynthesis. *Qualitative Health Research*, 12, 453–472.

Beck, C. T. (2006). Postpartum depression: It isn't just the blues. *American Journal of Nursing*, 106(5), 40–50.

Beck, C. T. (2008). Impact of birth trauma on breastfeeding: A tale of two pathways. *Nursing Research*, 57, 229–236.

Beck, C. T. (2009). An adult survivor of child sexual abuse and her breastfeeding experience: A case study. *MCN American Journal of Maternal Child Nursing*, 34(2), 91–97.

Beck, C. T. (2011). A metaethnography of traumatic childbirth and its aftermath: Amplifying causal looping. *Qualitative Health Research*, 21, 301–311.

Beck, C. T. (2015). Middle range theory of traumatic childbirth: The ever-widening ripple effect. *Global Qualitative Nursing Research,* doi:10.1177/2333393615575313.

Beck, C. T., & Gable, R. K. (2000). Postpartum Depression Screening Scale: Development and psychometric testing. *Nursing Research*, 49, 272–282.

Beck, C. T., & Gable, R. K. (2001a). Comparative analysis of the performance of the Postpartum Depression Screening Scale with two other depression instruments. *Nursing Research*, 50, 242–250.

Beck, C. T., & Gable, R. K. (2001b). Further validation of the Postpartum Depression Screening Scale. *Nursing Research*, 50, 155–164.

Beck, C. T., & Watson, S. (2008). Impact of birth trauma on breast-feeding. *Nursing Research*, 57, 228–236.

Beck, C. T., Froman, R. D., & Bernal, H. (2005). Acculturation level and postpartum depression in Hispanic mothers. *MCN*, 30, 299–304.

Beck, C. T., Gable, R. K., Sakala, C., & Declercq, E. R. (2011). Posttraumatic stress disorder in new mothers: Results from a two-stage U.S. national survey. *Birth*, 38, 216–227.

Beeghly, M., Weinberg, M. K., Olson, K. L., Kernan, H., Riley, J., & Tronick, E. Z. (2002). Stability and change in level of maternal depressive symptomatology during the first postpartum year. *Journal of Affective Disorders*, 71, 169–180.

Bei, B., Milgrom, J., Ericksen, J., & Trinder, J. (2010). Subjective perception of sleep, but not its objective quality, is associated with immediate postpartum mood disturbances in healthy women. *Sleep*, 33, 531–538.

Beilin, B., Shavit, Y., Trabekin, E., Mordashev, B., Mayburd, E., Zeidel, A., & Bessler, H. (2003). The effects of postoperative pain management on immune response to surgery. *Anesthesia & Analgesia*, 97, 822–827.

Belleville, G., Guay, S., & Marchand, A. (2011). Persistence of sleep disturbances follow-ing cognitive–behavior therapy for posttraumatic stress disorder. *Journal of Psychosomatic Research*, 70, 318–327.

Berk, M., Williams, L. J., Jacka, F. N., O'Neil, A., Pasco, J. A., Moylan, S., Allen, N. B., Stuart, A. Z., Hayley, A. C., & Maes, M. (2013). So depression is an inflammatory disease, but where does the inflammation come from? *BMC Medicine*, 11, 200. www.biomedcentral.com/1741–7015/11/200

Berman, H., Mason, R., Hall, J., Rodger, S., Classen, C. C., Evans, M. K., Ross, L. E., Mulcahy, G. A., Carranza, L., & Al-Zoubi, F. (2014). Laboring to mother in the context of past trauma: The transition to motherhood. *Qualitative Health Research*, 24, 1253–1264. doi:10.1177/1049732314521902

Bigelow, A., Power, M., MacLellan-Peters, J., Alex, M., & McDonald, C. (2012). Effect of mother/infant skin-to-skin contact on postpartum depressive symptoms and maternal physiological stress. *Journal of Obstetric, Gynecologic, and Neonatal Nursing*, 41, 369–382.

Bilszta, J. L. C., Tsuchiya, S., Han, K., Buist, A., & Einarson, A. (2011). Primary care physician's attitudes and practices regarding antidepressant use during pregnancy: A survey of two coun-tries. *Archives of Women's Mental Health*, 14, 71–75.

Black, M. M., Papas, M. A., Hussey, J. M., Dubowitz, H., Kotch, J. B.-., & Starr, R. H. (2002). Behavior problems among preschool children born to adolescent mothers: Effects of maternal depression and perceptions of partner relationships. *Journal of Clinical Child & Adolescent Psychology*, 31, 16–26.

Bloch, M., Schmidt, P. J., Danaceau, M., Murphy, J., Niemann, L., & Rubinow, D. R. (2000). Effects of gonadal steroids in women with a history of postpartum depression. *American Journal of Psychiatry*, 157, 924–930.

Blumenthal, J. A., Babyak, M. A., Doraiswamy, P. M., Watkins, L., Hoffman, B. M., Barbour, K. A., Herman, S., et al. (2007). Exercise and pharmacotherapy in the treatment of major depressive disorder. *Psychosomatic Medicine*, 69, 587–596.

Blyton, D. M., Sullivan, C. E., & Edwards, N. (2002). Lactation is associated with an increase in slow-wave sleep in women. *Journal of Sleep Research*, 11, 297–303.

Boath, E., Bradley, E., & Henshaw, C. (2004). Women's views of antidepressants in the treatment of postnatal depression. *Journal of Psychosomatic Obstetrics & Gynecology*, 25, 221–233.

Bobo, W. V., Epstein, R. A., Hayes, R. M., Shelton, R. C., Hartert, T. V., Mitchel, E., Horner, J., & Wu, P. (2014). The effect of regulatory advisories on maternal antidepressant prescribing, 1995–2007: An interrupted time series study on 228,876 pregnancies. *Archives of Women's Mental Health*, 17, 17–26.

Bond, M. J., Prager, M. A., Tiggemann, M., & Tao, B. (2001). Infant crying, maternal well-being and perceptions of caregiving. *Journal of Applied Health Behavior*, 3, 3–9.

Borja-Hart, N. L., & Marino, J. (2010). Role of omega-3 fatty acids for prevention or treatment of perinatal depression. *Pharmacotherapy*, 30, 210–216.

Borra, C., Iacovou, M., & Sevilla, A. (2015). New evidence on breastfeeding and postpartum depression: The importance of understanding women's intentions. *Maternal & Child Health Journal*, 19, 897–907. doi:10.//s10995-014-1591-z

Boufidou, F., Lambrinoudaki, I., Argeitis, J., Zervas, I. M., Pliatsika, P., Leonardou, A. A., Petropoulos, G., et al. (2009). CSF and plasma cytokines at delivery and postpartum mood disorders. *Journal of Affective Disorders*, 115, 287–292.

Bowen, E., Heron, J., Waylen, A., Wolke, D., & ALSPAC Study Team (2005). Domestic violence risk during and after pregnancy: Findings from a British longitudinal study. *British Journal of Obstetrics and Gynecology*, 112, 1083–1089.

Boyce, P., & Condon, J. (2001). Providing good clinical care means listening to women's concerns. *British Medical Journal*, 322, 928.

Bozoky, I., & Corwin, E. J. (2002). Fatigue as a predictor of postpartum depression. *Journal of Obstetric, Gynecologic, and Neonatal Nursing*, 31, 436–443.

Brand, S. R., Brennan, P. A., Newport, D. J., Smith, A. K., Weiss, T., & Stowe, Z. (2010). The impact of maternal childhood abuse on maternal and infant HPA axis function in the postpartum period. *Psychoneuroendocrinology*, 35, 686–693.

Brand, S. R., Engel, S. M., Canfield, R. L., & Yehuda, R. (2006). The effect of maternal PTSD following *in utero* trauma exposure on behavior and temperament in the 9-month-old infant. *Annals of the New York Academy of Sciences*, 1071, 454–458.

Brandon, A. R., Ceccotti, N., Hynan, L. S., Shivakumar, G., Johnson, N., & Jarrett, R. B. (2012). Proof of concept: Partner-assisted interpersonal psychotherapy for perinatal depression. *Archives of Women's Mental Health*, 15, 469–480.

Brandon, D. H., Tully, K. P., Silva, S. G., Malcolm, W. F., Murtha, A. P., & Turner, B. S. (2011). Emotional responses of mothers of late-preterm and term infants. *Journal of Obstetric, Gynecologic, and Neonatal Nursing*, 40, 719–731.

Bratman, S., & Girman, A. M. (2003). *Handbook of herbs and supplements and their therapeutic uses*. St Louis, MO: Mosby.

Brennan, P. A., Hammen, C., Anderson, M. J., Bor, W., Najman, J. M., & Williams, G. M. (2000). Chronicity, severity, and timing of maternal depressive symptoms: Relationships with child outcomes at age 5. *Developmental Psychology*, 36, 759–766.

Britton, J. R. (2007). Postpartum anxiety and breast feeding. *Journal of Reproductive Medicine*, 52, 689–695.

REFERENCES

Britton, W. B., Shahar, B., Szepsenwol, O., & Jacobs, W. J. (2012). Mindfulness-based cognitive therapy improves emotional reactivity to social stress: Results from a randomized controlled trial. *Behavior Therapy*, 365–380.

Brummelte, S., & Galea, L. A. M. (2016). Postpartum depression: Etiology, treatment, and consequences for maternal care. *Hormones & Behaviors*, 77, 153–166. http://dx.doi.org/10.1016/j.yhbeh.2015.08.008

Brummelte, S., Grunau, R. E., Zaidman-Zait, A., Weinberg, J., Nordstokke, D., & Cepeda, I. L. (2011). Cortisol levels in relation to maternal interaction and child internalizing behavior in preterm and full-term children at 18 month corrected age. *Developmental Psychobiology*, 53, 184–195.

Buck, M. L., Amir, L. H., Cullinane, M., Donath, S. M., & the CASTLE Study Team. (2014). Nipple pain, damage, and vasospasm in the first 8 weeks postpartum. *Breastfeeding Medicine*, 9, 56–62. doi:10.1089/bfm.2013.0106

Bugental, D. B., Beaulieu, D., & Schwartz, A. (2008). Hormonal sensitivity of preterm versus full-term infants to the effects of maternal depression. *Infant Behavior & Development*, 31, 51–61.

Buss, C., Davis, E. P., Shahbaba, B., Pruessner, J. C., Head, K., & Sandman, C. A. (2012). Maternal cortisol over the course of pregnancy and subsequent child amygdala and hippocampus volumes and affecive problems. *Proceedings of the National Academy of Sciences USA*, 109(20), E1312–E1319.

Buttner, M. M., Brock, R. L., O'Hara, M. W., & Stuart, S. (2015). Efficacy of yoga for depressed postpartum women: A randomized controlled trial. *Complementary Therapies in Clinical Practice*, 21, 94–100.

Buttner, M. M., Mott, S. L., Pearlstein, T., Stuart, S., Zlotnick, C., & O'Hara, M. W. (2013). Examination of premenstrual symptoms as a risk factor for depression in postpartum women. *Archives of Women's Mental Health*, 16, 219–225.

Byatt, N., Biebel, K., Friedman, L., Debordes-Jackson, G., & Ziedonis, D. (2013). Women's perspectives on postpartum depression screening in pediatric settings: A preliminary study. *Archives of Women's Mental Health*, 16, 429–432.

Cacciatore, J., Schnebly, S., & Froen, J. F. (2009). The effects of social support on maternal anxiety and depression after stillbirth. *Health & Social Care in the Community*, 17, 167–176.

Caldwell, B. A., & Redeker, N. S. (2009). Sleep patterns and psychological distress in women living in an inner city. *Research in Nursing & Health*, 32, 177–190.

Canivet, C., Jakobsson, I., & Hagander, B. (2002). Colicky infants according to maternal reports in telephone interviews and diaries: A large Scandinavian study. *Journal of Developmental & Behavioral Pediatrics*, 23, 1–8.

Centers for Disease Control and Prevention. (2006). Understanding intimate partner violence fact sheet. www.cdc.gov/injury

Centers for Disease Control and Prevention. (2008). Prevalence of postpartum depressive symptoms: 17 states, 2004–2005. *Morbidity & Mortality Weekly Report*, 57, 361–367.

Centers for Disease Control and Prevention. (2015). *Mental health among women of reproductive age*. www.cdc.gov/reproductivehealth/depression/pdfs/mental_health_women_repo_age.pdf

Cerulli, C., Talbot, N. L., Tang, W., & Chaudron, L. H. (2011). Co-occurring intimate partner violence and mental health diagnoses in perinatal women. *Journal of Women's Health*, 20, 1797–1803.

Chabrol, H., & Teissedre, J. (2004). Relation between Edinburgh Postnatal Depression Scale scores at 2–3 days and 4–6 weeks postpartum. *Journal of Reproductive and Infant Psychology*, 22, 33–39.

Chabrol, H., Teissedre, J., Armitage, M. D., & Walburg, V. (2004). Acceptability of psychotherapy and antidepressants for postnatal depression among newly delivered mothers. *Journal of Reproductive and Infant Psychology*, 22, 5–12.

Chandra, P. S., Vankatasubramanian, G., & Thomas, T. (2002). Infanticidal ideas and infanticial behavior in Indian women with severe postpartum psychiatric disorders. *Journal of Nervous & Mental Disease*, 190, 457–461.

Chang, S.-R., Chen, K.-H., Ho, H.-N., Lai, Y.-H., Lin, M.-I., Lee, C.-N., & Lin, W.-A. (2015). Depressive symptoms, pain, and sexual dysfunction over the first year following vaginal or cesarean delivery: A prospective longitudinal study. *International Journal of Nursing Studies*, 52, 1433–1444.

Chaudron, L. H. (2007). Treating pregnant women with antidepressants: The gray zone. *Journal of Women's Health*, 16, 551–553.

Chaudron, L. H., Kitzman, H. J., Peifer, K. L., Morrow, S., Perez, L. M., & Newman, M. C. (2005). Prevalence of maternal depressive symptoms in low-income Hispanic women. *Journal of Clinical Psychiatry*, 66, 418–423.

Chaudron, L. H., Klein, M. H., Remington, P., Palta, M., Allen, C., & Essex, M. J. (2001). Predictors, prodromes, and incidence of postpartum depression. *Journal of Psychosomatic Obstetrics & Gynecology*, 22, 103–112.

Chaudron, L. H., Szilagyi, P. G., Campbell, A. T., Mounts, K. O., & McInerny, T. K. (2007). Legal and ethical considerations: Risk and benefits of postpartum depression screening at well-child visits. *Pediatrics*, 119, 123–128.

Chen, E., Bloomberg, G. R., Fisher, E. B., & Strunk, R. C. (2003). Predictors of repeat hospitalizations in children with asthma: The role of psychosocial and socioenvironmental factors. *Health Psychology*, 22, 12–18.

Chi, T. C., & Hinshaw, S. P. (2002). Mother–child relationships of children with ADHD: The role of maternal depressive symptoms and depression-related distortions. *Journal of Abnormal Child Psychology*, 30, 387–400.

Cho, H. J., Kwon, J. H., & Lee, J. J. (2008). Antenatal cognitive-behavioral therapy for prevention of postpartum depression: A pilot study. *Yonsei Medical Journal*, 49, 553–562.

Choi, K. R., & Seng, J. S. (2016). Predisposing and precipitating factors for dissociation during labor in a cohort study of posttraumatic stress disorder and childbearing outcomes. *Journal of Midwifery and Women's Health*, 61, 68–76.

Chojenta, C. L., Lucke, J. C., Forder, P. M., & Loxton, D. J. (2016). Maternal health factors as risks for postnatal depression: A prospective longitudinal study. *PLoS ONE*, 11(1), e0147246. doi:10.1371/journal.pone.0147246

Chong, M. F. F., Ong, Y.-L., Calder, P. C., Colega, M., Wong, J. X. Y., Tan, C. S., Lim, A. L., et al. (2015). Long-chain polyunsaturated fatty acid status during pregnancy and maternal mental health in pregnancy and the postpartum period: Results from the GUSTO study. *Journal of Clinical Psychiatry*, 76, e848–e856.

Christl, B., Reilly, N., Smith, M., Sims, D., Chavasse, F., & Austin, M.-P. (2013). The mental health of mothers of unsettled infants: Is there value in routine psychosocial assessment in this context? *Archives of Women's Mental Health*, 16, 391–399.

Cigoli, V., Gilli, G., & Saita, E. (2006). Relational factors in psychopathological responses to childbirth. *Journal of Psychosomatic Obstetrics & Gynecology*, 27(2), 91–97.

Cipriani, A., Geddes, J. R., Furukawa, T. A., & Barbui, C. (2007). Metareview on short-term effectiveness and safety of antidepressants for depression: An evidence-based approach to inform clinical practice. *Canadian Journal of Psychiatry*, 52, 553–562.

Claridge, A. M. (2014). Efficacy of systemically oriented psychotherapies in the treatment of perinatal depression: A meta-analysis. *Archives of Women's Mental Health*, 17, 3–15.

Clout, D., & Brown, R. (2015). Sociodemographic, pregnancy, obstetric, and postnatal predictors of postpartum stress, anxiety, and depression in new mothers. *Journal of Affective Disorders*, 188, 60–67.

Collins, C. H., Zimmerman, C., & Howard, L. M. (2011). Refugee, asylum seeker, immigrant women and postnatal depression: Rates and risk factors. *Archives of Women's Mental Health*, 14, 3–11.

Conrad, P., & Adams, C. (2012). The effects of clinical aromatherapy for anxiety and depression in the high risk postpartum woman—A pilot study. *Complementary Therapies in Clinical Practice*, 18, 164–168. doi:10.1016/j.ctcp.2012.05.002

REFERENCES

Cooney, G. M., Dwan, K., Greig, C. A., Lawlor, D. A., Rimer, J., Waugh, F. R., McMurdo, M., & Mead, G. E. (2013). Exercise for depression. *Cochrane Database of Systematic Review, Issue* 9, CD004366.

Cooper, P. J., Landman, M., Tomlinson, M., Molteno, C., Swartz, L., & Murray, L. (2002). Impact of a mother–infant intervention in an indigent peri-urban South African context: Pilot study. *British Journal of Psychiatry*, 180, 76–81.

Cornish, A. M., McMahon, C. A., Ungerer, B., Barnett, B., Kowalenko, N., & Tennant, C. (2005). Postnatal depression and infant cognitive and motor development in the second postnatal year: The infant of depression chronicity and infant gender. *Infant Behavior & Development*, 28, 407–417.

Corral, M., Kuan, A., & Kostaras, D. (2000). Bright light therapy's effect on postpartum depression. *American Journal of Psychiatry*, 157, 303–304.

Corral, M., Wardrop, A. A., Zhang, H., Grewal, A. K., & Patton, S. (2007). Morning light therapy for postpartum depression. *Archives of Women's Mental Health*, 10, 221–224.

Corwin, E. J., & Arbour, M. (2007). Postpartum fatigue and evidence-based interventions. *MCN*, 32, 215–220.

Corwin, E. J., & Johnston, N. (2008). Symptoms of postpartum depression associated with elevated levels of Interleukin-1 beta during the first month postpartum. *Biological Research for Nursing*, 10, 128–133.

Corwin, E. J., & Pajer, K. (2008). The psychoneuroimmunology of postpartum depression. *Journal of Women's Health*, 17, 1529–1534.

Corwin, E. J., Bozoky, I., Pugh, L. C., & Johnston, N. (2003). Interleukin-1 beta elevation during the postpartum period. *Annals of Behavioral Medicine*, 25, 41–47.

Corwin, E. J., Guo, Y., Pajer, K., Lowe, N., McCarthy, D., Schmiege, S., Weber, M., Pace, T., & Stafford, B. (2013). Immune dysregulation and glucocorticoid resistance in minority and low income pregnant women. *Psychoneuroendocrinology*, 38, 1786–1796.

Corwin, E. J., Kohen, R., Jarrett, M., & Stafford, B. (2010). The heritability of postpartum depression. *Biological Research for Nursing*, 12, 73–83.

Corwin, E. J., Pajer, K., Paul, S., Lowe, N., Weber, M., & McCarthy, D. O. (2015). Bidirectional psychoneuroimmune interactions in the early postpartum period influence risk of postpartum depression. *Brain, Behavior & Immunity*, 49, 86–93. doi:10.1016/j.bbi2015.04.012

Coussons-Read, M. E., Lobel, M., Carey, J. C., Kreither, M. O., D'Anna, K., Argys, L., Ross, R. G., Brandt, C., & Cole, S. (2012). The occurrence of preterm delivery is linked to pregnancy-specific distress and elevated inflammatory markers across gestation. *Brain, Behavior & Immunity*, 26, 650–659.

Coussons-Read, M. E., Okun, M. L., Schmitt, M. P., & Giese, S. (2005). Prenatal stress alters cytokine levels in a manner that may endanger human pregnancy. *Psychosomatic Medicine*, 67, 625–631.

Cox, J. L., Holden, J. M., & Sagovsky, R. (1987). Detection of postnatal depression: Development of the 10-item Edinburgh Postnatal Depression Scale. *British Journal of Psychiatry*, 150, 782–786.

Crouch, J. L., Skowronski, J. J., Milner, J. S., & Harris, B. (2008). Parental responses to infant crying: The influence of child physical abuse risk and hostile priming. *Child Abuse & Neglect*, 32, 702–710.

Crowley, S. K., & Youngstedt, S. D. (2012). Efficacy of light therapy for perinatal depression: A review. *Journal of Physiological Anthropology*, 31, 15. wwwjphysiolanthropol.com/content/31/1/15 Retrieved from wwwjphysiolanthropol.com/content/31/1/15

Cryan, E., Keogh, F., Connolly, E., Cody, S., Quinlan, A., & Daly, I. (2001). Depression among postnatal women in an urban Irish community. *Irish Journal of Psychological Medicine*, 18, 5–10.

Currie, M. L., & Rademacher, R. (2004). The pediatrician's role in recognizing and intervening in postpartum depression. *Pediatric Clinics of North America*, 51, 785–801.

Cutler, C. B., Legano, L. A., Dreyer, B. P., Fierman, A. H., Berkule, S. B., Lusskin, S. I., Tomopoulos, S., Roth, M., & Mendelsohn, A. L. (2007). Screening for maternal depression in a low education population using a two-item questionnaire. *Archives of Women's Mental Health*, 10, 277–283.

Da Costa, D., Dritsa, M., Verreault, N., Balaa, C., Kudzman, J., & Khalife, S. (2010). Sleep problems and depressed mood negatively impact health-related quality of life during pregnancy. *Archives of Women's Mental Health*, 13, 249–257.

Da Costa, D., Larouche, J., Dritsa, M., & Brender, W. (2000). Psychosocial correlates of prepartum and postpartum depressed mood. *Journal of Affective Disorders*, 59, 31–40.

Dagher, R. K., & Shenassa, E. D. (2012). Prenatal health behaviors and postpartum depression: Is there an association? *Archives of Women's Mental Health*, 15, 31–37.

Dagher, R. K., McGovern, P. M., Alexander, B. H., Dowd, B. E., Ukestad, L. K., & McCaffrey, D. J. (2009). The psychosocial work environment and maternal postpartum depression. *International Journal of Behavioral Medicine*, 16, 339–346.

Daley, A. J., Foster, L., Long, G., Palmer, C., Robinson, O., Walmsley, H., & Ward, R. (2015). The effectiveness of exercise for the prevention and treatment of antenatal depression: Systematic review with meta-analysis. *British Journal of Obstetrics & Gynecology*, 122, 57–63.

Daley, A. J., Macarthur, C., & Winter, H. (2007). The role of exercise in treating postpartum depression: A review of the literature. *Journal of Midwifery and Women's Health*, 52, 56–62.

Daley, A. J., Winter, H., Grimmett, C., McGuinness, M., McManus, R., & Macarthur, C. (2008). Feasibility of an exercise intervention for women with postnatal depression: A pilot randomised controlled trial. *British Journal of General Practice*, 58, 178–183.

Danaci, A. E., Dinc, G., Deveci, A., Sen, F. S., & Icelli, I. (2002). Postnatal depression in Turkey: Epidemiological and cultural aspects. *Social Psychiatry & Psychiatric Epidemiology*, 37, 125–129.

Danese, A., Pariante, C. M., Caspi, A., Taylor, A., & Poulton, R. (2007). Childhood maltreatment predicts adult inflammation in a life-course study. *Proceedings of the National Academy of Sciences U S A*, 104, 1319–1324. doi:0610362104 [pii]10.1073/pnas.0610362104

Dave, S., Petersen, I., Sherr, L., & Nazareth, I. (2010). Incidence of maternal and paternal depression in primary care: A cohort study using a primary care database. *Archives of Pediatric & Adolescent Medicine*, 164, 1038–1044.

Davis, E. P., Glynn, L. M., Waffarn, F., & Sandman, C. A. (2011). Prenatal maternal stress programs infant stress regulation. *Journal of Child Psychology and Psychiatry*, 52, 119–129.

Davis, K., Pearlstein, T., Stuart, S., O'Hara, M. W., & Zlotnick, C. (2013). Analysis of brief screening tools for the detection of postpartum depression: Comparisons of the PRAMS 6-item instrument, PHQ-9, and structured interviews. *Archives of Women's Mental Health*, 16, 271–277.

Dawson, A. L., Ailes, E. C., Gilboa, S. M., Simeone, R. M., Lind, J. N., Farr, S. L., Broussard, C. S., et al. (2016). Antidepressant prescription claims among reproductive-aged women with private employer-sponsored insurance—United States 2008–2013. *Morbidity & Mortality Weekly Report*, 65(3), 41–46. Retrieved from http://dx.doi.org/10.15585/mmwr.mm6503a1

Dayan, J., Creveuil, C., Marks, M. N., Conroy, S., Herlicoviez, M., Dreyfus, M., & Tordjman, S. (2006). Prenatal depression, prenatal anxiety, and spontaneous preterm birth: A prospective cohort study among women with early and regular care. *Psychosomatic Medicine*, 68, 938–946.

de Jonge, P., van den Brink, R. H., Spijkerman, T. A., & Ormel, J. (2006). Only incident depressive episodes after myocardial infarction are associated with new cardiovascular events. *Journal of the American College of Cardiology*, 48, 2204–2208. doi:S0735-1097(06)02325-4 [pii]10.1016/j.jacc.2006.06.077

De Schepper, S., Vercauteren, T., Tersago, J., Jacquemyn, Y., Raes, F., & Franck, E. (2016). Post-traumatic stress disorder after childbirth and the influence of maternity team care during labour and birth: A cohort study. *Midwifery*, 32, 87–92.

Declercq, E. R., Sakala, C., Corry, M. P., & Applebaum, S. (2008). *New mothers speak out: National survey results highlight women's postpartum experiences*. New York, NY: Childbirth Connection.

REFERENCES

Delatte, R., Cao, H., Meltzer-Brody, S., & Menard, M. K. (2009). Universal screening for postpartum depression: An inquiry into provider attitudes and practice. *American Journal of Obstetrics and Gynecology*, 200(5), e63–e64.

Deligiannidis, K. M., & Freeman, M. P. (2014). Complementary and alternative medicine therapies for depression. *Best Practice & Research Clinical Obstetrics & Gynecology*, 28, 85–95.

Dell'Aica, I., Caniato, R., Biggin, S., & Garbisa, S. (2007). Matrix proteases, green tea, and St. John's wort: Biomedical research catches up with folk medicine. *Clinical Chimica Acta*, 381, 69–77.

Demissie, Z., Siega-Riz, A. M., Evenson, K. R., Herring, A. H., Dole, N., & Gaynes, B. N. (2011a). Associations between physical activity and postpartum depressive symptoms. *Journal of Women's Health*, 20, 1025–1034.

Demissie, Z., Siega-Riz, A. M., Evenson, K. R., Herring, A. H., Dole, N., & Gaynes, B. N. (2011b). Physical activity and depressive symptoms among pregnant women: The PIN3 study. *Archives of Women's Mental Health*, 14, 145–157.

deMontigny, F., Girard, M.-E., Lacharite, C., Dubeau, D., & Devault, A. (2013). Psychosocial factors associated with paternal postnatal depression. *Journal of Affective Disorders*, 150, 44–49.

Dennis, C.-L. (2004a). Can we identify mothers at risk for postpartum depression in the immediate postpartum period using the Edinburgh Postnatal Depression Scale? *Journal of Affective Disorders*, 78, 163–169.

Dennis, C.-L. (2004b). Influence of depressive symptomatology on maternal health service utilization and general health. *Archives of Women's Mental Health*, 7, 183–191.

Dennis, C.-L. (2005). Psychosocial and psychological interventions for prevention of postnatal depression: Systematic review. *British Medical Journal*, 331, 15. doi:10.1136/bmj.1331.7505.1115.

Dennis, C.-L., & Allen, K. (2008). Interventions (other than pharmacological, psychosocial or psychological) for treating antenatal depression. *Cochrane Database Systematic Review*(4), CD006795. doi:006710.001002/14651858.CD14006795.pub14651852.

Dennis, C.-L., & Chung-Lee, L. (2006). Postpartum depression help-seeking barriers and maternal treatment preferences: A qualitative systematic review. *Birth*, 33, 323–331.

Dennis, C.-L., & Kingston, D. (2008). A systematic review of telephone support for women during pregnancy and the early postpartum period. *Journal of Obstetric, Gynecologic and Neonatal Nursing*, 37, 301–314.

Dennis, C.-L., & McQueen, K. (2007). Does maternal postpartum depressive symptomatology influence infant feeding outcomes? *Acta Paediatrica*, 96, 590–594.

Dennis, C.-L., & McQueen, K. (2009). The relationship between infant-feeding outcomes and postpartum depression: A qualitative systematic review. *Pediatrics*, 123, e736–e751.

Dennis, C.-L., & Ross, L. E. (2005). Relationships among infant sleep patterns, maternal fatigue, and development of depressive symptomatology. *Birth*, 32, 187–193.

Dennis, C.-L., & Ross, L. E. (2006a). The clinical utility of maternal self-reported personal and familial psychiatric history in identifying women at risk for postpartum depression. *Acta Obstetricia et Gynecologica*, 85, 1179–1185.

Dennis, C.-L., & Ross, L. E. (2006b). Women's perceptions of partner support and conflict in the development of postpartum depressive symptoms. *Journal of Advanced Nursing*, 56, 588–599.

Dennis, C.-L., Hodnett, E., Kenton, L., Weston, J., Zupancic, J., Stewart, D. E., & Kiss, A. (2009). Effect of peer support on prevention of postnatal depression among high-risk women: Multisite randomised controlled trial. *British Medical Journal*, 338, a3064. doi:3010.1136/bmj.a3064.

Dennis, C.-L., Janssen, P. A., & Singer, J. (2004). Identifying women at-risk for postpartum depression in the immediate postpartum period. *Acta Psychiatrica Scandanavica*, 110, 338–346.

des Rivieres-Pigeon, C., Seguin, L., Goulet, L., & Descarries, F. (2001). Unraveling the complexities of the relationship between employment status and postpartum depressive symptomatology. *Women & Health*, 34, 61–79.

Desan, P. H., Weinstein, A.J., Michalak, E.E., Tam, E.M., Meesters, Y., Ruiter, M.J., Horn, E., et al. (2007). A controlled trial of the Litebook light-emitting diode (LED) light therapy device for treatment of Seasonal Affective Disorder (SAD). *BMC Psychiatry*, 7, 38. doi:10.1186/1 471-1244X/1187/1138.

di Scalea, T. L., Hanusa, B. H., & Wisner, K. L. (2009). Sexual function in postpartum women treated for depression: Results from a randomized trial of nortriptyline versus sertraline. *Journal of Clincal Psychiatry*, 70, 423–428.

Diego, M. A., Field, T., & Hernandez-Reif, M. (2005). Prepartum, postpartum and chronic depression effects on neonatal behavior. *Infant Behavior & Development*, 28, 155–164.

Dietert, R. R. (2013). Natural childbirth and breastfeeding as preventive measures of immune-microbiome dysbiosis and misregulated inflammation. *Journal of Ancient Diseases & Preventive Remedies*, 1(2). http://dx.doi.org/10.4172/jadpr.1000103

Ding, T., Wang, D. X., Chen, Q., & Zhu, S. N. (2014). Epidural labor analgesia is associated with a decreased risk of postpartum depression: A prospective cohort study. *Anesthesia & Analgesia*, 119, 383–392. doi:10.1213/ANE.0000000000000107

Doan, T., Gardiner, A., Gay, C. L., & Lee, K. A. (2007). Breastfeeding increases sleep duration of new parents. *Journal of Perinatal & Neonatal Nursing*, 21, 200–206.

Doering, L. V., Cross, R., Vredevoe, D., Martinez-Maza, O., & Cowan, M. J. (2007). Infection, depression and immunity in women after coronary artery bypass: A pilot study of cognitive behavioral therapy. *Alternative Therapy, Health & Medicine*, 13, 18–21.

Doering, L. V., Martinez-Maza, O., Vredevoe, D. L., & Cowan, M. J. (2008). Relation of depression, natural killer cell function, and infections after coronary artery bypass in women. *European Journal of Cardiovascular Nursing*, 7, 52–58.

Dombrowski, M. A., Anderson, G. C., Santori, C., & Burkhammer, M. (2001). Kangaroo (skin-to-skin) care with a postpartum woman who felt depressed. *MCN: American Journal of Maternal Child Nursing*, 26, 214–216.

Dorheim, S. K., Bondevik, G. T., Eberhard-Gran, M., & Bjorvatn, B. (2009). Sleep and depression in postpartum women: A population-based study. *Sleep*, 32, 847–855.

Douglas, A. R. (2000). Reported anxieties concerning intimate parenting in women sexually abused as children. *Child Abuse & Neglect*, 24, 425–434.

Downs, D. S., DiNallo, J. M., & Kirner, T. L. (2008). Determinants of pregnancy and postpartum depression: Prospective influences of depressive symptoms, body image satisfaction, and exercise behavior. *Annals of Behavioral Medicine*, 36, 54–63.

Dowrick, C., Dunn, G., Ayuso-Mateos, J. L., Dalgard, O. S., Page, H., Lehtinen, V., Casey, P., et al. (2000). Problem solving treatment and group psychoeducation for depression: Multicentre randomised controlled trial. *British Medical Journal*, 321, 1450.

Dubois, B. (2003). Overcoming the past. *New Beginnings*, March–April, 50–51.

Dubowitz, H., Black, M. M., Kerr, M. A., Hussey, J. M., Morrel, T. M., Everson, M. D., & Starr, R. H. (2001). Type and timing of mothers' victimization: Effects on mothers and children. *Pediatrics*, 107, 728–735.

Dudley, M., Roy, K., Kelk, N., & Bernard, D. (2001). Psychological correlates of depression in fathers and mothers in the first postnatal year. *Journal of Reproductive and Infant Psychology*, 19, 187–202.

Dugoua, J.-J., Mills, E., Perri, D., & Koren, G. (2006). Safety and efficacy of St. John's wort (*Hypericum*) during pregnancy and lactation. *Canadian Journal of Clinical Pharmacology*, 13, e268–e276.

Dunham, C. (1992). *Mamatoto: A celebration of birth*. New York, NY: Viking Penguin.

Dunn, C., Hanieh, E., Roberts, R., & Powrie, R. (2012). Mindful pregnancy and childbirth: Effects of a mindfulness-based intervention on women's psychological distress and well-being in the perinatal period. *Archives of Women's Mental Health*, 15, 139–143.

Dunstan, J. A., Mori, T. A., Barden, A., Beilin, L. J., Holt, P. G., Calder, P. C., Taylor, A. L., & Prescott, S. L. (2004a). Effects of n-3 polyunsaturated fatty acid supplementation in pregnancy on maternal and fetal erythrocyte fatty acid composition. *European Journal of Clinical Nutrition*, 58, 429–437.

REFERENCES

Dunstan, J. A., Roper, J., Mitoulas, L., Hartmann, P. E., Simmer, K., & Prescott, S. L. (2004b). The effect of supplementation with fish oil during pregnancy on breast milk immunoglobulin A, soluble CD14, cytokine levels and fatty acid composition. *Clinical & Experimental Allergy*, 34, 1237–1242.

Dutton, M. A., Bermudez, D., Matas, A., Majid, H., & Myers, N. L. (2013). Mindfulness-based stress reduction for low-income, predominantly African American women with PTSD and a history of intimate partner violence. *Cognitive & Behavioral Practice*, 20, 23–32.

Earls, M. F., & Committee on Psychosocial Aspects of Child and Family Health American Academy of Pediatrics (2010). Clinical report incorporating recognition and management of perinatal and postpartum depression into pediatric practice. *Pediatrics*, 126, 1032–1039. doi:doi10.1542/peds.2010–2348

Eberhard-Gran, M., Garthus-Niegel, S., Garthus-Niegel, K., & Eskild, A. (2010). Postnatal care: A cross-cultural and historical perspective. *Archives of Women's Mental Health*, 13, 459–466.

Eberhard-Gran, M., Tambs, K., Opjordsmoen, S., Skrondal, A., & Eskild, A. (2004). Depression during pregnancy and after delivery: A repeated measurement study. *Journal of Psychosomatic Obstetrics & Gynecology*, 25, 15–21.

Einarson, A., Choi, J., Einarson, T. R., & Koren, G. (2009). Rates of spontaneous and therapeutic abortions following use of antidepressants in pregnancy: Results from a large prospective database. *Journal of Obstetrics & Gynaecology Canadian*, 31, 452–456.

Eisenach, J. C., Pan, P. H., Smiley, R., Lavand'homme, P., Landau, R., & Houle, T. T. (2008). Severity of acute pain after childbirth, but not type of delivery, predicts persistent pain and postpartum depression. *Pain*, 140, 87–94.

El Marroun, H., Jaddoe, V. V. W., Hudziak, J. J., Roza, S. J., Steegers, E. A. P., Hofman, A., Verhulst, F. C., et al. (2012). Maternal use of selective serotonin reuptake inhibitors, fetal growth, and risk of adverse birth outcomes. *Archives of General Psychiatry*, 69, 706–714.

Elliot, S. A., & Leverton, T. J. (2000). Is the EPDS a magic wand? "Myths" and the evidence base. *Journal of Reproductive and Infant Psychology*, 18, 297–307.

Elliot, S. A., Leverton, T. J., Sanjack, M., Turner, H., Cowmeadow, P., Hopkins, J., & Bushnell, D. (2000). Promoting mental health after childbirth: A controlled trial of primary prevention of postnatal depression. *British Journal of Clinical Psychology*, 39, 223–241.

Ellis, K. K., Chang, C., Bhandari, S., Ball, K., Geden, E., Everett, K. D., & Bullock, L. F. (2008). Rural mothers experiencing the stress of intimate partner violence or not: Their newborn health concerns. *Journal of Midwifery and Women's Health*, 53, 556–562.

Elmir, R., Schmied, V., Wilkes, L., & Jackson, D. (2010). Women's perceptions and experiences of a traumatic birth: A meta-ethnography. *Journal of Advanced Nursing*, 66, 2142–2153.

Emery, C. F., Kiecolt-Glaser, J. K., Glaser, R., Malarky, W. B., & Frid, D. J. (2005). Exercise accelerates wound healing among health older adults: A preliminary investigation. *The Journals of Gerontology: Medical Sciences*, 60A, 1432–1436.

Enlow, M. B., Kitts, R. L., Blood, E., Bizarro, A., Hofmeister, M., & Wright, R. J. (2011). Maternal posttraumatic stress symptoms and infant emotional reactivity and emotion regulation. *Infant Behavior & Development*, 34, 487–503.

Epperson, N., Czarkowski, K. A., Ward-O'Brien, D., Weiss, E., Gueorguieva, R., Jatlow, P., & Anderson, G. M. (2001). Maternal sertraline treatment and serotonin transport in breastfeeding mother–infant pairs. *American Journal of Psychiatry*, 158, 1631–1637.

Erman, M. K. (2007). Pharmacologic therapy: Melatonin, antidepressants, and other agents. *Primary Psychiatry*, 14, 21–24.

Ernst, E. (2002). The risk–benefit profile of commonly used herbal therapies: Ginkgo, St. John's wort, ginseng, echinacea, saw palmetto, and kava. *Annals of Internal Medicine*, 136, 42–53.

Ertel, K. A., Koenen, K. C., Rich-Edwards, J. W., & Gillman, M. W. (2010). Antenatal and postpartum depressive symptoms are differentially associated with early childhood weight and adiposity. *Paediatric & Perinatal Epidemiology*, 24, 179–189. doi:10.1111/j.1365-3016.2010.01098.x.

Etain, B., Henry, C., Bellivier, F., Mathieu, F., & Leboyer, M. (2008). Beyond genetics: Childhood affective trauma in bipolar disorder. *Bipolar Disorders*, 10, 867–876.

Evans, J., Heron, J., Francomb, H., Oke, S., & Golding, J. (2001). Cohort study of depressed mood during pregnancy and after childbirth. *British Medical Journal*, 323, 257–260.

Evans, J., Heron, J., Patel, R.R., & Wiles, N. (2007). Depressive symptoms during pregnancy and low birth weight at term. *British Journal of Psychiatry*, 191, 84–85.

Evans, M., Donelle, L., & Hume-Loveland, L. (2012). Social support and online postpartum depression discussion groups: A content analysis. *Patient Education and Counseling*, 87, 405–410.

Falah-Hassani, K., Shiri, R., Vigod, S., & Dennis, C.-L. (2015). Prevalence of postpartum depression among immigrant women: A systematic review and meta-analysis. *Journal of Psychiatric Research*, 70, 67–82.

Fan, F., Zou, Y., Ma, A., Yue, Y., Mao, W., & Ma, X. (2009). Hormonal changes and somatopsychologic manifestations in the first trimester of pregnancy and postpartum. *International Journal of Gynecology and Obstetrics*, 105, 46–49.

Feeley, N., Zelkowitz, P., Cormier, C., Charbonneau, L., Lacroix, A., & Papgeorgiou, A. (2011). Posttraumatic stress among mother of very low birthweight infants 6 months after discharge from the neonatal intensive care unit. *Applied Nursing Research*, 24, 114–117.

Feldman, R., Eidelman, A. I., Sirota, L., & Weller, A. (2002). Comparison of skin-to-skin (kangaroo) and traditional care: Parenting outcomes and preterm infant development. *Pediatrics*, 110(1 Pt 1), 16–26. Retrieved from www.ncbi.nlm.nih.gov/entrez/query.fcgi?cmd=Retrieve&db=PubMed&dopt=Citation&list_uids=12093942

Feldman, R., Granat, A., Pariente, C., Kanety, H., Kuint, J., & Gilboa-Schechtman, E. (2009). Maternal depression and anxiety across the postpartum year and infant social engagement, fear regulation, and stress reactivity. *Journal of the American Academy of Child and Adolescent Psychiatry*, 48, 919–927.

Ferber, S. G., Granot, M., & Zimmer, E. Z. (2005). Catastrophizing labor pain compromises later maternity adjustments. *American Journal of Obstetrics & Gynecology*, 192, 826–831.

Fernandez y Garcia, E., Joseph, J., Wilson, M. D., Hinton, L., Simon, G., Ludman, E., Scott, F., & Kravitz, R. L. (2015). Pediatric-based intervention to motivate mothers to seek follow-up for depression screens: The Motivating Our Mothers (MOM) trial. *Academic Pediatrics*, 15, 311–318.

Ferrucci, L., Cherubini, A., Bandinelli, S., Bartali, B., Corsi, A., Lauretani, F., Martin, A., et al. (2006). Relationship of plasma polyunsaturated fatty acids to circulating inflammatory markers. *Journal of Clinical Endocrinology & Metabolism*, 91, 439–446.

Field, T. (2010). Postpartum depression effects on early interactions, parenting, and safety practices: A review. *Infant Behavior & Development*, 33(1), 1–6. doi:10.1016/j.infbeh.2009.10.005

Field, T., Diego, M., & Hernandez-Reif, M. (2006a). Prenatal depression effects on the fetus and newborn: A review. *Infant Behavior & Development*, 29, 445–455.

Field, T., Diego, M., Hernandez-Reif, M., Figueiredo, B., Schanberg, S., & Kuhn, C. (2007). Sleep disturbance in depressed pregnant women and their newborns. *Infant Behavior & Development*, 30, 127–133.

Field, T., Diego, M., Hernandez-Reif, M., Schanberg, S., & Kuhn, C. (2002). Relative right versus left frontal EEG in neonates. *Developmental Psychobiology*, 41, 147–155.

Field, T., Hernandez, M., Diego, M., Figueiredo, B., Schanberg, S., & Kuhn, C. (2006b). Prenatal cortisol, prematurity, and low birthweight. *Infant Behavior & Development*, 29, 268–275.

Figueira, P., Malloy-Diniz, L. F., Romano-Silva, M. A., Neves, F. S., & Correa, H. (2009). Postpartum depression and comorbid disorders: Frequency and relevance to clinical management. *Archives of Women's Mental Health*, 12, 451.

Figueiredo, B., & Costa, R. (2009). Mother's stress, mood and emotional involvement with the infant: 3 months before and 3 months after childbirth. *Archives of Women's Mental Health*, 12, 143–153.

Figueiredo, B., Dias, C. C., Brandao, S., Canario, C., & Nunes-Costa, R. (2013). Breastfeeding and postpartum depression: State of the art review. *Jornal de Pediatria*, 89, 332–338.

REFERENCES

Finucane, A., & Mercer, S. W. (2006). An exploratory mixed methods study of the acceptability and effectiveness of mindfulness-based cognitive therapy for patients with active depression and anxiety in primary care. *BMC Psychiatry*, 6, 14. doi:10.11186/1471-244X-6-14.

Fiorelli, M., Aceti, F., Marini, I., Giacchetti, N., Macci, E., Tinelli, E., Calistri, V., et al. (2015). Magnetic resonance imaging studies of postpartum depression: An overview. *Behavioural Neurology*, 2015, 913843. http://dx.doi.org/10.1155/2015/913843

Fisher, J. R., Feekery, C. J., Amir, L. H., & Sneedon, M. (2002). Health and social circumstances of women admitted to a private mother baby unit. A descriptive cohort study. *Australian Family Physician*, 31, 966–970.

Fisher, S. D., Kopelman, R., & O'Hara, M. W. (2012). Partner report of paternal depression using the Edinburgh Postnatal Depression Scale-Partner. *Archives of Women's Mental Health*, 15, 283–288.

Foa, E. B., & Cahill, S. P. (2002). Specialized treatment for PTSD: Matching survivors to the appropriate modality. In R. Yehuda (Ed.), *Treating trauma survivors with PTSD* (pp. 43–62). Washington, DC: American Psychiatric Association Press.

Forcada-Guex, M., Borghini, A., Pierrehumbert, B., Ansermet, F., & Muller-Nix, C. (2011). Prematurity, maternal posttraumatic stress and consequences on the mother–infant relationship. *Early Human Development*, 87, 21–26.

Ford, E., & Ayers, S. (2009). Stressful events and support during birth: The effect on anxiety, mood, and perceived control. *Journal of Anxiety Disorders*, 23, 260–268.

Ford, E., & Ayers, S. (2012). Support during birth interacts with prior trauma and birth intervention to predict postnatal post-traumatic stress symptoms. *Psychology & Health*, 26, 1553–1570.

Foss, G. F. (2001). Maternal sensitivity, posttraumatic stress, and acculturation in Vietnamese and Hmong mothers. *Maternal & Child Nursing*, 26, 257–263.

Frangou, S., Lewis, M., & McCrone, P. (2006). Efficacy of ethyl-eicosapentaenoic acid in bipolar depression: Randomized double-blind placebo-controlled study. *British Journal of Psychiatry*, 188, 46–50.

Franko, D. L., Blais, M. A., Becker, A. E., Delinsky, S. S., Greenwood, D. N., Flores, A. T., Ekeblad, E. R., et al. (2001). Pregnancy complications and neonatal outcomes in women with eating disorders. *American Journal of Psychiatry*, 158, 1461–1466.

Frasure-Smith, N., & Lesperance, F. (2005). Reflections on depression as a cardiac risk factor. *Psychosomatic Medicine*, 67, S19–S25.

Freeman, M. P. (2009). Complementary and alternative medicine for perinatal depression. *Journal of Affective Disorders*, 112, 1–10.

Freeman, M. P., & Sinha, P. (2007). Tolerability of omega-3 fatty acid supplements in perinatal women. *Prostaglandins, Leukotrienes, and Essential Fatty Acids*, 77, 203–208.

Freeman, M. P., Davis, M., Sinha, P., Wisner, K. L., Hibbeln, J. R., & Gelenberg, A. J. (2008). Omega-3 fatty acids and supportive psychotherapy for perinatal depression: A randomized placebo-controlled study. *Journal of Affective Disorders*, 110, 142–148.

Freeman, M. P., Hibbeln, J. R., Wisner, K. L., Davis, J. M., Mischoulon, D., Peet, M., Keck, P. E., Jr., et al. (2006a). Omega-3 fatty acids: Evidence basis for treatment and future research in psychiatry. *Journal of Clinical Psychiatry*, 67, 1954–1967.

Freeman, M. P., Hibbeln, J. R., Wisner, K. L., Brumbach, B. H., Watchman, M., & Gelenberg, A. J. (2006b). Randomized dose-ranging pilot trial of omega-3 fatty acids for postpartum depression. *Acta Psychiatrica Scandanavica*, 113, 31–35.

Freeman, M. P., Smith, K. W., Freeman, S. A., McElroy, S. L., Kmetz, G. F., Wright, R., & Keck, P. E., Jr. (2002). The impact of reproductive events on the course of bipolar disorder in women. *Journal of Clinical Psychiatry*, 63, 284–287.

Freeman, M. P., Wright, R., Watchman, M., Wahl, R. A., Sisk, D. J., Fraleigh, L., & Weibrecht, J. M. (2005). Postpartum depression assessments at well-baby visits: Screening feasibility, prevalence, and risk factors. *Journal of Women's Health*, 14, 929–935.

Friedman, M. J. (2001). *Posttraumatic stress disorder: The latest assessment and treatment strategies*. Kansas City, MO: Compact Clinicals.

Friedman, M. J., Cohen, J. A., Foa, E. B., & Keane, T. M. (2009). Integration and summary. In E. B. Foa, T. M. Keane, M. J. Friedman, & J. A. Cohen (Eds.), *Effective treatments for PTSD: Practice guidelines from the International Society for Traumatic Stress Studies* (pp. 617–642). New York, NY: Guilford.

Friedman, M. J., Resick, P. A., Bryant, R. A., & Brewin, C. R. (2011). Considering PTSD for DSM-5. *Depression & Anxiety*, 28, 750–769.

Furman, L., Minich, N., & Hack, M. (2002). Correlates of lactation in mothers of very low birth-weight infants. *Pediatrics*, 109, e57.

Furuta, M., Sandall, J., Cooper, D., & Bick, D. (2014). The relationship between severe maternal morbidity and psychological health symptoms at 6–8 weeks postpartum: A prospective cohort study in one English maternity unit. *BMC Pregnancy and Childbirth*, 14, 133. doi:10.1186/1471-2393-14-133

Gagnon, A. J., & Stewart, D. E. (2014). Resilience in international migrant women following violence associated with pregnancy. *Archives of Women's Mental Health*, 17, 303–310.

Galea, S., Vlahov, D., Resnick, H., Ahern, J., Susser, E., Gold, J., Bucuvalas, M., & Kilpatrick, D. (2003). Trends of probable post-traumatic stress disorder in New York City after the September 11 terrorist attacks. *American Journal of Epidemiology*, 158, 514–524.

Galler, J. R., Harrison, R. H., Ramsey, F., Chawla, S., & Taylor, J. (2006). Postpartum feeding attitudes, maternal depression, and breastfeeding in Barbados. *Infant Behavior & Development*, 29, 189–203.

Gamble, J. A., Creedy, D. K., Webster, J., & Moyle, W. (2002). A review of the literature on debriefing or non-directive counseling to prevent postpartum emotional distress. *Midwifery*, 8(1), 72–79.

Ganann, R., Sword, W., Thabane, L., Newbold, B., & Black, M. (2016). Predictors of postpartum depression among immigrant women in the year after childbirth. *Journal of Women's Health*, 25, 155–165.

Garthus-Niegel, S., von Soest, T., Knoph, C., Simonsen, T. B., Torgersen, L., & Eberhard-Gran, M. (2014). The influence of women's preferences and actual mode of delivery on post-traumatic stress symptoms following childbirth: A population-based, longitudinal study. *BMC Pregnancy and Childbirth*, 14, 191. www.biomedcentral.com/1471-2393/14/191

Gausia, K., Fisher, C., Ali, M., & Oosthuizen, J. (2009). Antenatal depression and suicidal ideation among rural Bangladeshi women: A community-based study. *Archives of Women's Mental Health*, 12, 351–358.

Gawlik, S., Waldeier, L., Muller, M., Szabo, A., Sohn, C., & Reck, C. (2013). Subclinical depressive symptoms during pregnancy and birth outcome—A pilot study in a healthy German sample. *Archives of Women's Mental Health*, 16, 93–100.

Gay, C. L., Lee, K. A., & Lee, S.-Y. (2004). Sleep patterns and fatigue in new mothers and fathers. *Biological Nursing Research*, 5, 311–318.

Geddes, J. R., Furukawa, T. A., Cipriani, A., & Barbui, C. (2007). Depressive disorder needs an evidence base commensurate with its public health importance. *Canadian Journal of Psychiatry*, 52, 543–544.

Gelaye, B., Kajeepeta, S., Zhong, Q.-Y., Borba, C. P. C., Rondon, M. B., Sanchez, S. E., Henderson, D. C., & Williams, M. A. (2015). Childhood abuse is associated with stress-related sleep disturbance and poor sleep quality in pregnancy. *Sleep Medicine*, 16, 1274–1280.

George, L., & Elliot, S. A. (2004). Searching for antenatal predictors of postnatal depressive symptomatology: Unexpected findings from a study of obsessive–compulsive personality traits. *Journal of Reproductive and Infant Psychology*, 22, 25–31.

Geracioti, T. D. J., Carpenter, L. L., Owens, M. J., Baker, D. G., Ekhator, N. N., Horn, P. S., Strawn, J. R., et al. (2006). Elevated cerebrospinal fluid substance P concentrations in posttraumatic stress disorder and major depression. *American Journal of Psychiatry*, 63, 637–643.

REFERENCES

Ghosh, J. K. C., Wilhelm, M. H., Dunkel-Schetter, C., Lombardi, C. A., & Ritz, B. R. (2010). Paternal support and preterm birth, and the moderation of effects of chronic stress: A study in Los Angeles County mothers. *Archives of Women's Mental Health*, 13, 327–338.

Giallo, R., Cooklin, A., & Nicholson, J. M. (2014). Risk factors associated with trajectories of mothers' depressive symptoms across the early parenting period: An Australian population-based longitudinal study. *Archives of Women's Mental Health*, 17, 115–125.

Giardinelli, L., Innocenti, A., Benni, L., Stefanini, M. C., Lino, G., Lunardi, C., Svelto, V., et al. (2012). Depression and anxiety in perinatal period: Prevalence and risk factors in an Italian sample. *Archives of Women's Mental Health*, 15, 21–30.

Gilson, K. J., & Lancaster, S. (2008). Childhood sexual abuse in pregnant and parenting adolescents. *Child Abuse & Neglect*, 32, 869–877.

Gjerdingen, D., Crow, S., McGovern, P., Miner, M., & Center, B. (2009). Postpartum depression screening at well-child visits: Validity of a 2-question screen and the PHQ-9. *Annals of Family Medicine*, 7, 63–70.

Glover, V., Onozawa, K., & Hodgkinson, A. (2002). Benefits of infant massage for mothers with postnatal depression. *Seminars in Neonatalogy*, 7, 495–500.

Glynn, L. M., Davis, E. P., Schetter, C. D., Chicz-DeMet, A., Hobel, C. J., & Sandman, C. A. (2007). Postnatal maternal cortisol levels predict temperament in healthy breastfed infants. *Early Human Development*, 83, 675–681.

Glynn, L. M., Schetter, C. D., Hobel, C. J., & Sandman, C. A. (2008). Pattern of perceived stress and anxiety in pregnancy predicts preterm birth. *Health Psychology*, 27(1), 43–51.

Golden, R. N., Gaynes, B. N., Ekstrom, R. D., Hamer, R. M., Jacobsen, F. M., Suppes, T., Wisner, K. L., & Nemeroff, C. B. (2005). The efficacy of light therapy in the treatment of mood disorders: A review and meta-analysis of the evidence. *American Journal of Psychiatry*, 162, 656–662.

Goodman, J. H., Guarino, A., Chenausky, K., Klein, L., Prager, J., Petersen, R., Forget, A., & Freeman, M. (2014). CALM Pregnancy: Results of a pilot study of mindfulness-based cognitive therapy for perinatal anxiety. *Archives of Women's Mental Health*, 17, 373–387.

Goyal, D., Gay, C. L., & Lee, K. A. (2007). Patterns of sleep disruption and depressive symptoms in new mothers. *Journal of Perinatal & Neonatal Nursing*, 21, 123–129.

Goyal, D., Gay, C. L., & Lee, K. A. (2009). Fragmented maternal sleep is more strongly correlated wtih depressive symptoms than infant temperament at three months postpartum. *Archives of Women's Mental Health*, 12, 229–237.

Goyal, M., Singh, S., Sibinga, E. M. S., Gould, N. F., Rowland-Seymour, A., Sharma, R., Berger, Z., et al. (2014). *Meditation programs for psychological stress and well-being* (Vol. 13(14)-EHC116-EF). Rockville, MD: Agency for Healthcare Research and Quality.

Gracia, E., & Musitu, G. (2003). Social isolation from communities and child maltreatment: A cross-cultural comparison. *Child Abuse & Neglect*, 27, 153–168.

Grajeda, R., & Perez-Escamilla, R. (2002). Stress during labor and delivery is associated with delayed onset of lactation among urban Guatemalan women. *Journal of Nutrition*, 132, 3055–3060.

Grandjean, P., Bjerve, K. S., Weihe, P., & Steuerwald, U. (2001). Birthweight in a fishing community: Significance of essential fatty acids and marine food contaminants. *International Journal of Epidemiology*, 30, 1272–1278.

Grant, K. A., McMahon, C., Austin, M.-P., Reilly, N., Leader, L., & Ali, S. (2009). Maternal prenatal anxiety, postnatal caregiving and infants' cortisol response to the still-face procedure. *Developmental Psychobiology*, 51, 625–637.

Grazioli, R., & Terry, D. J. (2000). The role of cognitive vulnerability and stress in the prediction of postpartum depressive symptomatology. *British Journal of Clinical Psychology*, 39, 329–347.

Gregory, E. F., Butz, A. M., Ghazarian, S. R., Gross, S. M., & Johnson, S. B. (2015). Are unmet breastfeeding expectations associated with maternal depressive symptoms? *Academic Pediatrics*, 15, 319–325.

Grekin, R., & O'Hara, M. W. (2014). Prevalence and risk factors of postpartum posttraumatic stress disorder: A meta-analysis. *Clinical Psychology Review*, 34, 389–401.

Grigoriadis, S., & Ravitz, P. (2007). An approach to interpersonal psychotherapy for postpartum depression: Focusing on interpersonal changes. *Canadian Family Physician*, 53, 1469–1475.

Groër, M., Davis, K., & Casey, B. (2005). Neuroendocrine and immune relationships in postpartum fatigue. *MCN*, 30, 133–138.

Groer, M. W. (2005). Differences between exclusive breastfeeders, formula-feeders, and controls: A study of stress, mood, and endocrine variables. *Biological Nursing Research*, 7(2), 106–117.

Groër, M. W., & Morgan, K. (2007). Immune, health and endocrine characteristics of depressed postpartum mothers. *Psychoneuroendocrinology*, 32, 133–139.

Groer, M. W., Davis, M. W., & Hemphill, J. (2002). Postpartum stress: Current concepts and the possible protective role of breastfeeding. *Journal of Obstetric, Gynecologic, & Neonatal Nursing*, 31(4), 411–417. http://www.ncbi.nlm.nih.gov/entrez/query.fcgi?cmd=Retrieve&db=PubMed&dopt=Citation&list_uids=12146930

Groer, M. W., Thomas, S. P., Evans, G. W., Helton, S., & Weldon, A. (2006). Inflammatory effects and immune system correlates of rape. *Violence and Victims*, 21, 796–808. www.ncbi.nlm.nih.gov/entrez/query.fcgi?cmd=Retrieve&db=PubMed&dopt=Citation&list_uids=17220020

Grote, N. K., Bridge, J. A., Gavin, A. R., Melville, J. L., Iyengar, S., & Katon, W. J. (2010). A meta-analysis of depression during pregnancy and the risk of preterm birth, low birth weight, and intrauterine growth restriction. *Archives of General Psychiatry*, 67, 1012–1024.

Grote, N. K., Katon, W., Russo, J. E., Lohr, M. J., Curran, M., Galvin, E., & Carson, K. (2015). Collaborative care for perinatal depression in socioeconomically disadvantaged women: A randomized trial. *Depression & Anxiety*, 32, 821–834.

Grzeskowiak, L. E., Morrison, J. L., Henriksen, T. B., Bech, B. H., Obel, C., Olsen, J., & Pedersen, L. H. (2015). Prenatal antidepressant exposure and child behavioural outcomes at 7 years of age: A study within the Danish National Birth Cohort. *British Journal of Obstetrics & Gynecology*. doi:10.1111/1471-0528.13611

Guedeney, N., Fermanian, J., Guelfi, J. D., & Kumar, R. C. (2000). The Edinburgh Postnatal Depression Scale (EPDS) and the detection of major depressive disorders in early postpartum: Some concerns about false negatives. *Journal of Affective Disorders*, 61, 107–112.

Guo, S. F., Wu, J. L., Qu, C. Y., & Yan, R. Y. (2004). Physical and sexual abuse of women before, during and after pregnancy. *International Journal of Gynaecology and Obstetrics*, 84(3), 281–286.

Habel, C., Feeley, N., Hayton, B., Bell, L., & Zelkowitz, P. (2015). Causes of women's postpartum depression symptoms: Men's and women's perceptions. *Midwifery*, 31, 728–734.

Haga, S. M., Ulleberg, P., Slinning, K., Kraft, P., Steen, T. B., & Staff, A. (2012). A longitudinal study of postpartum depressive symptoms: Multilevel growth curve analyses of emotion regulation strategies, breastfeeding self-efficacy, and social support. *Archives of Women's Mental Health*, 15, 175–184.

Hagan, R., Evans, S. F., & Pope, S. (2004). Preventing postnatal depression in mothers of very preterm infants: A randomized controlled trial. *British Journal of Obstetrics & Gynecology*, 111, 641–647.

Hahn-Holbrook, J., Haselton, M. G., Schetter, C. D., & Glynn, L. M. (2013). Does breastfeeding offer protection against maternal depressive symptomatology? A prospective study from pregnancy to 2 years after birth. *Archives of Women's Mental Health*, 16, 411–422.

Hairston, I. S., Waxler, E., Seng, J. S., Fezzey, A. G., Rosenblum, K. L., & Muzik, M. (2011). The role of infant sleep in intergenerational transmission of trauma. *Sleep*, 34, 1373–1383.

Hale, T. W., & Rowe, H. (2014). *Medications and mothers' milk*, 16th Edition. Plano, TX: Hale Publishing.

Hale, T. W., Kendall-Tackett, K. A., Cong, Z., Votta, R., & McCurdy, F. (2010). Discontinuation syndrome in newborns whose mothers took antidepressants while pregnant or breastfeeding. *Breastfeeding Medicine*, 5, 283–288.

REFERENCES

Hall, M. F. (2014/2015). How to help women at risk for acute stress disorder after childbirth. *Nursing for Women's Health*, 18, 449–454.

Hallahan, B., & Garland, M. R. (2005). Essential fatty acids and mental health. *British Journal of Psychiatry*, 186, 275–277.

Hallahan, B., Hibbeln, J. R., Davis, J. M., & Garland, M. R. (2007). Omega-3 fatty acid supplementation in patients with recurrent self-harm. Single-centre double-blind randomized controlled trial. *British Journal of Psychiatry*, 190, 118–122.

Hamazaki, K., Itomura, M., Huan, M., Nishizawa, H., Sawazaki, S., Tanouchi, M., Watanabe, S., et al. (2005). Effect of omega-3 fatty acid-containing phospholipids on blood catecholamine concentrations in healthy volunteers: A randomized, placebo-controlled, double-blind trial. *Nutrition*, 21, 705–710.

Hamdan, A., & Tamim, H. (2011). Psychosocial risk and protective for postpartum depression in the United Arab Emirates. *Archives of Women's Mental Health*, 14, 125–133.

Hamer, M., & Steptoe, A. (2007). Association between physical fitness, parasympathetic control, and proinflammatory responses to mental stress. *Psychosomatic Medicine*, 69, 660–666.

Hammen, C., & Brennan, P. (2002). Interpersonal dysfunction in depressed women: Impairments independent of depressive symptoms. *Journal of Affective Disorders*, 72, 145–156.

Handal, M., Skurtveit, S., Furu, K., Hernandez-Diaz, S., Skovlund, E., Nystad, W., & Selmer, R. (2015). Motor development in children prenatally exposed to selective serotonin reuptake inhibitors: A large population-based pregnancy cohort study. *British Journal of Obstetrics & Gynecology*. doi:10.1111/1471-0528.13582

Handlin, L., Jonas, W., Pettersson, M., Ejdeback, M., Ransjo-Arvidson, A.-B., Nissen, E., & Uvnas-Moberg, K. (2009). Effects of sucking and skin-to-skin contact on maternal ACTH and cortisol levels during the second day postpartum—Influence of epidural analgesia and oxytocin in the perinatal period. *Breastfeeding Medicine*, 4, 207–220.

Hannibal, K. E., & Bishop, M. D. (2014). Chronic stress, cortisol dysfunction, and pain: A psychoneuroendocrine rationale for stress management in pain rehabilitation. *Physical Therapy*, 94, 1816–1825.

Harkness, R., & Bratman, S. (2003). *Handbook of drug–herb and drug–supplement interactions*. St. Louis, MO: Mosby.

Harrykissoon, S. D., Rickert, V. I., & Wiemann, C. M. (2002). Prevalence and patterns of intimate partner violence among adolescent mothers during the postpartum period. *Archives of Pediatric and Adolescent Medicine*, 156, 325–330.

Harville, E. W., Xiong, X., & Buekens, P. (2010). Disasters and perinatal health: A systematic review. *Obstetrical & Gynecological Survey*, 65, 713–728.

Harville, E. W., Xiong, X., Pridjian, G., Elkind-Hirsch, K., & Buekens, P. (2009). Postpartum mental health after Hurricane Katrina: A cohort study. *BMC Pregnancy and Childbirth*, 9, 21.

Haslam, D. M., Pakenham, K. I., & Smith, A. (2006). Social support and postpartum depressive symptomatogy: The mediating role of maternal self-efficacy. *Infant Mental Health Journal*, 27, 276–291.

Hatton, D. C., Harrison-Hohner, J., Coste, S., Dorato, V., Curet, L.B., & McCarron, D. A. (2005). Symptoms of postpartum depression and breastfeeding. *Journal of Human Lactation*, 21, 444–449.

Hay, D. F., Pawlby, S., Sharp, D., Asten, P., Mills, A., & Kumar, R. (2001). Intellectual problems shown by 11-year-old children whose mothers had postnatal depression. *Journal of Child Psychology and Psychiatry and Allied Disciplines*, 42, 871–889.

Hay, D. F., Pawlby, S., Water, C. S., & Sharp, D. (2008). Antepartum and postpartum exposure to maternal depression: Different effects on different adolescent outcomes. *The Journal of Child Psychology and Psychiatry*, 49, 1079–1088.

Hayes, B. A., Muller, R., & Bradley, B. S. (2001). Perinatal depression: A randomized controlled trial of an antenatal education intervention for primiparas. *Birth*, 28, 28–35.

Head, J. G., Storfer-Isser, A., O'Connor, K. G., Hoagwood, K. E., Kelleher, K. J., Heneghan, A. M., Park, E. R., et al. (2008). Does education influence pediatricians' perceptions of physician-specific barriers for maternal depression? *Clinical Pediatrics*, 47, 670–678.

Healey, C., Morriss, R., Henshaw, C., Wadoo, O., Sajjad, A., Scholefield, H., & Kinderman, P. (2013). Self-harm in postpartum depression and referrals to a perinatal mental health team: An audit study. *Archives of Women's Mental Health*, 16, 237–245.

Heath, N. M., Chesney, S. A., Gerhart, J. I., Goldsmith, R. E., Luborsky, J. L., Stevens, N. R., & Hobfoll, S. E. (2013). Interpersonal violence, PTSD, and inflammation: Potential psychogenic pathways to higher C-reactive protein levels. *Cytokine*, 63, 172–178.

Heh, S. S., Huang, L. H., Ho, S. M., Fu, Y. Y., & Wang, L. L. (2008). Effectiveness of an exercise support program in reducing the severity of postnatal depression in Taiwanese women. *Birth*, 35, 60–65.

Heinrichs, M., Meinlschmidt, G., Neumann, I., Wagner, S., Kirschbaum, C., Ehlert, U., & Hellhammer, D. H. (2001). Effects of suckling on hypothalamic–pituitary–adrenal axis responses to psychosocial stress in postpartum lactating women. *Journal of Clinical Endocrinology & Metabolism*, 86, 4798–4804.

Helland, I. B., Smith, L., Saarem, K., Saugstad, O. D., & Drevon, C. A. (2003). Maternal supplementation with very-long-chain n-3 fatty acids during pregnancy and lactation augments children's IQ at 4 years of age. *Pediatrics*, 111, e39–e44.

Helle, N., Barkmann, C., Bartz-Seel, J., Diehl, T., Ehrhardt, S., Hendel, A., Nestoriuc, Y., et al. (2015). Very low birth-weight as a risk factor for postpartum depression four to six weeks post-birth in mothers and fathers: Cross-sectional results from a controlled multicentre cohort study. *Journal of Affective Disorders*, 180, 154–161.

Heneghan, A. M., Chaudron, L. H., Storfer-Isser, A., Park, E. R., Kelleher, K. J., & Stein, R. E. K. (2007). Factors associated with identification and management or maternal depression by pediatricians. *Pediatrics*, 119, 444–454.

Hibbeln, J. R. (2002). Seafood consumption, the DHA content of mothers' milk and prevalence rates of postpartum depression: A cross-national, ecological analysis. *Journal of Affective Disorders*, 69, 15–29.

Highet, N., Stevenson, A. L., Purtell, C., & Coo, S. (2014). Qualitative insights into women's personal experiences of perinatal depression and anxiety. *Women & Birth*, 27, 179–184.

Hilt, R. J. (2015). Postpartum depression screening. *Pediatric Annals*, 44, 346–347.

Horowitz, J. A., Bell, M., Trybulski, J. A., Munro, B. H., Moser, D., Hartz, S. A., McCordic, L., & Sokol, E. S. (2001). Promoting responsiveness between mothers with depressive symptoms and their infants. *Journal of Nursing Scholarship*, 33, 323–329.

Houston, K. A., Kaimal, A. J., Nakagawa, S., Gregorich, S. E., Yee, L. M., & Kuppermann, M. (2015). Mode of delivery and postpartum depression: The role of patient preferences. *American Journal of Obstetrics and Gynecology*, 212, e1–e7.

Howard, L. M., Oram, S., Galley, H., Trevillion, K., & Feder, G. (2013). Domestic violence and perinatal mental disorders: A systematic review and meta-analysis. *PLoS Medicine*, 10(5), e1001452.

Howell, E. A., Bodnar-Deren, S., Balbierz, A., London, H., Mora, P. A., Zlotnick, C., Wang, J., & Leventhal, H. (2014). An intervention to reduce postpartum depressive symptoms: A randomized controlled trial. *Archives of Women's Mental Health*, 17, 57–63.

Hu, Z. P., Yang, X. X., Chan, S. Y., Xu, A.L., Duan, W., Zhu, Y. Z., Sheu, F. S., et al. (2006). St. John's wort attenuates irinotecan-induced diarrhea via down-regulation of intestinal pro-inflammatory cytokines and inhibition of intestinal epithelial apoptosis. *Toxicology & Applied Pharmacology*, 216, 225–237.

Huang, C.-M., Carter, P. A., & Guo, J.-L. (2004). A comparison of sleep and daytime sleepiness in depressed and non-depressed mothers during the early postpartum period. *Journal of Nursing Research*, 12, 287–295.

REFERENCES

Huang, H., Faisal-Cury, A., Chan, Y.-F., Tabb, K., Katon, W., & Menezes, P. R. (2012). Suicidal ideation during pregnancy: Prevalence and associated factors among low-income women in Sao Paulo, Brazil. *Archives of Women's Mental Health*, 15, 135–138.

Humphrey, S. (2007). Herbal therapeutics during lactation. In T. W. Hale & P. E. Hartmann (Eds.), *Textbook of human lactation* (pp. 629–654). Amarillo, TX: Hale Publishing.

Hunker, D. F., Patrick, T. E., Albrecht, S. A., & Wisner, K. L. (2009). Is difficult childbirth related to postpartum maternal outcomes in the early postpartum period? *Archives of Women's Mental Health*, 12, 211–219. doi:10.1007/s00737-009-0068-3.

Hutton, E. K., Hannah, M. E., Ross, S., Joseph, K. S., Ohlsson, A., Asztalos, E. V., Willan, A. R., et al. (2016). Maternal outcomes at 3 months after planned caesarean section versus planned vaginal birth for twin pregnancies in the Twin Birth Study: A randomised controlled trial. *British Journal of Obstetrics & Gynecology*, 123, 644. doi:10.1111/1471-0528.13597

Hypericum Depression Trial Study Group. (2002). Effect of *Hypericum perforatum* (St. John's Wort) in major depressive disorder. *Journal of the American Medical Association*, 287, 1807–1814.

Iido, M., Horiuchi, S., & Nagamori, K. (2014). A comparison of midwife-led care versus obstetrician-led care for low-risk women in Japan. *Women & Birth*, 27, 202–207.

Iles, J., Slade, P., & Spiby, H. (2011). Posttraumatic stress symptoms and postpartum depression in couples after childbirth: The role of partner support and attachment. *Journal of Anxiety Disorders*, 25, 520–530.

Illiadis, S. I., Comasco, E., Sylven, S., Hellgren, C., Poromaa, I. S., & Skalkidou, A. (2015). Prenatal and postpartum evening salivary cortisol levels in association with peripartum depressive symptoms. *PLoS ONE*. doi:10.1371/journal.pone.0135471

Irwin, M. R., Olmstead, R., Carrillo, C., Sadeghi, N., Breen, E. C., Witarama, T., Yokomizo, M., et al. (2014). Cognitive behavioral therapy vs. Tai Chi for late life insomnia and inflammatory risk: A randomized controlled comparative efficacy trial. *Sleep*, 37, 1543–1552.

Jackson, M. L., Sztendur, E. M., Diamond, N. T., Byles, J. E., & Bruck, D. (2014). Sleep difficulties and the development of depression and anxiety: A longitudinal study of young Australian women. *Archives of Women's Mental Health*, 17, 189–198.

Jones, I., & Craddock, N. (2001). Familiality of the puerperal trigger in bipolar disorder: Results of a family study. *American Journal of Psychiatry*, 158, 913–917.

Jones, N. A., McFall, B. A., & Diego, M. A. (2004). Patterns of brain electrical activity in infants of depressed mothers who breastfeed and bottle feed: The mediating role of infant temperament. *Biological Psychology*, 67, 103–124.

Jotzo, M., & Poets, C. F. (2005). Helping parents cope with the trauma of premature birth: An evaluation of a trauma-preventive psychological intervention. *Pediatrics*, 115, 915–919.

Kabir, K., Sheeder, J., & Kelly, L. S. (2008). Identifying postpartum depression: Are 3 questions as good as 10? *Pediatrics*, 122, e696–e702.

Kallen, B. (2004). Neonate characteristics after maternal use of antidepressants in late pregnancy. *Archives of Pediatric & Adolescent Medicine*, 158, 312–316.

Kargar Jahromi, M., Zare, A., Taghizadeganzadeh, M., & Rahmanian Koshkaki, A. (2014). A study of marital satisfaction among non-depressed and depressed mothers after childbirth in Jahrom, Iran, 2014. *Global Journal of Health Science*, 26(7), 140–146.

Karlstrom, A., Engstrom-Olofsson, R., Norbergh, K. G., Sjoling, M., & Hidlingsson, I. (2007). Postoperative pain after cesarean birth affects breastfeeding and infant care. *Journal of Obstetric, Gynecologic and Neonatal Nursing*, 36, 430–440.

Kashaninia, Z., Sajedi, F., Rahgozar, M., & Noghabi, F. A. (2008). The effect of Kangaroo Care on behavioral responses to pain of an intramuscular injection in neonates. *JSPN*, 13, 275–280.

Kawano, A., & Emori, Y. (2015). The relationship between maternal postpartum psychological state and breast milk secretory immunoglobulin A level. *Journal of the American Psychiatric Nurses Association*, 21, 23–30.

Kearney, D. J., McDermott, K., Malte, C., Martinez, M., & Simpson, T. L. (2013). Effects of participation in a mindfulness program for veterans with posttraumatic stress disorder: A randomized controlled pilot study. *Journal of Clinical Psychology*, 69, 14–27.

Kendall-Tackett, K. A. (2007). A new paradigm for depression in new mothers: The central role of inflammation and how breastfeeding and anti-inflammatory treatments protect maternal mental health. *International Breastfeeding Journal*, 2, 6. doi:10.1186/1746-4358-2-6

Kendall-Tackett, K. A. (2010). Long-chain omega-3 fatty acids and women's mental health in the perinatal period. *Journal of Midwifery and Women's Health*, 55, 561–567.

Kendall-Tackett, K. A. (2014a). Childbirth-related posttraumatic stress disorder symptoms and implications for breastfeeding. *Clinical Lactation*, 5(2), 51–55.

Kendall-Tackett, K. A. (2014b). Intervention for mothers who have experienced childbirth-related trauma and posttraumatic stress disorder. *Clinical Lactation*, 5(2), 56–61.

Kendall-Tackett, K. A., & Hale, T. W. (2010). The use of antidepressants in pregnant and breast-feeding women: A review of recent studies. *Journal of Human Lactation*, 26(2), 187–196.

Kendall-Tackett, K. A., Cong, Z., & Hale, T. W. (2010). Mother–infant sleep locations and night-time feeding behavior: U.S. data from the Survey of Mothers' Sleep and Fatigue. *Clinical Lactation*, 1(1), 27–30.

Kendall-Tackett, K. A., Cong, Z., & Hale, T. W. (2011). The effect of feeding method on sleep duration, maternal well-being, and postpartum depression. *Clinical Lactation*, 2(2), 22–26.

Kendall-Tackett, K. A., Cong, Z., & Hale, T. W. (2013). Depression, sleep quality, and maternal well-being in postpartum women with a history of sexual assault: A comparison of breastfeeding, mixed-feeding, and formula-feeding mothers. *Breastfeeding Medicine*, 8, 16–22.

Kendall-Tackett, K. A., Cong, Z., & Hale, T. W. (2015). Birth interventions related to lower rates of exclusive breastfeeding and increased risk of postpartum depression in a large sample. *Clinical Lactation*, 6(3), 87–97.

Kendall-Tackett, K. A., Cong, Z., & Hale, T. W. (2016, in press-a). Factors that influence where babies sleep in the U.S.: The impact of feeding method, mother's race/ethnicity, partner status, employment, education, and income. *Clinical Lactation*.

Kendall-Tackett, K. A., Cong, Z., & Hale, T. W. (2016, in press-b). Feeding method and sleep location's impact on maternal depression and well-being. *Clinical Lactation*.

Keogh, E., Hughes, S., Ellery, D., Daniel, C., & Holdcroft, A. (2006). Psychosocial influences on women's experience of planned elective cesarean section. *Psychosomatic Medicine*, 68, 167–174. doi:68/1/167 [pii] 10.1097/01.psy.0000197742.50988.9e

Kersting, A., Dorsch, M., Kreulich, C., Reutemann, M., Ohrmann, P., Baez, E., & Arolt, V. (2005). Trauma and grief 2–7 years after termination of pregnancy because of fetal anomalies—A pilot study. *Journal of Psychosomatic Obstetrics & Gynecology*, 26, 9–14.

Kersting, A., Dorsch, M., Wesselman, U., Ludorff, K., Witthaut, J., Ohrmann, P., Hoernig-Franz, I., et al. (2004). Maternal posttraumatic stress response after the birth of a very low-birth-weight infant. *Journal of Psychosomatic Research*, 57, 473–476.

Kersting, A., Kroker, K., Steinhard, J., Hoernig-Franz, I., Wesselmann, U., Luedorff, K., Ohrmann, P., et al. (2009). Psychological impact on women after second and third trimester termination of pregnancy due to fetal anomalies versus women after preterm birth—a 14-month follow up study. *Archives of Women's Mental Health*, 12, 193–201.

Khajehei, M., Doherty, M., Tilley, P. J., & Sauer, K. (2015). Prevalence and risk factors of sexual dysfunction in postpartum Australian women. *Journal of Sexual Medicine*, 12, 1415–1426.

Khalifa, D. S., Glavin, K., Bjertness, E., & Lien, L. (2015). Postnatal depression among Sudanese women: Prevalence and validation of the Edinburgh Postnatal Depression Scale at 3 months postpartum. *International Journal of Women's Health*, 7, 677–684.

Kiecolt-Glaser, J. K., Belury, M. A., Porter, K., Beversdoft, D., Lemeshow, S., & Glaser, R. (2007). Depressive symptoms, omega-6:omega-3 fatty acids, and inflammation in older adults. *Psychosomatic Medicine*, 69, 217–224.

Kiecolt-Glaser, J. K., Christian, L., Preston, H., Houts, C., Malarkey, W. B., Emery, C. F., & Glaser, R. (2010). Stress, inflammation, and yoga practice. *Psychosomatic Medicine*, 72, 113–121.

Kiecolt-Glaser, J. K., Derry, H. M., & Fagundes, C. P. (2015). Inflammation: Depression fans the flames and feast in the heat. *American Journal of Psychiatry*, 172, 1075–1091.

REFERENCES

Kiecolt-Glaser, J. K., Loving, T. J., Stowell, J. R., Malarky, W. B., Lemeshow, S., Dickinson, S. L., & Glaser, R. (2005). Hostile marital interactions, proinflammatory cytokine production, and wound healing. *Archives of General Psychiatry*, 62, 1377–1384.

Kiecolt-Glaser, J. K., Preacher, K. J., MacCallum, R. C., Atkinson, C., Malarkey, W. B., & Glaser, R. (2003). Chronic stress and age-related increases in the proinflammatory cytokine IL-6. *Proceedings of the National Academy of Sciences U S A*, 100, 9090–9095.

Kiernan, K., & Pickett, K. E. (2006). Marital status disparities in maternal smoking during pregnancy, breastfeeding and maternal depression. *Social Science & Medicine*, 63, 335–346.

Kim, D. R., Sockol, L. E., Sammel, M. D., Kelly, C., Moseley, M., & Epperson, C. N. (2013). Elevated risk of adverse obstetric outcomes in pregnant women with depression. *Archives of Women's Mental Health*, 16, 475–482.

Kim, J. J., Choi, S. S., & Ha, K. (2008). A closer look at depression in mothers who kill their children: Is it unipolar or bipolar depression? *Journal of Clincal Psychiatry*, 69, 1625–1631.

Kim, J. J., La Porte, L. M., Adams, M. G., Gordon, T. E. J., Kuendig, J. M., & Silver, R. K. (2009). Obstetric care provider engagement in a perinatal depression screening program. *Archives of Women's Mental Health*, 12, 167–172.

Kim, S. H., Schneider, S. M., Kravitz, L., Mermier, C., & Burge, M. R. (2013). Mind–body practices for posttraumatic stress disorder. *Journal of Investigative Medicine*, 61, 827–834.

Kim, Y.-D., Heo, I., Shin, B.-C., Crawford, C., Kang, H.-W., & Lim, J.-H. (2013). Acupuncture for posttraumatic stress disorder: A systematic review of randomized controlled trials and prospective clinical trials. *Evidence-Based Complementary and Alternative Medicine*. http://dx.doi.org/10.1155/2013/615857

Kim, Y., & Ahn, S. (2015). A review of postpartum depression: Focused on psychoneuroimmunological interaction. *Korean Journal of Women's Health Nursing*, 21(2), 106–114.

King, P. A. L. (2012). Replicability of structural models of the Edinburgh Postnatal Depression Scale (EPDS) in a community sample of postpartum African American women with low socioeconomic status. *Archives of Women's Mental Health*, 15, 77–86.

Kirpinar, I., Gozum, S., & Pasinlioglu, T. (2010). Prospective study of postpartum depression in eastern Turkey prevalence, socio-demographic and obstetric correlates, prenatal anxiety and early awareness. *Journal of Clinical Nursing*, 19, 422–431.

Klier, C. M., Muzik, M., Rosenblum, K. L., & Lenz, G. (2001). Interpersonal psychotherapy adapted for the group setting in the treatment of postpartum depression. *Journal of Psychotherapy Practice and Research*, 10, 124–131.

Klier, C. M., Schafer, M. R., Schmid-Siegel, B., Lenz, G., & Mannel, M. (2002). St. John's wort (*Hypericum perforatum*)—Is it safe during breastfeeding? *Pharmacopsychiatry*, 35, 29–30.

Klier, C. M., Schmid-Siegel, B., Schafer, M. R., Lenz, G., Saria, A., Lee, A., & Zernig, G. (2006). St. John's wort (*Hypericum perforatum*) and breastfeeding: Plasma and breast milk concentrations of hyperforin for 5 mothers and 2 infants. *Journal of Clinical Psychiatry*, 67, 305–309.

Knipscheer, J. W., & Kleber, R. J. (2006). The relative contribution of posttraumatic and acculturative stress to subjective mental health among Bosnian refugees. *Journal of Clinical Psychology*, 62, 339–353.

Ko, Y.-L., Yang, C.-L., Fang, C.-L., Lee, M.-Y., & Lin, P.-C. (2013). Community-based postpartum exercise program. *Journal of Clinical Nursing*, 22, 2122–2131.

Kobayashi, K., Kuki, C., Oyama, S., & Kumara, H. (2016). Pro-inflammatory cytokine TNF-alpha is a key inhibitory factor for lactose synthesis pathway in lactating mammary epithelial cells. *Experimental Cell Research*, 340(2), 295–304.

Kokubu, M., Okano, T., & Sugiyama, T. (2012). Postnatal depression, maternal bonding failure, and negative attitudes towards pregnancy: A longitudinal study of pregnant women in Japan. *Archives of Women's Mental Health*, 15, 211–216.

Koleva, H., & Stuart, S. (2014). Risk factors for depressive symptoms in adolescent pregnancy in a late-teen subsample. *Archives of Women's Mental Health*, 17, 155–159.

Koopman, C., Ismailji, T., Holmes, D., Classen, C. C., Palesh, O., & Wales, T. (2005). The effects of expressive writing on pain, depression and posttraumatic stress disorder symptoms in survivors of intimate partner violence. *Journal of Health Psychology*, 10, 211–221.

Kritsotakis, G., Vassilaki, M., Melaki, V., Georgiou, V., Philalithis, A. E., Bitsios, P., Kogevinas, M., et al. (2013). Social capital in pregnancy and postpartum depressive symptoms: A prospective mother–child cohort study (the Rhea study). *International Journal of Nursing Studies*, 50, 63–72.

Krol, K. M., Rajhans, P., Missana, M., & Grossman, T. (2015). Duration of exclusive breastfeeding is associated with differences in infants' brain responses to emotional body expressions. *Frontiers in Behavioral Neuroscience*, 8, 459. doi:10.3389/fnbeh.2014.00459

Kubera, M., Kenis, G., Bosmans, E., Kajta, M., Basta-Kalm, A., Scharpe, S., … Maes, M. (2004). Stimulatory effect of antidepressants on the productioni of IL-6. *International Immunopharmacology*, 4(2), 185–192.

Kubera, M., Lin, A., Kenis, G., Bosmans, E., van Bockstaele, D., & Maes, M. (2001). Anti-inflammatory effects of antidepressants through suppression of the interferon-gamma/interleukin-10 production ratio. *Journal of Clinical Psychopharmacology*, 21, 199–206.

Kuhn, M. A., & Winston, D. (2000). *Herbal therapy and supplements: A scientific and traditional approach*. Philadelphia, PA: Lippincott.

Kuo, S.-Y., Chen, S.-R., & Tzeng, Y.-L. (2014). Depression and anxiety trajectories among women who undergo an elective cesarean section. *PLoS ONE*, 9(1), e86653. doi:10.1371/journal.pone.0086653

Lam, R. W., Levitt, A. J., Levitan, R. D., Enns, M. W., Morehouse, R., Michalak, E. E., & Tam, E. M. (2006). The CAN-SAD Study: A randomized controlled trial of the effectiveness of light therapy and fluoxetine in patients with winter seasonal affective disorder. *American Journal of Psychiatry*, 163, 805–812.

Lam, R. W., Song, C., & Yatham, L. N. (2004). Does neuroimmune dysfunction mediate seasonal mood changes in winter depression? *Medical Hypotheses*, 63, 567–573.

Lane, A. M., Crone-Grant, D., & Lane, H. (2002). Mood changes following exercise. *Perceptual & Motor Skills*, 94, 732–734.

Lang, A. J., Rodgers, C. S., & Lebeck, M. M. (2006). Associations between maternal childhood maltreatment and psychopathology and aggression during pregnancy and postpartum. *Child Abuse & Neglect*, 30, 17–25.

Lappin, J. (2001). Time points for assessing perinatal mood must be optimized. *British Medical Journal*, 323, 1367a.

Lau, Y., & Chan, K. S. (2007). Influence of intimate partner violence during pregnancy and early postpartum depressive symptoms on breastfeeding among Chinese women in Hong Kong. *Journal of Midwifery and Women's Health*, 52(2), e15–e20.

Lauderdale, D. S. (2006). Birth outcomes for Arabic-named women in California before and after September 11. *Demography*, 43, 185–201.

Lawvere, S., & Mahoney, M. C. (2005). St. John's wort. *American Family Physician*, 72, 2249–2254.

LeCheminant, J. D., Hinman, T., Pratt, K. B., Earl, N., Bailey, B. W., Thackeray, R., & Tucker, L. A. (2014). Effect of resistance training on body composition, self-efficacy, depression, and activity in postpartum women. *Scandinavian Journal of Medical Science of Sports*, 24, 414–421.

Lecrubier, Y., Clerc, G., Didi, R., & Kieser, M. (2002). Efficacy of St. John's wort extract WS 5570 in major depression: A double-blind, placebo-controlled trial. *American Journal of Psychiatry*, 159, 1361–1366.

Lee, C., Crawford, C., Wallerstedt, D., York, A., Duncan, A., Smith, J., Sprengel, M., et al. (2012). The effectiveness of acupuncture research across components of the trauma spectrum response (tsr): A systematic review of reviews. *Systematic Reviews*, 1, 46. www.systematicreviewsjournal.com/content/1/1/46

Lee, J. H., O'Keefe, J. H., Bell, D., Hensrud, D. D., & Holick, M. F. (2008). Vitamin D deficiency. *Journal of the American College of Cardiology*, 52, 1949–1956.

REFERENCES

Lee, J. Y., & Hwang, J. Y. (2015). A study on postpartum symptoms and their related factors in Korea. *Taiwanese Journal of Obstetrics & Gynecology*, 54, 355–363.

Lee, S.-Y., Aycock, D. M., & Moloney, M. F. (2012). Bright light therapy to promote sleep in mothers of low birthweight infants: A pilot study. *Biological Research for Nursing*, 15, 398–406.

Lee, S.-Y., Lee, K. A., Rankin, S. H., Weiss, S. J., & Alkon, A. (2007). Sleep disturbance, fatigue, and stress among Chinese-American parents with ICU hospitalized infants. *Issues in Mental Health Nursing*, 28, 593–605.

Lee, Y.-J., Yi, D.-H., Lee, S.-S., Sohn, W.-S., & Kim, I.-J. (2015). Correlation between postpartum depression and premenstrual dysphoric disorder: Single center study. *Obstetrics & Gynecology Science*, 58, 353–358.

Leeners, B., Rath, W., Block, E., Gorres, G., & Tshudin, S. (2014). Risk factors for unfavorable pregnancy outcome in women with adverse childhood experiences. *Journal of Perinatal Medicine*, 42, 171–178. doi:10.1515/jpm20130003

Leibenluft, E. (2000). Women and bipolar disorder: An update. *Bulletin of the Menninger Clinic*, 64, 5–17.

Leonard, B. E. (2010). The concept of depression as a dysfunction of the immune system. *Current Immunology Review*, 6, 205–212.

Lesperance, F., & Frasure-Smith, N. (2000). Depression in patients with cardiac disease: A practical review. *Journal of Psychosomatic Research*, 48, 379–391.

Letourneau, N., Duffett-Leger, L., Stewart, M., Hegadoren, K., Dennis, C.-L., Rinaldi, C. M., & Stoppard, J. (2007). Canadian mothers' perceived support needs during postpartum depression. *Journal of Obstetric, Gynecologic, and Neonatal Nursing*, 36, 441–449.

Leu, S. J., Shiah, I. S., Yatham, L. N., Cheu, Y. M., & Lam, R. W. (2001). Immune-inflammatory markers in patients with seasonal affective disorder: Effects of light therapy. *Journal of Affective Disorders*, 63, 27–34.

Lev-Wiesel, R., & Daphna-Tekoah, S. (2007). Prenatal posttraumatic stress symptomatology in pregnant survivors of childhood sexual abuse: A brief report. *Journal of Loss & Trauma*, 12, 145–153.

Lev-Wiesel, R., Chen, R., Daphna-Tekoah, S., & Hod, M. (2009). Past traumatic events: Are they a risk factor for high-risk pregnancy, delivery complications, and postpartum posttraumatic symptoms? *Journal of Women's Health*, 18, 119–125.

Lev-Wiesel, R., Daphna-Tekoah, S., & Hallak, M. (2009). Childhood sexual abuse as a predictor of birth-related posttraumatic stress and postpartum posttraumatic stress. *Child Abuse & Neglect*, 33, 877–887.

Li, A., Tu, M. T., Sousa, A. C., Alvarado, B., Kone, G. K., Guralnik, J., & Zunzunegui, M. V. (2015). Early life adversity and C-reactive protein in diverse populations of older adults: A cross-sectional analysis from the International Mobility in Aging Study (IMIAS). *BMC Geriatrics*, 15, 102. doi:10.1186/s12877-015-0104-2

Lieb, R., Isensee, B., Hofler, M., Pfister, H., & Wittchen, H.-U. (2002). Parental major depression and the risk of depression and other mental disorders in offspring. *Archives of General Psychiatry*, 59, 365–374.

Lin, P., & Su, K.-P. (2007). A meta-analysis review of double-blinded, placebo-controlled trials of antidepressant efficacy of omega-3 fatty acids. *Journal of Clinical Psychiatry*, 68, 1056–1061.

Lobato, G., Brunner, M. A. C., Dias, M. A. B., Moraes, C. L., & Reichenheim, M. E. (2012). Higher rates of postpartum depression among women lacking care after childbirth: Clinical and epidemiological importance of missed postnatal visits. *Archives of Women's Mental Health*, 15, 145–146.

Lobel, M., DeVincent, C. J., Kaminer, A., & Meyer, B. A. (2000). The impact of prenatal maternal stress and optimistic disposition on birth outcomes in medically high-risk women. *Health Psychology*, 19, 544–553.

Logsdon, M. C., & Usui, W. (2001). Psychosocial predictors of postpartum depression in diverse groups of women. *Western Journal of Nursing Research*, 23, 563–574.

Logsdon, M. C., Usui, W. M., & Nering, M. (2009a). Validation of Edinburgh Postnatal Depression Scale for adolescent mothers. *Archives of Women's Mental Health*, 12, 433–440.

Logsdon, M. C., Wisner, K. L., & Hanusa, B. H. (2009b). Does maternal role functioning improve with antidepressant treatment in women with postpartum depression. *Journal of Women's Health*, 18, 85–90.

Looper, K. J. (2007). Potential medical and surgical complications of sertonergic antidepressant medications. *Psychosomatics*, 48, 1–9.

Louik, C., Lin, A. E., Werler, M. M., Hernandez-Diaz, S., & Mitchell, A. A. (2007). First-trimester use of selective serotonin-reuptake inhibitors and the risk of birth defects. *New England Journal of Medicine*, 356, 2675–2683.

Lucas, A., Pizarro, E., Granada, M. L., Salinas, I., & Santmarti, A. (2001). Postpartum thyroid dysfunction and postpartum depression: Are they two linked disorders? *Clinical Endocrinology*, 55, 809–814.

Luoma, I., Tamminen, T., Kaukonen, P., Laippala, P., Puura, K., Salelin, R., & Almqvist, F. (2001). Longitudinal study of maternal depressive symptoms and child well-being. *Journal of the American Academy of Child and Adolescent Psychiatry*, 40, 1367–1374.

Lupien, S. J., Parent, S., Evans, A. C., Tremblay, R. E., Zelazo, P., Corbo, V., Pruessner, J. C., & Seguin, J. R. (2011). Larger amygdala but no change in hippocampal volume in 10-year-old children exposed to maternal depressive symptomatology since birth. *Proceedings of the National Academy of Sciences USA*, 108, 14324–14329.

Lutz, K. F. (2005). Abuse experiences, perceptions, and associated decisions during the childbearing cycle. *Western Journal of Nursing*, 27, 802–824.

Lutz, W. J., & Hock, E. (2002). Parental emotions following the birth of the first child: Gender differences in depressive symptoms. *American Journal of Orthopsychiatry*, 72, 415–421.

MacArthur, C., Winter, H. R., Bick, D. E., Knowles, H., Lilford, R., Henderson, C., Lancashire, R. J., Braunholtz, D. A., & Gee, H. (2002). Effects of redesigned community postnatal care on women's health 4 months after birth: A cluster randomized controlled trial. *Lancet*, 359, 378–385.

Machado, M. C., Assis, K. F., Oliveira Fde, C., Ribeiro, A. Q., Araujo, R. M., Cury, A. F., Priore, S. E., & Franceschini Sdo, C. (2014). Determinants of the exclusive breastfeeding abandonment: Psychosocial factors. *Revista Saude Publica*, 48, 985–994.

Maclean, L. I., McDermott, M. R., & May, C. P. (2000). Method of delivery and subjective distress: Women's emotional responses to childbirth practices. *Journal of Reproductive and Infant Psychology*, 18, 153–162.

Maes, M. (2001a). The immunoregulatory effects of antidepressants. *Human Psychopharmacology*, 16, 95–103.

Maes, M. (2001b). Psychological stress and the inflammatory response system. *Clinical Science*, 101, 193–194.

Maes, M., & Smith, R. S. (1998). Fatty acids, cytokines, and major depression. *Biological Psychiatry*, 43, 313–314.

Maes, M., Christophe, A., Bosmans, E., Lin, A., & Neels, H. (2000a). In humans, serum polyunsaturated fatty acid levels predict the response of proinflammatory cytokines to psychologic stress. *Biological Psychiatry*, 47, 910–920.

Maes, M., Lin, A., Ombelet, W., Stevens, K., Kenis, G., DeJongh, R., Cox, J., & Bosmans, E. (2000b). Immune activation in the early puerperium is related to postpartum anxiety and depressive symptoms. *Psychoneuroendocrinology*, 25, 121–137.

Maes, M., Ombelet, W., DeJongh, R., Kenis, G., & Bosmans, E. (2001). The inflammatory response following delivery is amplified in women who previously suffered from major depression, suggesting that major depression is accompanied by a sensitization of the inflammatory response system. *Journal of Affective Disorders*, 63, 85–92.

Maes, M., Yirmyia, R., Noraberg, J., Brene, S., Hibblen, J., Perini, G., Kubera, M., et al. (2009). The inflammatory & neurodegenerative (I&ND) hypothesis of depression: Leads for future research and new drug developments in depression. *Metabolic Brain Disease*, 24, 27–53.

REFERENCES

Maia, B. R., Pereira, A. T., Marques, M., Bos, S., Soares, M. J., Valente, J., Gomes, A. A., et al. (2012). The role of perfectionism in postpartum depression and symptomatology. *Archives of Women's Mental Health*, 15, 459–468.

Maimburg, R. D., & Vaeth, M. (2015). Postpartum depression among first-time mothers—Results from a parallel randomised trial. *Sexual & Reproductive Healthcare*, 6, 95–100.

Maina, G., Rosso, G., Aguglia, A., & Bogetto, F. (2014). Recurrence rates of bipolar disorder during the postpartum period: A study on 276 medication-free Italian women. *Archives of Women's Mental Health*, 17, 367–372.

Makrides, M., Gibson, R. A., McPhee, A. J., Yelland, L., Quinlivan, J., Ryan, P., & DOMInO Investigative Team. (2010). Effect of DHA supplementation during pregnancy on maternal depression and neurodevelopment of young children. *JAMA*, 304, 1675–1683.

Malm, H., Sourander, A., Gissler, M., Gyllenberg, D., Hinkka-Yli-Salomaki, S., McKeague, I. W., Artama, M., & Brown, A. S. (2015). Pregnancy complications following prenatal exposure to SSRIs or maternal psychiatric disorders: Results from population-based national register data. *American Journal of Psychiatry*, 172, 1224–1232.

Manber, R., Schnyer, R. N., Allen, J. J. B., Rush, A. J., & Blasey, C. M. (2004). Acupuncture: A promising treatment for depression. *Journal of Affective Disorders*, 83, 89–95.

Manber, R., Schnyer, R. N., Lyell, D., Chambers, A. S., Caughey, A. B., Druzin, M., Carlyle, E., et al. (2010). Acupuncture for depression during pregnancy: A randomized controlled trial. *Obstetrics & Gynecology*, 115, 511–520.

Mann, J. R., McKeown, R. E., Bacon, J., Vesselinov, R., & Bush, F. (2008a). Do antenatal religious and spiritual factors impact the risk of postpartum depressive symptoms? *Journal of Women's Health*, 17, 745–755.

Mann, J. R., McKeown, R. E., Bacon, J., Vesselinov, R., & Bush, F. (2008b). Religiosity, spirituality and antenatal anxiety in Southern U.S. women. *Archives of Women's Mental Health*, 11, 19–26.

Marangell, L. B., Martinez, J. M., Zboyan, H. A., Chong, H., & Puryear, L. J. (2004). Omega-3 fatty acids for the prevention of postpartum depression: Negative data from a preliminary, open-label pilot study. *Depression & Anxiety*, 19, 20–23.

Marchesi, C. (2008). Pharmacological management of panic disorder. *Neuropsychiatric Disease and Treatment*, 4, 93–106.

Marchesi, C., Ossola, P., Amerio, A., Daniel, B. D., Tonna, M., & De Panfilis, C. (2016). Clinical management of perinatal anxiety disorders: A systematic review. *Journal of Affective Disorders*, 190, 543–550.

Markhus, M. W., Skotheim, S., Graff, I. E., Froyland, L., Braarud, H. C., Stormark, K. M., & Malde, M. K. (2013). Low omega-3 index in pregnancy is a possible biological risk factor for postpartum depression. *PLoS ONE*, 8(7), e67617.

Martin, S. L., Mackie, L., Kupper, L. L., Buescher, P. A., & Moracco, K. E. (2001). Physical abuse of women before, during, and after pregnancy. *Journal of the American Medical Association*, 285, 1581–1584.

Maschi, S., Clavenna, A., Campi, R., Schiavetti, B., Bernat, M., & Bonati, M. (2008). Neonatal outcome following pregnancy exposure to antidepressants: A prospective controlled cohort study. *British Journal of Obstetrics & Gynecology*, 115, 283–289.

Matijasevich, A., Murray, J., Cooper, P. J., Anselmi, L., Barros, A. J. D., Barros, F. C. F., & Santos, I. S. (2015). Trajectories of maternal depression and offspring psychopathology at 6 years: 2004 Pelotas cohort study. *Journal of Affective Disorders*, 174, 424–431.

Matthey, S., Lee, C., Crrncec, R., & Trapolini, T. (2013). Errors in scoring the Edinburgh Postnatal Depression Scale. *Archives of Women's Mental Health*, 16, 117–122.

Matthey, S., White, T., & Rice, S. (2010). Women's responses to postnatal self-report mood and experience measures: Does anonymity make a difference? *Archives of Women's Mental Health*, 13, 477–484.

Mauri, M., Oppo, A., Borri, C., & Banti, S. (2012). Suicidality in the perinatal period: Comparison of two self-report instruments. Results from PND-ReScU. *Archives of Women's Mental Health*, 15, 39–47.

Mbah, A. K., Salihu, H. M., Dagne, G., Wilson, R. E., & Bruder, K. (2013). Exposure to environmental tobacco smoke and risk of antenatal depression: Application of latent variable modeling. *Archives of Women's Mental Health*, 16, 293–302.

McCarter-Spaulding, D., & Horowitz, J. A. (2007). How does postpartum depression affect breastfeeding? *MCN*, 32, 10–17.

McCoy, S. J., Beal, M., Shipman, S. B. M., Payton, M. E., & Watson, G. H. (2006). Risk factors for postpartum depression: A retrospective investigation at 4-weeks postnatal and a review of the literature. *Journal of the American Osteopathic Association*, 106, 193–198.

McEwen, B. S. (2003). Mood disorders and allostatic load. *Biological Psychiatry*, 54, 200–207.

McGarry, J., Kim, H., Sheng, X., Egger, M., & Baksh, L. (2009). Postpartum depression and help-seeking behavior. *Journal of Midwifery and Women's Health*, 54, 50–59.

McGovern, P., Dowd, B. E., Gjerdingen, D., Gross, C. R., Kenney, S., Ukestad, L., McCaffrey, D., & Lundberg, U. (2006). Postpartum health of employed mothers 5 weeks after childbirth. *Annals of Family Medicine*, 4, 159–167.

McGrath, J. M., Records, K., & Rice, M. (2008). Maternal depression and infant temperament characteristics. *Infant Behavior & Development*, 31, 71–80.

McKee, M. D., Cunningham, M., Jankowski, K. R., & Zayas, L. (2001). Health-related functional status in pregnancy: Relationship to depression and social support in a multi-ethnic population. *Obstetrics & Gynecology*, 97, 988–993.

McLearn, K. T., Minkovitz, C. S., Strobino, D. M., Marks, E., & Hou, W. (2006a). The timing of maternal depressive symptoms and mothers' parenting practices with young children: Implications for pediatric practice. *Pediatrics*, 118, e174–e182.

McLearn, K. T., Minkovitz, C. S., Strobion, D. M., Marks, E., & Hou, W. (2006b). Maternal depressive symptoms at 2 to 4 months postpartum and early parenting practices. *Archives of Pediatrics and Adolescent Medicine*, 160, 279–284.

McLennan, J. D., & Kotelchuck, M. (2000). Parental prevention practices for young children in the context of maternal depression. *Pediatrics*, 105, 1090–1095.

McLennan, J. D., & Offord, D. R. (2002). Should postpartum depression be targeted to improve child mental health? *Journal of the American Academy of Child and Adolescent Psychiatry*, 41, 28–35.

McLennan, J. D., Kotelchuck, M., & Cho, H. (2001). Prevalence, persistence, and correlates of depressive symptoms in a national sample of mothers of toddlers. *Journal of the American Academy of Child and Adolescent Psychiatry*, 40, 1316–1323.

McNamara, R. K. (2009). Evaluation of docosahexaenoic acid deficiency as a preventable risk factor for recurrent affective disorders: Current status, future directions, and dietary recommendations. *Prostaglandins, Leukotrienes, and Essential Fatty Acids*, 81, 223–231.

Meades, R., Pond, C., Ayers, S., & Warren, F. (2011). Postnatal debriefing: Have we thrown the baby out with the bath water? *Behavior Research and Therapy*, 49, 367–372.

Mellor, R., Chua, S. C., & Boyce, P. (2014). Antenatal depression: An artefact of sleep disturbance? *Archives of Women's Mental Health*, 17, 291–302.

Meltzer-Brody, S., Boschloo, L., Jones, I., Sullivan, P. F., & Penninx, B. W. (2013). The EPDS-Lifetime: Assessment of lifetime prevalence and risk factors for perinatal depression in a large cohort of depressed women. *Archives of Women's Mental Health*, 16, 465–473.

Meyer, C. L., & Oberman, M. (2001). *Mothers who kill their children: Understanding the acts of moms from Susan Smith to the "Prom Mom"*. New York, NY: NYU Press.

Mezzacappa, E. S., & Endicott, J. (2007). Parity mediates the association between infant feeding method and maternal depressive symptoms in the postpartum. *Archives of Women's Mental Health*, 10, 259–266.

Miceli, P. J., Goeke-Morey, M. C., Whitman, T. L., Kolberg, K. S., Miller-Loncar, C., & White, R. D. (2000). Birth status, medical complication, and social environment: Individual differences in development of preterm, very low birth weight infants. *Journal of Pediatric Psychology*, 25, 353–358.

REFERENCES

Mick, E., Biederman, J., Prince, J., Fischer, B. A., & Faraone, S. V. (2002). Impact of low birth-weight on attention-deficit hyperactivity disorder. *Journal of Developmental & Behavioral Pediatrics*, 23, 16–22.

Milgrom, J., Negri, L. M., Gemmill, A. W., McNeil, M., & Martin, P. R. (2005). A randomized controlled trial of psychological interventions for postnatal depression. *British Journal of Clinical Psychology*, 44, 529–542.

Miller, A. M., Hogue, C. J., Knight, B. T., Stowe, Z., & Newport, D. J. (2012). Maternal expectations of postpartum social support: Validation of the postpartum social support questionnaire during pregnancy. *Archives of Women's Mental Health*, 15, 307–311.

Miller, E. S., Hoxha, D., Wisner, K. L., & Gossett, D. R. (2015). Obsessions and compulsions in postpartum women without obsessive compulsive disorder. *Journal of Women's Health*, 24, 825–830.

Miller, L. J. (2002). Postpartum depression. *Journal of the American Medical Association*, 287, 762–765.

Miniati, M., Callari, A., Calugi, S., Rucci, P., Savino, M., Mauri, M., & Dell'Osso, L. (2014). Interpersonal psychotherapy for postpartum depression: A systematic review. *Archives of Women's Mental Health*, 17, 257–268.

Mirowsky, J., & Ross, C. E. (2002). Depression, parenthood, and age at first birth. *Social Science & Medicine*, 54, 1281–1298.

Misri, S., Albert, G., Abizadeh, J., Kendrick, K., Carter, D., Ryan, D., & Oberlander, T. F. (2012). Biopsychosocial determinants of treatment outcome for mood and anxiety disorders up to 8 months postpartum. *Archives of Women's Mental Health*, 15, 313–316.

Misri, S., Kim, J., Riggs, K. W., & Kostaras, X. (2000a). Paroxetine levels in postpartum depressed women, breast milk, and infant serum. *Journal of Clinical Psychiatry*, 61, 828–832.

Misri, S., Kostaras, X., Fox, D., & Kostaras, D. (2000b). The impact of partner support in the treatment of postpartum depression. *Canadian Journal of Psychiatry*, 45, 554–558.

Misri, S., Reebye, P., Corral, M., & Mills, L. (2004). The use of paroxetine and cognitive-behavioral therapy in postpartum depression and anxiety: A randomized controlled trial. *Journal of Clinical Psychiatry*, 65, 1236–1241.

Misri, S., Reebye, P., Milis, L., & Shah, S. (2006). The impact of treatment intervention on parenting stress in postpartum depressed women: A prospective study. *American Journal of Orthopsychiatry*, 76, 115–119.

Miszkurka, M., Zunzunegui, M. V., & Goulet, L. (2012). Immigrant status, antenatal depressive symptoms, and frequency and source of violence: What's the relationship? *Archives of Women's Mental Health*, 15, 387–396.

Mitchell, J. E., Trangle, M., Degnan, B., Gabert, T., Haight, B., Kessler, D., Mack, N., et al. (2013). *Adult depression in primary care*. Bloomington, MN: Institute for Clinical Systems Improvement.

Miyake, Y., Sasaki, S., Yokoyama, T., Tanaka, K., Ohya, Y., Fukushima, W., Saito, K., et al. (2006). Risk of postpartum depression in relation to dietary fish and fat intake in Japan: The Osaka Maternal and Child Health Study. *Psychological Medicine*, 36, 1727–1735.

Modarres, M., Afrasiabi, S., Rahnama, P., & Montazeri, A. (2012). Prevalence and risk factors of childbirth-related post-traumatic stress symptoms. *BMC Pregnancy and Childbirth*, 12(88). doi: www.biomedcentral.com/1471–2393/12/88

Montgomery, S. M., Ehlin, A., & Sacker, A. (2006). Breast feeding and resilience against psychosocial stress. *Archives of Diseases of Childhood*, 91, 990–994.

Monti, F., Agostini, F., Fagandini, P., La Sala, G. B., & Blickstein, I. (2009). Depressive symptoms during late pregnancy and early parenthood following assisted reproductive technology. *Fertility & Sterility*, 91, 851–857.

Mora, P. A., Bennett, I. M., Elo, I. T., Mathew, L., Coyne, J. C., & Culhane, J. F. (2009). Distinct trajectories of perinatal depressive symptomatology: Evidence from growth mixing modeling. *American Journal of Epidemiology*, 169, 24–32.

Morgan, J. F., Lacey, J. H., & Chung, E. (2006). Risk of postnatal depression, miscarriage, and preterm birth in bulimia nervosa: Retrospective contolled study. *Psychosomatic Medicine*, 68, 487–492.

Morrell, C. J., Spiby, H., Stewart, P., Walters, S., & Morgan, A. (2000). Costs and effectiveness of community postnatal support workers: Randomised controlled trial. *British Medical Journal*, 321, 593–598.

Morris-Rush, J. K., & Bernstein, P. S. (2002). Postpartum depression. www.medscape.com/viewarticle/433013

Moses-Kolko, E. L., & Roth, E. K. (2004). Antepartum and postpartum depression: Healthy mom, healthy baby. *Journal of the American Medical Women's Association*, 59, 181–191.

Moses-Kolko, E. L., Berga, S. L., Kalro, B., Sit, D. K. Y., & Wisner, K. L. (2009). Transdermal estradiol for postpartum: A promising treatment option. *Clinical Obstetrics & Gynecology*, 52, 516–529.

Moss, K. M., Skouteris, H., Wertheim, E. H., Paxton, S. J., & Milgrom, J. (2009). Depressive and anxiety symptoms through late pregnancy and the first year post birth: An examination of prospective relationships. *Archives of Women's Mental Health*, 12, 345–349.

Mozurkewich, E. L., Clinton, C. M., Chilimigras, J. L., Hamilton, S. E., Allbaugh, L. J., Berman, D. R., Marcus, S. M., et al. (2013). The Mothers, Omega-3, and Mental Health Study: A double-blind, randomized controlled trial. *American Journal of Obstetrics and Gynecology*, 208, 313. doi:10.1016/j.ajog2013.01.038

Mu, P.-F., Wong, T.-T., Chang, K.-P., & Kwan, S.-Y. (2001). Predictors of maternal depression for families having a child with epilepsy. *Journal of Nursing Research*, 9, 116–126.

Mufson, L., Dorta, K. P., Wickramaratne, P., Nomura, Y., Olfson, M., & Weissman, M. M. (2004). A randomized effectiveness trial of interpersonal psychotherapy for depressed adolescents. *Archives of General Psychiatry*, 61, 577–584.

Muller, W. E. (2003). Current St. John's wort research from mode of action to clinical efficacy. *Pharmacology Research*, 47, 101–109.

Munk-Olsen, T., Laursen, T. M., Mendelson, T., & Pedersen, C. B. (2010). Perinatal mental disorders in native Danes and immigrant women. *Archives of Women's Mental Health*, 13, 319–326.

Murray, L., Dunne, M. P., Vo, T. V., Anh, P. N. T., Khawaja, N. G., & Cao, T. N. (2015). Postnatal depressive symptoms amongst women in Central Vietnam: A cross-sectional study investigating prevalence and associations with social, cultural, and infant factors. *BMC Pregnancy and Childbirth*, 15, 234. doi:10.1186/s12884-015-0662-5

Murray, L., Woolgar, M., Cooper, P., & Hipwell, A. (2001). Cognitive abilities to depression in 5-year-old children of depression mothers. *Journal of Child Psychology and Psychiatry*, 42, 891–899.

Muzik, M., Bocknek, E. L., Broderick, A., Richardson, P., Rosenblum, K. L., Thelen, K., & Seng, J. S. (2013). Mother–infant bonding impairment across the first 6 months postpartum: The primacy of psychopathology in women with childhood abuse and neglect histories. *Archives of Women's Mental Health*, 16, 29–38.

Najman, J. M., Williams, G. M., Nikles, J., Spence, S., Bor, W., O'Callaghan, M., Le Brocque, R., & Andersen, M. J. (2000). Mothers' mental illness and child behavior problems: Cause–effect association or observation bias? *Journal of the American Academy of Child and Adolescent Psychiatry*, 39, 592–602.

National Alliance on Mental Illness (NAMI). (2007). Seasonal affective disorder. www.nami.org.

National Center for PTSD. (2010). Mindfulness practice in the treatment of traumatic stress. Retrieved from www.ptsd.va.gov/public/pages/mindful-ptsd.asp

National Center for PTSD. (2014a). DSM-5 criteria for PTSD. Retrieved from www.ptsd.va.gov/professional/PTSD-overview/dsm5_criteria_ptsd.asp

National Center for PTSD. (2014b). Treatment for PTSD. Retrieved from www.ptsd.va.gov/public/treatment/therapy-med/treatment-ptsd.asp

REFERENCES

Navarro, P., Garcia-Esteve, L., Ascaso, C., Aguado, J., Gelabert, E., & Martin-Santos, R. (2008). Non-psychotic psychiatric disorders after childbirth: Prevalence and comorbidity in a community sample. *Journal of Affective Disorders*, 109, 171–176.

Newport, D. J., Hostetter, A., Arnold, A., & Stowe, Z. (2002). The treatment of postpartum depression: minimizing infant exposures. *Journal of Clinical Psychiatry*, 63(Suppl 7), 31–44.

Ngai, F.-W., & Ngu, S.-F. (2015). Predictors of maternal and paternal depressive symptoms at postpartum. *Journal of Psychosomatic Research*, 78, 156–161.

Nicklas, J. M., Miller, L. J., Zera, C. A., Davis, R. B., Levkoff, S. E., & Seely, E. W. (2013). Factors associated with depressive symptoms in the early postpartum period among women with recent gestational diabetes mellitus. *Maternal & Child Health Journal*, 17, 1665–1672. doi:10.1007/s10995-012-1180-y

Nicolson, S., Judd, F., Thomson-Salo, F., & Mitchell, S. (2013). Supporting the adolescent mother–infant relationship: Preliminary trial of a brief perinatal attachment intervention. *Archives of Women's Mental Health*, 16, 511–520.

Nishimura, A., Fujita, Y., Katsuta, M., Ishihara, A., & Ohashi, K. (2015). Paternal postnatal depression in Japan: An investigation of correlated factors including relationship with partner. *BMC Pregnancy and Childbirth*, 15, 128. doi:10.1186/s12884-015-0552-x

Noaghiul, S., & Hibbeln, J. R. (2003). Cross-national comparisons of seafood consumption and rates of bipolar disorders. *American Journal of Psychiatry*, 160, 2222–2227.

Noorbakhshnia, M., Dehkordi, N. G., Ghaedi, K., Esmaeili, A., & Dabaghi, M. (2015). Omega-3 fatty acids prevent LPS-induced passive avoidance learning and memory and CaMKII-gene expression impairments in hippocampus of rat. *Pharmacological Reports*, 67, 370–375.

Norman, E., Sherburn, M., Osborne, R., & Galea, M. P. (2010). An exercise and education program improves well-being of new mothers: A randomized controlled trial. *Physical Therapy*, 90, 348–355.

Nylen, K. J., O'Hara, M. W., Brock, R., Moel, J., Gorman, L., & Stuart, S. (2010). Predictors of the longitudinal course of postpartum depression following interpersonal psychotherapy. *Journal of Consulting & Clinical Psychology*, 78, 757–763.

O'Brien, S. M., Scott, L. V., & Dinan, T. G. (2004). Cytokines: Abnormalities in major depression and implications for pharmacological treatment. *Human Psychopharmacology*, 19, 397–403.

O'Brien, S. M., Scott, L. V., & Dinan, T. G. (2006). Antidepressant therapy and C-reactive protein levels. *British Journal of Psychiatry*, 188, 449–452. doi:188/5/449 [pii] 10.1192/bjp.bp.105.011015

O'Donovan, A., Alcorn, K. L., Patrick, J. C., Creedy, D. K., Dawe, S., & Devilly, G. J. (2014). Predicting posttraumatic stress disorder after childbirth. *Midwifery*, 30, 935–941.

O'Hara, M. W. (2009). Postpartum depression: What we know. *Journal of Clinical Psychology*, 65, 1258–1269.

O'Hara, M. W., Stuart, S., Gorman, L. L., & Wenzel, A. (2000). Efficacy of interpersonal psychotherapy for postpartum depression. *Archives of General Psychiatry*, 57, 1039–1045.

O'Higgins, M., St. James Roberts, I., Glover, M., & Taylor, A. (2013). Mother–child bonding at 1 year: Associations with symptoms of postnatal depression and bonding in the first few weeks. *Archives of Women's Mental Health*, 16, 381–389.

O'Leary, J. (2005). The trauma of ultrasound during a pregnancy following perinatal loss. *Journal of Loss and Trauma*, 10, 183–204.

Oberlander, T. F., Grunau, R. E., Fitzgerald, C. E., Papsdorf, M., Rurak, D., & Riggs, W. (2005). Pain reactivity in 2-month-old infants after prenatal and postnatal serotonin reuptake inhibitor medication exposure. *Pediatrics*, 115, 411–425.

Oberlander, T. F., Misri, S., Fitzgerald, C. E., Kostaras, X., Rurak, D., & Riggs, W. (2004). Pharmacologic factors associated with transient neonatal symptoms following prenatal psychotropic medication exposure. *Journal Clinical Psychiatry*, 65, 230–237.

Oberlander, T. F., Reebye, P., Misri, S., Papsdorf, M., Kim, J., & Grunau, R. E. (2007). Externalizing and attentional behaviors in children of depressed mothers treated with selective serotonin reuptake inhibitor antidepressant during pregnancy. *Archives of Pediatric & Adolescent Medicine*, 161, 22–29.

Oberlander, T. F., Warburton, W., Misri, S., Aghajanian, J., & Hertzman, C. (2006). Neonatal outcomes after prenatal exposure to selective serotonin reuptake inhibitor antidepressants and maternal depression using population-based linked health data. *Archives of General Psychiatry*, 63, 898–906.

Okun, M. L., Schetter, C. D., & Glynn, L. M. (2011). Poor sleep quality is associated with preterm birth. *Sleep*, 34, 1493–1498.

Olafsdottir, A. S., Skuladottir, G. V., Thorsdottir, I., Hauksson, A., Thorgeirsdottir, H., & Steingrimsdottir, L. (2006). Relationship between high consumption of marine fatty acids in early pregnancy and hypertensive disorders in pregnancy. *British Journal of Obstetrics & Gynecology*, 113, 301–309.

Olfson, M., Marcus, S. C., Tedeschi, M., & Wan, G. J. (2006). Continuity of antidepressant treatment for adults with depression in the United States. *American Journal of Psychiatry*, 163, 101–108.

Onoye, J. M., Goebert, D., Morland, L., & Matsu, C. (2009). PTSD and postpartum mental health in a sample of Caucasian, Asian, and Pacific Islander women. *Archives of Women's Mental Health*, 12, 393–400.

Onoye, J. M., Shafer, L. A., Goebert, D. A., Morland, L. A., Matsu, C. R., & Hamagami, F. (2013). Changes in PTSD symptomatology and mental health during pregnancy and postpartum. *Archives of Women's Mental Health*, 16, 453–463.

Onozawa, K., Glover, V., Adams, D., Modi, N., & Kumar, R. C. (2001). Infant massage improves mother–infant interaction for mothers with postnatal depression. *Journal of Affective Disorders*, 63, 201–207.

Oppo, A., Mauri, M., Ramacciotti, D., Camilleri, V., Banti, S., Borri, C., Rambelli, C., et al. (2009). Risk factors for postpartum depression: The role of the Postpartum Depression Predictors Inventory-Revised (PDPI-R). *Archives of Women's Mental Health*, 12, 239–249.

Oren, D. A., Wisner, K. L., Spinelli, M., Epperson, C. N., Peindl, K. S., Terman, J. S., & Terman, M. (2002). An open trial of morning light therapy for treatment of antepartum depression. *American Journal of Psychiatry*, 159, 666–669.

Orhon, F. S., Ulukol, B., & Soykan, A. (2007). Postpartum mood disorders and maternal perceptions of infant patterns in well-child follow-up visits. *Acta Paediatrica*, 96, 1777–1783.

Orr, S. T., Reiter, J. P., Blazer, D. G., & James, S. A. (2007). Maternal prenatal pregnancy-related anxiety and spontaneous preterm birth in Baltimore, Maryland. *Psychosomatic Medicine*, 69, 566–570.

Osborne, L., Birndorf, C. A., Szkodny, L. E., & Wisner, K. L. (2014). Returning to tricyclic antidepressants for depression during childbearing: Clinical and dosing challenges. *Archives of Women's Mental Health*, 17, 239–246.

Pace, T. W., Hu, F., & Miller, A. H. (2007). Cytokine-effects on glucocorticoid receptor function: Relevance to glucocorticoid resistance and the pathophysiology and treatment of major depression. *Brain, Behavior and Immunity*, 21, 9–19.

Pajulo, M., Savonlahti, E., Sourander, A., Ahlqvist, S., Helenius, H., & Piha, J. (2001a). An early report on the mother–baby interactive capacity of substance-abusing mothers. *Journal of Substance Abuse Treatment*, 20, 143–151.

Pajulo, M., Savonlahti, E., Sourander, A., Helenius, H., & Piha, J. (2001b). Antenatal depression, substance dependency, and social support. *Journal of Affective Disorders*, 65, 9–17.

Papakostas, G. I., Mischoulon, D., Shyu, I., Alpert, J. E., & Fava, M. (2010). S-adenosyl methionine (SAMe) augmentation of serortonin reuptake inhibitors for antidepressant nonresponders with major depressive disorder: A double-blind, randomized clinical trial. *American Journal of Psychiatry*, 167, 942–948.

Paris, R., Bolton, R. E., & Weinberg, M. K. (2009). Postpartum depression, suicidality, and mother–infant interactions. *Archives of Women's Mental Health*, 12, 309–321.

Park, E. M., Meltzer-Brody, S., & Stickgold, R. (2013). Poor sleep maintenance and subjective sleep quality are associated with postpartum maternal depression symptom severity. *Archives of Women's Mental Health*, 16, 539–547.

271

REFERENCES

Park, E. R., Storfer-Isser, A., Kelleher, K. J., Stein, M. B., Heneghan, A. M., Chaudron, L. H., Hoagwood, K. E., et al. (2007). In the moment: Attitudinal measure of pediatrician management of maternal depression. *Ambulatory Pediatrics*, 7, 239–246.

Park, J.-H., Karmaus, W., & Zhang, H. (2015). Prevalence of and risk factors for depressive symptoms in Korean women throughout pregnancy and in postpartum period. *Asian Nursing Research*, 9, 219–225.

Parker, G., Gibson, N.A., Brotchie, H., Heruc, G., Rees, A-M., & Hadzi-Pavlovic, D. (2006). Omega-3 fatty acids and mood disorders. *American Journal of Psychiatry*, 163, 969–978.

Parmar, V. R., Kumar, A., Kaur, R., Parmar, S., Kaur, D., Basu, S., Jain, S., & Narula, S. (2009). Experience with Kangaroo Mother Care in a neonatal intensive care unit (NICU) in Chandigarh, India. *Indian Journal of Pediatrics*, 76, 25–28.

Patel, V., & Prince, M. (2006). Maternal psychological morbidity and low birth weight in India. *British Journal of Psychiatry*, 188, 284–285.

Patel, V., Rodrigues, M., & DeSouza, N. (2002). Gender, poverty, and postnatal depression: A study of mothers in Goa, India. *American Journal of Psychiatry*, 159, 43–47.

Pauli-Pott, U., Becker, K., Mertesacker, T., & Beckmann, D. (2000). Infants with "colic"—Mothers' perspectives on the crying problem. *Journal of Psychosomatic Research*, 48, 125–132.

Paxson, C., Fussell, E., Rhodes, J., & Waters, M. (2010). Five years later: Recovery from post traumatic stress and psychological distress among low-income mothers affected by Hurricane Katrina. *Social Science & Medicine*, 74, 150–157.

Pearson, R. M., Lightman, S. L., & Evans, J. (2012). Symptoms of depression during pregnancy are associated with increased systolic blood pressure responses towards infant distress. *Archives of Women's Mental Health*, 15, 95–105.

Pedersen, C. A., Johnson, J. L., Silva, S., Bunevicius, R., Meltzer-Brody, S., Hamer, M., & Leserman, J. (2007). Antenatal thyroid correlates of postpartum depression. *Psychoneuroendocrinology*, 32, 235–245.

Peeler, S., Chung, M. C., Stedmon, J., & Skirton, H. (2013). A review assessing current treatment strategies for postnatal psychological morbidity with a focus on post-traumatic stress disorder. *Midwifery*, 29, 377–388. doi:10.1016/j.midw.2012.03.004

Pelaez, M., Field, T., Pickens, J. N., & Hart, S. (2008). Disengaged and authoritarian parenting behavior of depressed mothers with their toddlers. *Infant Behavior & Development*, 31, 145–148.

Penckofer, S., Kouba, J., Wallis, D. E., & Emanuele, M. A. (2008). Vitamin D and diabetes. *Nutrition Update*, 34, 939–954.

Perez-Blasco, J., Viguer, P., & Rodrigo, M. F. (2013). Effects of a mindfulness-based intervention on psychological distress, well-being, and maternal self-efficacy in breast-feeding mothers: Results of a pilot study. *Archives of Women's Mental Health*, 16, 227–236.

Perren, S., von Wyl, A., Burgin, D., Simoni, H., & von Klitzing, K. (2005). Depressive symptoms and psychosocial stress across the transition to parenthood: Associations with parental psychopathology and child difficulty. *Journal of Psychosomatic Obstetrics & Gynecology*, 26, 173–183.

Peter, E. A., Janssen, P. A., Grange, C. S., & Douglas, M. J. (2001). Ibuprofen versus acetaminophen with codeine for the relief of perineal pain after childbirth: A randomized controlled trial. *Canadian Medical Association Journal*, 165, 1203–1209.

Plaza, A., Garcia-Esteve, L., Ascaso, C., Navarro, P., Gelabert, E., Halperin, I., Valdes, M., & Martin-Santos, R. (2010). Childhood sexual abuse and hypothalamus–pituitary–thyroid axis in postpartum major depression. *Journal of Affective Disorders*, 122, 159–163.

Pope, C. J., Xie, B., Sharma, V., & Campbell, M. K. (2013). A prospective study of thoughts of self-harm and suicidal ideation during the postpartum period in women with mood disorders. *Archives of Women's Mental Health*, 16, 483–488.

Porcel, J., Feigal, C., Poye, L., Postma, I. R., Zeeman, G. G., Olowoyeye, A., Tsigas, E., & Wilson, M. (2013). Hypertensive disorders of pregnancy and risk of screening positive for posttraumatic stress disorder: A cross-sectional study. *Pregnancy Hypertension*, 3, 254–260.

Posmontier, B. (2008a). Functional status outcomes in mothers with and without postpartum depression. *Journal of Midwifery and Women's Health*, 53(4), 310–318.

Posmontier, B. (2008b). Sleep quality in women with and without postpartum depression. *Journal of Obstetric, Gynecologic and Neonatal Nursing*, 37(6), 722–737.

Prentice, J. C., Lu, M. C., Lange, L., & Halfon, N. (2002). The association between reported childhood sexual abuse and breastfeeding initiation. *Journal of Human Lactation*, 18, 291–226.

Preston, J., & Johnson, J. (2009). *Clinical psychopharmacology made ridiculously simple*, 6th ed. Miami, FL: MedMaster.

Priddis, H., Schmied, V., & Dahlen, H. (2014). Women's experiences following severe perineal trauma: A qualitative study. *BMC Women's Health*, 14(32). www.biomedcentral.com/1472–6874/14/32

Prochaska, E. (2015). Human rights in maternity care. *Midwifery*, 31, 1015–1016.

Punamaki, R.-L., Repokari, L., Vilska, S., Poikkeus, P., Tiitinen, A., Sinkkonen, J., & Tulppala, M. (2006). Maternal mental health and medical predictors of infant development and health problems from pregnancy to one year: Does former infertility matter? *Infant Behavior & Development*, 29, 230–242.

Qu, Z., Wang, X., Tian, D., Zhao, Y., Zhang, Q., He, H., Zhang, X., et al. (2012). Posttraumatic stress disorder and depression among new mothers at 8 months later of the 2008 Sichuan earthquake in China. *Archives of Women's Mental Health*, 15, 49–55.

Quillin, S. I. M., & Glenn, L. L. (2004). Interaction between feeding method and co-sleeping on maternal–newborn sleep. *Journal of Obstetric, Gynecologic, and Neonatal Nursing*, 33, 580–588.

Quinn, T. J., & Carey, G. B. (1999). Does exercise intensity or diet influence lactic acid accumulation in breast milk? *Medicine and Science in Sports and Exercise*, 31, 105–110.

Rampono, J., Hackett, L. P., Kristensen, J. H., Kohan, R., Page-Sharp, M., & Ilett, K. F. (2006). Transfer of escitalopram and its metabolite demethylescitalopram into breastmilk. *British Journal of Clinical Pharmacology*, 62, 316–322.

Rampono, J., Teoh, S., Hackett, L. P., Kohan, R., & Illet, K. F. (2011). Estimation of desvenlafaxine transfer into milk and infant exposure during its use in lactating women with postnatal depression. *Archives of Women's Mental Health*, 14, 49–53.

Rapkin, A. J., Mikacich, J. A., Moatakef-Imani, B., & Rasgon, N. (2002). The clinical nature and formal diagnosis of premenstrual, postpartum, and perimenopausal affective disorders. *Current Psychiatry Reports*, 4, 419–428.

Reading, R., & Reynolds, S. (2001). Debt, social disadvantage, and maternal depression. *Social Science & Medicine*, 53, 441–453.

Reay, R., Fisher, Y., Robertson, M., Adams, E., Owen, C., & Kumar, R. (2006). Group interpersonal psychotherapy for postnatal depression: A pilot study. *Archives of Women's Mental Health*, 9, 31–39.

Reay, R. E., Owen, C., Shadbolt, B., Raphael, B., Mulcahy, R., & Wilkinson, R. B. (2012). Trajectories of long-term outcomes for postnatally depressed mothers treated with group interpersonal psychotherapy. *Archives of Women's Mental Health*, 15, 217–228.

Rees, A.-M., Austin, M.-P., & Parker, G. (2005). Role of omega-3 fatty acids as a treatment for depression in the perinatal period. *Australia & New Zealand Journal of Psychiatry*, 39, 274–280.

Regmi, C., Sligl, W., Carter, D., Grut, W., & Seear, M. (2002). A controlled study of postpartum depression among Nepalese women: Validation of the Edinburgh Postnatal Depression Scale in Kathmandu. *Tropical Medicine and International Health*, 7, 378–382.

Reid, K. M., & Taylor, M. G. (2015). Social support, stress, and maternal postpartum depression: A comparison of supportive relationships. *Social Science Research*, 54, 246–262.

Remick, R. A. (2002). Diagnosis and management of depression in primary care. *Canadian Journal of Nursing Research*, 33, 19–34.

Ribeiro, J. D., Pease, J. L., Gutierrez, P. M., Silva, C., Bernert, R. A., Rudd, M. D., & Joiner, T. E. (2012). Sleep problems outperform depression and hopelessness as cross-sectional and longitudinal predictors of suicidal ideation and behavior in young adults in the military. *Journal of Affective Disorders*, 136, 743–750.

Rich-Edwards, J. W., James-Todd, T., Mohllajee, A., Kleinman, K., Burke, A., Gillman, M. W., & Wright, R. J. (2011). Lifetime maternal experiences of abuse and risk of prenatal depression in two demographically distinct populations in Boston. *International Journal of Epidemiology*, 40, 375–384. doi:10.1093/ije/dyq247

Rini, C., Manne, S., DuHamel, K., Austin, J., Ostroff, J., Boulad, F., Parsons, S. K., et al. (2008). Social support from family and friends as a buffer of low spousal support among mothers of critically ill children: A multilevel modeling approach. *Health Psychology*, 27, 593–603.

Ritter, C., Hobfoll, S. E., Lavin, J., Cameron, R. P., & Hulsizer, M. R. (2000). Stress, psychosocial resources, and depressive symptomatology during pregnancy in low-income, inner-city women. *Health Psychology*, 19, 576–585.

Roberts, J., Sword, W. S., Gafni, A., Krueger, P., Sheehan, D., & Soon-Lee, K. (2001). Costs of post-partum care: Examining associations from the Ontario mothers and infant survey. *Canadian Journal of Nursing Research*, 33, 19–34.

Robinson, M., Whitehouse, A. J. O., Newnham, J. P., Gorman, S., Jacoby, P., Holt, B. J., Serralha, M., et al. (2014). Low maternal serum vitamin D during pregnancy and the risk for postpartum depression symptoms. *Archives of Women's Mental Health*, 17, 213–219.

Rohleder, N., Chen, E., Wolf, J. M., & Miller, G. E. (2008). The psychobiology of trait shame in young women: Extending the social self preservation theory. *Health Psychology*, 27, 523–532.

Roman, L. A., Gardiner, J. C., Lindsay, J. K., Moore, J. S., Luo, Z., Baer, L. J., Goddeeris, J. H., et al. (2009). Alleviating perinatal depressive symptoms and stress: A nurse-community health work randomized trial. *Archives of Women's Mental Health*, 12, 379–391.

Romieu, I., Torrent, M., Garcia-Esteban, R., Ferrer, C., Ribas-Fito, N., Anto, J. M., & Sunyer, J. (2007). Maternal fish intake during pregnancy and atopy and asthma in infancy. *Clinical & Experimental Allergy*, 37, 518–525.

Rondo, P. H. C., & Souza, M. R. (2007). Maternal distress and intended breastfeeding duration. *Journal of Psychosomatic Obstetrics & Gynecology*, 28, 55–60.

Rosen, D., Seng, J. S., Tolman, R. M., & Mallinger, G. (2007). Intimate partner violence, depression, and posttraumatic stress disorder as additional predictors of low birth weight infants among low-income mothers. *Journal of Interpersonal Violence*, 22, 1305–1314.

Rosenblum, K. L., McDonough, S., Muzik, M., Miller, A., & Sameroff, A. (2002). Maternal representations of the infant: Associations with infant response to the still face. *Child Development*, 73, 999–1015.

Ross, L. E., & Dennis, C.-L. (2009). The prevalence of postpartum depression among women with substance use, an abuse history, or chronic illness: A systematic review. *Journal of Women's Health*, 18, 475–486.

Ross, L. E., & McLean, L. M. (2006). Anxiety disorders during pregnancy and the postpartum period: A systematic review. *Journal of Clinical Psychiatry*, 67, 1285–1298.

Ross, L. E., Murray, B. J., & Steiner, M. (2005). Sleep and perinatal mood disorders: A critical review. *Journal of Psychiatry & Neuroscience*, 30, 247–256.

Roubenoff, R. (2003). Exercise and inflammatory disease. *Arthritis Care & Research*, 49, 263–266.

Roumestan, C., Michel, A., Bichon, F., Portet, K., Detoc, M., Henriquet, C., Jaffuel, D., & Mathieu, M. (2007). Anti-inflammatory properties of desipramine and fluoxetine. *Respiratory Research*, 8, 35. doi:1465-9921-8-35 [pii] 10.1186/1465-9921-8-35

Roux, G., Anderson, C., & Roan, C. (2002). Postpartum depression, marital dysfunction, and infant outcome: A longitudinal study. *Journal of Perinatal Education*, 11, 25–36.

Rowan, C., Bick, D., & da Sliva Bastos, M. H. (2007). Postnatal debriefing intervention to prevent maternal mental health problems after birth: Exploring the gap between the evidence and UK policy and practice. *Worldviews on Evidence-Based Nursing*, 4(2), 97–105.

Rowan, P., Greisinger, A., Brehm, B., Smith, F., & McReynolds, E. (2012). Outcomes from implementing systematic antepartum depression screening in obstetrics. *Archives of Women's Mental Health*, 15, 115–129.

Rowe, H., Sperlich, M. A., Cameron, H., & Seng, J. S. (2014). A quasi-experimental analysis of a psychoeducation intervention for pregnant women with abuse-related posttraumatic stress disorder. *Journal of Obstetric, Gynecologic, and Neonatal Nursing*, 43, 282–293.

Rowe-Murray, H. J., & Fisher, J. R. W. (2001). Operative intervention in delivery is associated with compromised early mother–infant interaction. *British Journal of Obstetrics & Gynecology*, 108, 1068–1075.

Rowlands, I. J., & Redshaw, M. (2012). Mode of birth and women's psychological and physical wellbeing in the postnatal period. *BMC Pregnancy and Childbirth*, 12, 138. doi:www.biomed-central.com/1471-2393/12/138

Roy, A., Janal, M. N., & Roy, M. (2010). Childhood trauma and prevalence of cardiovascular disease in patients with Type 1 diabetes. *Psychosomatic Medicine*, 72, 833–838.

Ruglass, L., & Kendall-Tackett, K. A. (2015). *The psychology of trauma 101*. New York, NY: Springer.

Ruiz, R. J., Marti, C. N., Pickler, R., Murphey, C., Wommack, J., & Brown, C. E. L. (2012). Acculturation, depressive symptoms, estriol, progesterone, and preterm birth in Hispanic women. *Archives of Women's Mental Health*, 15, 57–67.

Runsten, S., Korkeila, K., Koskenvuo, M., Rautava, P., Vainio, O., & Korkeila, J. (2014). Can social support alleviate inflammation associated with childhood adversities? *Nordic Journal of Psychiatry*, 68, 137–144.

Rupke, S. J., Blecke, D., & Renfrow, M. (2006). Cognitive therapy for depression. *American Family Physician*, 73, 83–86.

Rychnovsky, J., & Hunter, L. P. (2009). The relationship between sleep characteristics and fatigue in healthy postpartum women. *Women's Health Issues*, 19, 36–44.

Saisto, T., Salmela-Aro, K., Nurmi, J. F., & Halmesmaki, E. (2001). Psychosocial predictors of disappointment with delivery and puerperal depression: A longitudinal study. *Acta Obstetrica Gynecologica Scandanavica*, 80, 39–45.

Salovey, P., Rothman, A. J., Detweiler, J. B., & Steward, W. T. (2000). Emotional states and physical health. *American Psychologist*, 55, 110–121.

Sanderson, C. A., Cowden, B., Hall, D. M. B., Taylor, E. M., Carpenter, R. G., & Cox, J. L. (2002). Is postnatal depression a risk factor for sudden infant death? *British Journal of General Practice*, 52, 636–640.

Sanguanklin, N., McFarlin, B. L., Finnegan, L., Park, C. G., Giurgescu, C., White-Traut, R., & Engstrom, J. L. (2014). Job strain and psychological distress among employed pregnant Thai women: Role of social support and coping strategies. *Archives of Women's Mental Health*, 17, 317–326.

Santucci, A. K., Singer, L. T., Wisniewski, S., Luther, J. F., Eng, H. F., Dills, J. L., Sit, D. K., et al. (2014). Impact of prenatal exposure to serotonin reuptake inhibitors or maternal major depressive disorder on infant developmental outcomes. *Journal of Clinical Psychiatry*, 75, 1088–1095.

Sargent, C. (2015). *Birth trauma in New Zealand: Some major concerns*. New Zealand: Voice for Parents.

Sarris, J. (2007). Herbal medicines in the treatment of psychiatric disorders: A systematic review. *Phytotherapy Research*, 21, 703–716.

Saunders, T. A., Lobel, M., Veloso, C., & Meyer, B. A. (2006). Prenatal maternal stress is associated with delivery analgesia and unplanned cesareans. *Journal of Psychosomatic Obstetrics & Gynecology*, 27, 141–146.

Sawada, N., Gagne, F. M., Seguin, L., Kramer, M. S., McNamara, H., Platt, R. W., Goulet, L., et al. (2015). Maternal prenatal felt security and infant health at birth interact to predict infant fussing and crying at 12 months postpartum. *Health Psychology*, 34, 811–819.

Sayar, K., Arikan, M., & Yontem, T. (2002). Sleep quality in chronic pain patients. *Canadian Journal of Psychiatry*, 47, 844–848.

Schiller, C. E., O'Hara, M. W., Rubinow, D., & Johnson, A. K. (2013). Estradiol modulates anhedonia and behavioral despair in rats and negative affect in a subgroup of women at high risk for postpartum depression. *Physiology & Behavior*, 119, 137–144.

REFERENCES

Schneider, S., Houweling, J. E. G., Gommlich-Schneider, S., Klein, C., Nundel, B., & Wolke, D. (2009). Effect of maternal panic disorder on mother–child interaction and relation to child anxiety and child self-efficacy. *Archives of Women's Mental Health*, 12, 251–259.

Schuetze, P., & Das Eiden, R. (2005). The relationship between sexual abuse during childhood and parenting outcomes: Modeling direct and indirect pathways. *Child Abuse & Neglect*, 29, 645–659.

Schultz, V. (2006). Safety of St. John's wort extract compared to synthetic antidepressants. *Phytomedicine*, 13, 199–204.

Schwartz, E. B., Ray, R. M., Stuebe, A. M., Allison, M. A., Ness, R. B., Freiberg, M. S., & Cauley, J. A. (2009). Duration of lactation and risk factors for maternal cardiovascular disease. *Obstetrics & Gynecology*, 113, 974–982.

Scorza, P., Owusu-Agyei, S., Asampong, E., & Wainberg, M. L. (2015). The expression of perinatal depression in rural Ghana. *International Journal of Cultural Mental Health*, 8, 370–381.

Seng, J. S., Kohn-Wood, L. P., McPherson, M. D., & Sperlich, M. A. (2011a). Disparity in posttraumatic stress disorder diagnosis among African American pregnant women. *Archives of Women's Mental Health*, 14, 295–306.

Seng, J. S., Low, L. K., Sperlich, M. A., Ronis, D. L., & Liberzon, I. (2011b). Posttraumatic stress disorder, child abuse history, birth weight, and gestational age: A prospective cohort study. *British Journal of Obstetrics & Gynecology*, 118, 1329–1339.

Seng, J. S., Low, L. M. K., Sperlich, M. A., Ronis, D. L., & Liberzon, I. (2009). Prevalence, trauma history, and risk for posttraumatic stress disorder among nulliparous women in maternity care. *Obstetrics & Gynecology*, 114, 839–847.

Seng, J. S., Sperlich, M. A., Low, L. K., Ronis, D. L., Muzik, M., & Liberzon, I. (2013). Childhood abuse history, posttraumatic stress disorder, postpartum mental health, and bonding: A prospective cohort study. *Journal of Midwifery and Women's Health*, 58, 57–68.

Setse, R., Grogan, R., Pham, L., Cooper, L. A., Strobino, D., Powe, N. R., & Nicholson, W. (2009). Longitudinal study of depressive symptoms and health-related quality of life during pregnancy and after delivery: The Health Status in Pregnancy (HIP) Study. *Maternal Child Health Journal*, 13, 577–587.

Sharma, V., & Mazmanian, D. (2014). The DSM-5 peripartum specifier: Prospects and pitfalls. *Archives of Women's Mental Health*, 17, 171–173.

Shaw, R. J., Bernard, R. S., DeBlois, T., Ikuta, L. M., Ginzburg, K., & Koopman, C. (2009). The relationship between acute stress disorder and posttraumatic stress disorder in the neonatal intensive care unit. *Psychosomatics*, 50, 131–137.

Shaw, R. J., Deblois, T., Ikuta, L., Ginzburg, K., Fleisher, B., & Koopman, C. (2006). Acute stress disorder among parents of infants in the neonatal intensive care nursery. *Psychosomatics*, 47, 206–212. doi:47/3/206 [pii] 10.1176/appi.psy.47.3.206

Shaw, R. J., st. John, N., Lilo, E., Jo, B., Benitz, W., Stevenson, D. K., & Horwitz, S. M. (2014). Prevention of traumatic stress in mothers of preterms: 6-month outcomes. *Pediatrics*, 134(2), e481–e488.

Shields, B. (2005). *Down came the rain: My journal through postpartum depression*. New York, NY: Hyperion.

Shoji, H., Franke, C., Campoy, C., Rivero, M., Demmelmair, H., & Koletzko, B. (2006). Effect of docosahexaenoic acid and eicosapentaenoic acid supplementation on oxidative stress levels during pregnancy. *Free Radical Research*, 40, 379–384.

Sidebottom, A. C., Harrison, P. A., Godecker, A., & Kim, H. (2012). Validation of the Patient Health Questionnaire (PHQ)-9 for prenatal depression screening. *Archives of Women's Mental Health*, 12, 367–374.

Sie, S. D., Wennink, J. M. B., van Driel, J. J., te Winkel, A. G. W., Boer, K., Casteelen, G., & van Weissenbruch, M. M. (2012). Maternal use of SSRIs, SNRIs, and NaSSAs: Practical recommendations during pregnancy and lactation. *Archives of Disease of Childhood, Fetal, Neonatal Edition*, 97, F472–F476.

Silverman, M. E., & Loudon, H. (2010). Antenatal reports of pre-pregnancy abuse is associated with symptoms of depression in the postpartum period. *Archives of Women's Mental Health*, 13, 411–415.

Simkin, P. (1991). Just another day in a woman's life? Women's long-term perceptions of their first birth experience. Part I. *Birth*, 18, 203–210.

Simkin, P. (1992). Just another day in a woman's life? Part II: Nature and consistency of women's long-term memories of their first birth experiences. *Birth*, 19, 64–81.

Sit, D., Luther, J., Buysse, D., Dills, J. L., Eng, H., Okun, M., Wisniewski, S., & Wisner, K. L. (2015). Suicidal ideation in depressed postpartum women: Associations wtih childhood trauma, sleep disturbance, and anxiety. *Journal of Psychiatric Research*, 66–67, 95–104.

Siu, A. L., & US Preventive Services Task Force (USPSTF). (2016). Screening for depression in adults: US Preventive Services Task Force recommendation statement. *Journal of the American Medical Association*, 315, 380–387.

Sivertsen, B., Hysing, M., Dorheim, S. K., & Eberhard-Gran, M. (2015). Trajectories of maternal sleep problems before and after childbirth: A longitudinal population-based study. *BMC Pregnancy and Childbirth*, 15, 129. doi:10.1186/s12884-015-0577-1

Skouteris, H., Wertheim, E. H., Rallis, S., Milgrom, J., & Paxton, S. J. (2009). Depression and anxiety through pregnancy and the early postpartum: An examination of prospective relationships. *Journal of Affective Disorders*, 113, 303–308.

Skurtveit, S., Selmer, R., Roth, C., Hernandez-Diaz, S., & Handal, M. (2014). Prenatal exposure to antidepressants and language competence at age three: Results from a large population-based pregnancy cohort in Norway. *British Journal of Obstetrics & Gynecology*, 121, 1621–1631. doi:10.1111/1471-0528.12821

Slade, P. (2006). Towards a conceptual framework for understanding post-traumatic stress symptoms following childbirth and implications for further research. *Journal of Psychosomatic Obstetrics & Gynecology*, 27, 99–105.

Small, R., Lumley, J., Donohue, L., Potter, A., & Waldenstrom, U. (2000). Randomised controlled trial of midwife led debriefing to reduce maternal depression after operative childbirth. *British Medical Journal*, 321, 1043–1047.

Smith, T. W., Uchino, B. N., Bosch, J. A., & Kent, R. G. (2014). Trait hostility is associated with systemic inflammation in married couples: An actor-partner analysis. *Biological Psychiatry*, 102, 51–53.

Smyke, A. T., Boris, N. W., & Alexander, G. M. (2002). Fear of spoiling in at-risk African American mothers. *Child Psychiatry & Human Development*, 32, 295–307.

Sockol, L. E., Battle, C. L., Howard, M., & Davis, T. (2014). Correlates of impaired mother–infant bonding in a partial hospital program for perinatal women. *Archives of Women's Mental Health*, 17, 465–469.

Soderquist, I., Wijma, B., Thorbert, G., & Wijma, K. (2009). Risk factors in pregnancy for post-traumatic stress and depression after childbirth. *British Journal of Obstetrics & Gynecology*, 116, 672–680.

Somerville, S., Dedman, K., Hagan, R., Oxnam, E., Wettinger, M., Byrne, S., Coo, S., et al. (2014). The Perinatal Anxiety Screening Scale: Development and preliminary validation. *Archives of Women's Mental Health*, 17, 443–454.

Sorbo, M. F., Lukasse, M., Brantsaeter, A.-L., & Grimstad, H. (2015). Past and recent abuse is associated with early cessation of breast feeding: Results from a large prospective cohort in Norway. *BMJ Open*, 5, e009240.

Speisman, B. B., Storch, E. A., & Abramowitz, J. S. (2011). Postpartum obsessive–compulsive disorder. *Journal of Obstetric, Gynecologic, and Neonatal Nursing*, 40, 680–690.

Spinelli, M. G., & Endicott, J. (2003). Controlled clinical trial of interpersonal psychotherapy versus parenting education program for depressed pregnant women. *American Journal of Psychiatry*, 160, 555–562.

Spitzer, C., Barnow, S., Volzke, H., Wallaschotski, H., John, U., Freyberger, H. J., Löwe, B., & Grabe, H. J. (2010). Association of posttraumatic stress disorder with low-grade elevation of

C-reactive protein: Evidence from the general population. *Journal of Psychiatric Research*, 44(1), 15–21.

Spoormaker, V. I., & Montgomery, P. (2008). Disturbed sleep in posttraumaic stress disorder: Secondary symptom or core feature? *Sleep Medicine Reviews*, 12, 169–184.

Springate, B. A., & Chaudron, L. H. (2006). Mental health providers' self-reported expertise and treatment of perinatal depression. *Archives of Women's Mental Health*, 9, 60–61.

Stagnaro-Green, A. (2012). Approach to the patient with postpartum thyroiditis. *Journal of Clinical Endocrinology & Metabolism*, 97, 334–342.

Starkweather, A. R. (2007). The effects of exercise on perceived stress and IL-6 levels among older adults. *Biological Nursing Research*, 8, 1–9.

Stern, G., & Kruckman, L. (1983). Multi-disciplinary perspectives on postpartum depression: An anthropological critique. *Social Science & Medicine*, 17, 1027–1041.

Stewart, D. E., Gagnon, A. J., Merry, L. A., & Dennis, C.-L. (2012). Risk factors and health profiles of recent migrant women who experienced violence associated with pregnancy. *Journal of Women's Health*, 21, 1100–1106.

Stewart, R. C., Umar, E., Tomenson, B., & Creed, F. (2014). A cross-sectional study of antenatal depression and associated factors in Malawi. *Archives of Women's Mental Health*, 17, 145–154.

Stramrood, C. A., Paarlberg, K. M., Huis Veld, E. M., Berger, L. W. A. R., Vingerhoets, A. J. J. M., Schultz, W. C. M. W., & Van Pampus, M. G. (2011). Posttraumatic stress following childbirth in homelike- and hospital settings. *Journal of Psychosomatic Obstetrics & Gynecology*, 32, 88–97.

Stramrood, C. A., van der Velde, J., Doornbos, B., Paarlberg, K. M., Weijmar Schultz, W. C. M., & Van Pampus, M. G. (2012). The patient observer: Eye-Movement Desensitization and Reprocessing for the treatment of posttraumatic stress following childbirth. *Birth*, 39, 70–76.

Strathearn, L., Mamun, A. A., Najman, J. M., & O'Callaghan, M. J. (2009). Does breastfeeding protect against substantiated child abuse and neglect? A 15-year cohort study. *Pediatrics*, 123, 483–493. doi:123/2/483 [pii] 10.1542/peds.2007–3546

Stuebe, A. M., Grewen, K., Pedersen, C. A., Propper, C., & Meltzer-Brody, S. (2012). Failed lactation and perinatal depression: Common problems with shared neuroendocrine mechanisms? *Journal of Women's Health*, 21, 264–272.

Stuebe, A. M., Schwarz, E. B., Grewen, K., Rich-Edwards, J. W., Michels, K. B., Foster, E. M., Curhan, G., & Forman, J. (2011). Duration of lactation and incidenced of maternal hypertension: A longitudinal cohort study. *American Journal of Epidemiology*, 174, 1147–1158.

Su, D., Zhao, Y., Binna, C., Scott, J., & Oddy, W. (2007). Breast-feeding mothers can exercise: Results of a cohort study. *Public Health Nutrition*, 10, 1089–1093.

Su, K.-P., Huang, S.-Y., Chiu, T.-H., Huang, K.-C., Huang, C.-L., Chang, H.-C., & Pariante, C. M. (2008). Omega-3 fatty acids for major depressive disorder during pregnancy: Results from a randomized, double-blind, placebo trial. *Journal of Clinical Psychiatry*, 69, 644–651.

Suarez, E. C. (2006). Sex differences in the relation of depressive symptoms, hostility, and anger expression to indices of glucose metabolism in nondiabetic adults. *Health Psychology*, 25, 484–492.

Suarez, E. C., Lewis, J. G., Krishnan, R. R., & Young, K. H. (2004). Enhanced expression of cytokines and chemokines by blood monocytes to *in vitro* lipopolysaccharide stimulation are associated with hostility and severity of depressive symptoms in healthy women. *Psychoneuroendocrinology*, 29, 1119–1128.

Sullivan, B., & Payne, T. W. (2007). Affective disorders and cognitive failures: A comparison of seasonal and nonseasonal depression. *American Journal of Psychiatry*, 164, 1663–1667.

Suri, R., Altshuler, L., Hellemann, G., Burt, V. K., Aquino, A., & Mintz, J. (2007). Effects of antenatal depression and antidepressant treatment on gestational age at birth and risk of preterm birth. *American Journal of Psychiatry*, 164, 1206–1213.

Swain, A. M., Tasgin, E., Mayes, L. C., Feldman, R., Constable, R. T., & Leckman, J. F. (2008). Maternal brain response to own baby-cry is affected by cesarean section delivery. *Journal of Child Psychology and Psychiatry*, 49, 1042–1052.

Swalm, D., Brooks, J., Doherty, D., Nathan, E., & Jacques, A. (2010). Using the Edinburgh post-natal depression scale to screen for perinatal anxiety. *Archives of Women's Mental Health*, 13, 515–522.

Sword, W., Busser, D., Ganann, R., McMillan, T., & Swinton, M. (2008). Women's care-seeking experiences after referral for postpartum depression. *Qualitative Health Research*, 18, 1161–1173.

Szajewska, H., Horvath, A., & Koletzko, B. (2006). Effect of n-3 long-chain polyunsaturated fatty acide supplementation of women with low-risk pregnancies on pregnancy outcomes and growth measures at birth: A meta-analysis of randomized controlled trials. *American Journal of Clinical Nutrition*, 83, 1337–1344.

Szegedi, A., Kohnen, R., Dienel, A., & Kieser, M. (2005). Acute treatment of moderate to severe depression with hypericum extract WS 5570 (St. John's wort): Randomised controlled double blind non-inferiority trial versus paroxetine. *British Medical Journal*, 330, 503. doi:10.1136/bmj.38356.655266.82

Taj, R., & Sikander, K. S. (2003). Effects of maternal depression on breastfeeding. *Journal of the Pakistani Medical Association*, 53, 8–11.

Tam, L. W., Newton, R. P., Dern, M., & Parry, B. L. (2002). Screening women for postpartum depression at well baby visits: Resistance encountered and recommendations. *Archives of Women's Mental Health*, 5, 79–82.

Tammentie, T., Paavilainen, E., Astedt-Kurki, P., & Tarkka, M.-T. (2004). Family dynamics of postnatally depressed mothers: Discrepancy between expectations and reality. *Journal of Clinical Nursing*, 13, 65–74.

Taveras, E. M., Rifas-Shiman, S. L., Rich-Edwards, J. W., Gunderson, E. P., Stuebe, A. M., & Mantzoros, C. S. (2011a). Association of maternal short sleep duration with adiposity and cardio-metabolic status at 3 years postpartum. *Obesity*, 19, 171–178. doi:10.1038/oby.2010.117.

Taveras, E. M., Rifas-Shiman, S. L., Rich-Edwards, J. W., & Mantzoros, C. S. (2011b). Maternal short sleep duration is associated with increased levels of inflammatory markers at 3 years post-partum. *Metabolism*, 60, 982–986. doi:10.1016/j.metabol.2010.09.008.

Tees, M. T., Harville, E. W., Xiong, X., Buekens, P., Pridjian, G., & Elkind-Hirsch, K. (2010). Hurricane Katrina-related maternal stress, maternal mental health, and early infant temperament. *Maternal & Child Health Journal*, 14, 511–518.

Tegethoff, M., Greene, N., Olsen, J., Meyer, A. H., & Meinlschmidt, G. (2010). Maternal psycho-social adversity during pregnancy is associated with length of gestation and offspring size at birth: Evidence from a population-based cohort study. *Psychosomatic Medicine*, 72, 419–426.

Terman, M., & Terman, J. S. (2006). Controlled trial of naturalistic dawn simulation and negative air ionization for Seasonal Affective Disorder. *American Journal of Psychiatry*, 163, 2126.

Terman, M., & Terman, J. S. (2005). Light therapy for seasonal and nonseasonal depression: Efficacy, protocol, safety, and side effects. *CNS Spectrums*, 10, 647–663.

Teychenne, M., & York, R. (2013). Physical activity, sedentary behavior, and postnatal depressive symptoms: A review. *American Journal of Preventive Medicine*, 45, 217–227.

Tham, V., Ryding, E. L., & Christensson, K. (2010). Experience of support among mothers with and without post-traumatic symptoms following emergency caesarean section. *Sexual & Reproductive Healthcare*, 1, 175–190.

Thompson, J. F., Roberts, C. L., Currie, M., & Ellwood, D. A. (2002). Prevalence and persistence of health problems after childbirth: Associations with parity and method of birth. *Birth*, 29, 83–94.

Tietz, A., Zietlow, A.-L., & Reck, C. (2014). Maternal bonding in mothers with postpartum anxiety disorder: The crucial role of subclinical depressive symptoms and maternal avoidance behaviour. *Archives of Women's Mental Health*, 17, 433–442.

Tolman, A. O. (2001). *Depression in adults: The latest assessment and treatment strategies*. Kansas City, MO: Compact Clinicals.

Torchalla, I., Linden, I. A., Strehlau, V., Neilson, E. K., & Krausz, M. (2015). "Like a lots happened with my whole childhood": Violence, trauma, and addiction in pregnant and postpartum

REFERENCES

women from Vancouver's Downtown Eastside. *Harm Reduction Journal*, 12(1). Retrieved from www.harmreductionjournal.com/content/12/1/1

Torkan, B., Parsay, S., Lamyian, M., Kazemnejad, A., & Montazeri, A. (2009). Postnatal quality of life in women after normal vaginal delivery vs. caesarean section. *BMC Pregnancy and Childbirth*, 9, 4. doi:10.1186/1471-2393-9-4

Torvaldsen, S., Roberts, C. L., Simpson, J. M., Thompson, J. F., & Ellwood, D. A. (2006). Intrapartum epidural analgesia and breastfeeding: A prospective cohort study. *International Breastfeeding Journal*, 1, 24. doi:10.1186/1746-4358-1-24

Truijens, S. E. M., Wijnen, H. A., Pommer, A. M., Guid Oei, S., & Pop, V. J. M. (2014). Development of Childbirth Perception Scale (CPS): Perception of delivery and the first postpartum week. *Archives of Women's Mental Health*, 17, 411–421.

Turkcapar, A. F., Kadioglu, N., Aslan, E., Tunc, S., Zayifoglu, M., & Mollamahmutoglu, L. (2015). Sociodemographic and clinical features of postpartum depression among Turkish women: A prospective study. *BMC Pregnancy and Childbirth*, 15, 108. doi:10.1186/s12884-015-0532-1

Tzilos, G. K., Zlotnick, C., Raker, C., Kuo, C., & Phipps, M. G. (2012). Psychosocial factors associated with depression severity in pregnant adolescents. *Archives of Women's Mental Health*, 15, 397–401.

Valentine, J. M., Rodriguez, M. A., Lapeyrouse, L. M., & Zhang, M. (2011). Recent intimate partner violecne as a prenatal predictor of maternal depression in the first year postpartum among Latinas. *Archives of Women's Mental Health*, 14, 135–143.

van Bussel, J. C. H., Spitz, B., & Demyttenaere, K. (2009). Depressive symptomatology in pregnant and postpartum women. An exploratory study of the role of maternal antenatal orientations. *Archives of Women's Mental Health*, 12, 155–166.

van de Pol, G., De Leeuw, J. R. J., van Brummen, H. J., Bruinse, H. W., Heintz, A. P. M., & van der Vaart, C. H. (2006). Psychosocial factors and mode of delivery. *Journal of Psychosomatic Obstetrics & Gynecology*, 27, 231–238.

van der Hulst, L. A. M., Bonsel, G. J., Eskes, M., Birnie, E., van Teijlingen, E., & Bleker, O. P. (2006). Bad experience, good birthing: Dutch low-risk pregnant women with a history of sexual abuse. *Journal of Psychosomatic Obstetrics & Gynecology*, 27, 59–66.

van der Kolk, B. A. (2002). Assessment and treatment of complex PTSD. In R. Yehuda (Ed.), *Treating trauma survivors with PTSD* (pp. 127–156). Washington, DC: American Psychiatric Association Press.

Van Gurp, G., Meterissian, G. B., Haiek, L. N., McCusker, J., & Bellavance, F. (2002). St. John's wort or sertraline?: Randomized controlled trial in primary care. *Canadian Family Physician*, 48, 905–912.

van Pampus, M. G., Wolf, H., Weijmar Schultz, W. C. M., Neeleman, J., & Aarnoudse, J. G. (2004). Posttraumatic stress disorder following preeclampsia and HELLP syndrome. *Journal of Psychosomatic Obstetrics & Gynecology*, 25, 183–187.

Vanderbilt, D., Bushley, T., Young, R., & Frank, D. A. (2009). Acute posttraumatic stress symptoms among urban mothers with newborns in the neonatal intensive care unit: A preliminary study. *Journal of Developmental & Behavioral Pediatrics*, 30, 50–56.

Vericker, T. C. (2015). Maternal depression associated with less healthy dietary behaviors in young children. www.urban.org

Verkerk, G. J. M., Denollet, J., Van Heck, G. L., Van Son, M. J. M., & Pop, V. J. M. (2005). Personality factors as determinants of depression in postpartum women: A prospective 1-year follow-up study. *Psychosomatic Medicine*, 67, 632–637.

Verreault, N., Da Costa, D., Marchand, A., Ireland, K., Banack, H., Dritsa, M., & Khalife, S. (2012). PTSD following childbirth: A prospective study of incidence and risk factors in Canadian women. *Journal of Psychosomatic Research*, 73, 257–263.

Vesga-Lopez, O., Blanco, C., Keyes, K., Olfson, M., Grant, B. F., & Hasin, D. S. (2008). Psychiatric disorders in pregnant and postpartum women in the United States. *Archives of General Psychiatry*, 65, 805–815.

Vollmar, P., Haghikia, A., Dermietzel, R., & Faustmann, P. M. (2008). Venlafaxine exhibits an anti-inflammatory effect in an inflammatory co-culture model. *International Journal of Neuropsychopharmacology*, 11, 111–117. doi:S1461145707007729 [pii] 10.1017/S1461145707007729

Wagner, C. L. (2011). Vitamin D: Recommendations during pregnancy, lactation, and early infancy. *Clinical Lactation*, 2(1), 27–31.

Wagner, C. L., Hulsey, T. C., Fanning, D., Ebeling, M., & Hollis, B. W. (2006). High dose vitamin D3 supplementation in a cohort of breastfeeding mothers and their infants: A six-month follow-up pilot study. *Breastfeeding Medicine*, 1(2), 59–70.

Wakeel, F., Wisk, L. E., Gee, R., Chao, S. M., & Witt, W. P. (2013). The balance between stress and personal capital during pregnancy and the relationship with adverse obstetric outcomes: Findings from the 2007 Los Angeles Mommy and Baby (LAMB) study. *Archives of Women's Mental Health*, 16, 435–451.

Walker, E. R., McGee, R. E., & Druss, B. G. (2015). Mortality in mental disorders and Global Disease Burden Implications: A systematic review and meta-analysis. *JAMA Psychiatry*, 72, 334–341. doi:10.1001/jamapsychiatry.2014.2502

Walker, L. O., Gao, J., & Xie, B. (2015). Postpartum psychosocial and behavioral health: A systematic review of Self-Administered Scales validated for postpartum women in the United States. *Women's Health Issues*, 25, 586–600.

Walmer, R., Huynh, J., Wenger, J., Ankers, E., Mantha, A. B., Ecker, J., Thadhani, R., et al. (2015). Mental health disorders subsequent to gestational diabetes mellitus differ by race/ethnicity. *Depression & Anxiety*, 32, 774–782.

Wang, C., Chung, M., Lichtenstein, A., Balk, E., Kupelnick, B., DeVine, D., Lawrence, A., & Lau, J. (2004). *Effects of omega-3 fatty acids on cardiovascular disease* (Vol. AHRQ Publication No. 04-E009-1). Rockville, MD: Agency for Healthcare Research and Quality.

Wang, Y., Hu, Y.-P., Wang, W.-c., Pang, R.-z., & Zhang, A.-r. (2012). Clinical studies on treatment of earthquake-caused posttraumatic stress disorder using electroacupuncture. *Evidence-Based Complementary and Alternative Medicine*, 2012, 431279. doi:10.1155/2012/431279

Watkins, S., Meltzer-Brody, S., Zolnoun, D., & Stuebe, A. M. (2011). Early breastfeeding experiences and postpartum depression *Obstetrics & Gynecology*, 118, 214–221.

Webber, S. (1992). Supporting the postpartum family. *The Doula*, 23, 16–17.

Webster, J., Linnane, J. W. J., Dibley, L. M., Hinson, J. K., Starrenburg, S. E., & Roberts, J. A. (2000a). Measuring social support in pregnancy: Can it be simple and meaningful? *Birth*, 27, 97–101.

Webster, J., Linnane, J. W. J., Dibley, L. M., & Pritchard, M. (2000b). Improving antenatal recognition of women at risk for postnatal depression. *Australia and New Zealand Journal of Obstetrics and Gynaecology*, 40, 409–412.

Webster, J., Pritchard, M. A., Linnane, J., Roberts, J., Hinson, J. K., & Starrenburg, S. (2001). Postnatal depression: Use of health services and satisfaction with health-care providers. *Journal of Qualitative Clinical Practice*, 21, 144–148.

Wei, G., Greaver, L. B., Marson, S. M., Herndon, C. H., Rogers, J., & Robeson Healthcare Corporation (2008). Postpartum depression: Racial differences and ethnic disparities in a tri-racial and bi-ethnic population. *Maternal Child Health Journal*, 12, 699–707.

Weisman, O., Granat, A., Gilboa-Schechtman, E., Singer, M., Gordon, I., Azulay, H., Kuint, J., & Feldman, R. (2010). The experience of labor, maternal perception of the infant, and the mother's postpartum mood in a low-risk community cohort. *Archives of Women's Mental Health*, 13, 505–513.

Weissman, A. M., Levy, B. T., Hartz, A. J., Bentler, S., Donohue, M., Ellingrod, V. L., & Wisner, K. L. (2004). Pooled analysis of antidepressant levels in lactating mothers, breast milk, and nursing infants. *American Journal of Psychiatry*, 161, 1066–1078.

Weissman, M. M. (2007). Recent non-medication trials of interpersonal psychotherapy for depression. *International Journal of Neuropsychopharmacology*, 10, 117–122.

REFERENCES

Weissman, M. M., Pilowsky, D. J., Wickramaratne, P. J., Talati, A., Wisniewski, S. R., Fava, M., Hughes, C. W., et al. (2006). Remissions in maternal depression and child psychopathology. *JAMA*, 295, 1389–1398.

Werneke, U., Turner, T., & Priebe, S. (2006). Complementary medicines in psychiatry: Review of effectiveness and safety. *British Journal of Psychiatry*, 188, 109–121.

Williams, J. W., Gierisch, J. M., McDuffie, J., Strauss, J. L., & Nagi, A. (2011). *An overview of complementary and alternative medicine therapies for anxiety and depressive disorders: Supplement to efficacy of complementary and alternative medicine therapies for posttraumatic stress disorder*. Washington, DC: Health Service Research & Development Service.

Wilson, S., & Durbin, C. E. (2010). Effects of paternal depression on fathers' parenting behaviors: A meta-analytic review. *Clinical Psychology Review*, 30, 167–180.

Wisner, K. L., Logsdon, M. C., & Shanahan, B. R. (2008). Web-based education for postpartum depression: Conceptual development and impact. *Archives of Women's Mental Health*, 11, 377–385.

Wisner, K. L., Sit, D. K. Y., Hanusa, B. H., Moses-Kolko, E. L., Bogen, D. L., Hunker, D. F., Perel, J. M., et al. (2009). Major depression and antidepressant treatment: Impact of pregnancy and neonatal outcomes. *American Journal of Psychiatry*, 166, 557–566.

Witt, W. P., DeLeire, T., Hagen, E. W., Wichmann, M. A., Wisk, L. E., Spear, H. A., Cheng, E. R., et al. (2010). The prevalence and determinants of antepartum mental health problems among women in the USA: A nationally representative population-based study. *Archives of Women's Mental Health*, 13, 425–437.

Woelk, H. (2000). Comparison of St. John's wort and imipramine for treating depression: Randomised controlled trial. *British Medical Journal*, 321, 536–539.

Wolf, A. W., De Andraca, I., & Lozoff, B. (2002). Maternal depression in three Latin American samples. *Social Psychiatry & Psychiatric Epidemiology*, 37, 169–176.

Wolke, D., Rizzo, P., & Woods, S. (2002). Persistent infant crying and hyperactivity problems in middle childhood. *Pediatrics*, 109, 1054–1060.

Woods, A. B., Page, G. G., O'Campo, P., Pugh, L. C., Ford, D., & Campbell, J. C. (2005). The mediation effect of posttraumatic stress disorder symptoms on the relationship of intimate partner violence and IFN-gamma levels. *American Journal of Community Psychology*, 36, 159–175. doi:10.1007/s10464-005-6240-7

Woolhouse, H., Brown, S., Krastev, A., Perlen, S., & Gunn, J. (2009). Seeking help for anxiety and depression after childbirth: Results of the Maternal Health Study. *Archives of Women's Mental Health*, 12, 75–83.

Woolhouse, H., Gartland, D., Mensah, F., & Brown, S. J. (2015). Maternal depression from early pregnancy to 4 years postpartum in a prospective pregnancy cohort study: Implications for primary health care. *British Journal of Obstetrics & Gynecology*, 122, 312–321. doi:10.1111/1471-0528.12839.

World Health Organization. (2014). The prevention and elimination of disrespect and abuse during facility-based childbirth. Retrieved from http://apps.who.int/iris/bitstream/10665/134588/1/WHO_RHR_14.23_eng.pdf?ua=1&ua=1

Wu, J., Yeung, A. S., Schnyer, R. N., Wang, Y., & Micschoulon, D. (2012). Acupuncture for depression: A review of clinical applications. *Canadian Journal of Psychiatry*, 57, 397–405.

Wurglies, M., & Schubert-Zsilavecz, M. (2006). *Hypericum perforatum*: A "modern" herbal antidepressant: Pharmacokinetics of active ingredients. *Clinical Pharmacokinetics*, 45, 449–468.

Xiong, X., Harville, E. W., Mattison, D. R., Elkind-Hirsch, K., Pridjian, G., & Buekens, P. (2010). Hurricane Katrina experience and the risk of post-traumatic stress disorder and depression among pregnant women. *American Journal of Disaster Medicine*, 5, 181–187.

Xu, F., Austin, M.-P., Reilly, N., Hilder, L., & Sullivan, E. A. (2012). Major depressive disorder in the perinatal period: Using data linkage to inform perinatal mental health policy. *Archives of Women's Mental Health*, 15, 333–341.

Yang, F., Gardner, C. O., Bigdeli, T., Gao, J., Zhang, Z., Tao, M., Liu, Y., et al. (2015). Clinical features of and risk factors for major depression with history of postpartum episodes in Han Chinese women: A retrospective study. *Journal of Affective Disorders*, 183, 339–346.

Yatham, L. N., Kennedy, S. H., Schaffer, A., Parikh, S. V., Beaulieu, S., O'Donovan, C., MacQueen, G., et al. (2009). Canadian Network for Mood and Anxiety Treatments (CANMAT) and International Society for Bipolar Disorders (ISBD) collaborative update of CANMAT guidelines for the management of patients with bipolar disorder: Update 2009. *Bipolar Disorders*, 11, 225–255.

Yim, I. S., Glynn, L. M., Schetter, C. D., Hobel, C. J., Chicz-DeMet, A., & Sandman, C. A. (2009). Risk of postpartum depressive symptoms with elevated corticotropin-releasing hormone in human pregnancy. *Archives of General Psychiatry*, 66, 162–169.

Yonkers, K. A. (2007). The treatment of women suffering from depression who are either pregnant or breastfeeding. *American Journal of Psychiatry*, 164, 1457–1459.

Yonkers, K. A., Ramin, S. M., Rush, A. J., Navarrete, C. A., Carmody, T., March, D., Heartwell, S. F., & Leveno, K. J. (2001). Onset and persistence of postpartum depression in an inner-city maternal health clinic system. *American Journal of Psychiatry*, 158, 1856–1863.

Yonkers, K. A., Smith, M. V., Forray, A., Epperson, C. N., Costello, D., Lin, H., & Belanger, K. (2014). Pregnant women with posttraumatic stress disorder and risk of preterm birth. *JAMA Psychiatry*, 71, 897–904.

Yusuff, A. S. M., Tang, L., Binns, C. W., & Lee, A. H. (2016). Breastfeeding and postnatal depression: A prospective cohort study in Sabah, Malaysia. *Journal of Human Lactation*, 32(2), 277–281.

Zaers, S., Waschke, M., & Ehlert, U. (2008). Depressive symptoms and symptoms of post-traumatic stress disorder in women after childbirth. *Journal of Psychosomatic Obstetrics & Gynecology*, 29, 61–71.

Zafar, S., Jean-Baptiste, R., Rahman, A., Neilson, J. P., & van den Broek, N. (2015). Non-life threatening maternal morbidity: Cross sectional surveys from Malawi and Pakistan. *PLoS ONE*, 10. doi:10.1371/journal.pone.0138026

Zanoli, P. (2004). Role of hyperforin in the pharmacological activities of St. John's wort. *CNS*, 10, 203–218.

Zelkowitz, P., & Milet, T. H. (2001). The course of postpartum psychiatric disorders in women and their partners. *Journal of Nervous & Mental Disease*, 189, 575–582.

Zhao, Y., Kane, I., Wang, J., Shen, B., Luo, J., & Shi, S. (2015). Combined use of the postpartum depession screening scale (PDSS) and Edinburgh postnatal depression (EPDS) to identify antenatal depression among Chinese pregnant women with obstetric complications. *Psychiatry Research*, 226, 113–119.

Zhou, C., Tabb, M. M., Sadatrfiei, A., Grun, F., Sun, A., & Blumberg, B. (2004). Hyperforin, the active component of St. John's wort, induces IL-8 expression in human intestinal epithelial cells via MAPK-dependent, NF-kappaB-independent pathway. *Journal of Clinical Immunology*, 24, 623–636.

Zlotnick, C., Miller, I. W., Pearlstein, T., Howard, M., & Sweeney, P. (2006). A preventive intervention for pregnant women on public assistance at risk for postpartum depression. *American Journal of Psychiatry*, 163, 1443–1445.

Zlotnick, C., Tzilos, G. K., Miller, I., Seifer, R., & Stout, R. (2016). Randomized controlled trial to prevent postpartum depressioin in mothers on public assistance. *Journal of Affective Disorders*, 189, 263–268.

Index